Bayesian Meta-Analysis

"...this book is extremely timely...not just a technical exposition, but provides practical guidance about using different software platforms, as well as valuable advice about extracting summary statistics, eliciting prior information, communicating results, visualisation, and many other issues...reflects years of thoughtful experience, and should be of huge value to anyone faced with pooling studies into a coherent whole."

~From the Foreword by Professor Sir David Spiegelhalter

Meta-analysis is the statistical combination of previously conducted studies, often from summary statistics but sometimes with individual participant data. It is widespread in life sciences and is gaining popularity in economics and beyond. In many real-life meta-analyses, challenges in the source information, such as unreported statistics or biases, can be incorporated using Bayesian methods. *Bayesian Meta-Analysis: A Practical Introduction* provides an approachable introduction for researchers who are new to Bayes, meta-analysis, or both. There is an emphasis on hands-on learning using a variety of software packages.

Key Features

- Introductory chapters assume no prior experience or mathematical training and are aimed at non-statistical researchers.
- Examples of basic meta-analyses in seven different software alternatives: BUGS, JAGS, Stan, bayesmeta, brms, Stata, and JASP.
- Practical advice on extracting information from studies, eliciting expert opinions, managing project decisions, and writing up findings.
- Discussion of specific problems, including publication bias, unreported statistics, and a mixture of study designs, with code examples.
- Accompanying online blog and forum, with all code and data from the book, plus more translations to different software.

This book aims to bridge the gap between the researcher who wants to carry out tailored meta-analysis and the techniques they need, which have previously been available only in mathematically or computationally demanding publications.

Bayesian Meta-Analysis
A Practical Introduction

Robert Grant and Gian Luca Di Tanna

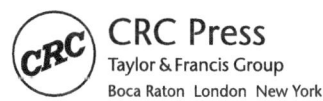

CRC Press
Taylor & Francis Group
Boca Raton London New York

CRC Press is an imprint of the
Taylor & Francis Group, an **informa** business

A CHAPMAN & HALL BOOK

Cover image: acrylic and coffee on card, Robert Grant, 2024

First edition published 2025
by CRC Press
2385 NW Executive Center Drive, Suite 320, Boca Raton FL 33431

and by CRC Press
4 Park Square, Milton Park, Abingdon, Oxon, OX14 4RN

CRC Press is an imprint of Taylor & Francis Group, LLC

Library of Congress Cataloging-in-Publication Data
Names: Grant, Robert (Statistician) author
Title: Bayesian meta-analysis : a practical introduction / Robert Grant and
    Gian Luca Di Tanna.
Description: First edition. | Boca Raton : CRC Press, 2025. | Includes
    bibliographical references and index. | Summary: "Meta-analysis is the
    statistical combination of previously conducted studies, often from
    summary statistics but sometimes with individual participant data. It is
    widespread in life sciences and is gaining popularity in economics and
    beyond. In many real-life meta-analyses, challenges in the source
    information, such as unreported statistics or biases, can be
    incorporated using Bayesian methods. This book provides an approachable
    introduction for researchers who are new to Bayes, meta-analysis, or
    both. There is an emphasis on hands-on learning using a variety of
    software packages"-- Provided by publisher.
Identifiers: LCCN 2024059598 (print) | LCCN 2024059599 (ebook) | ISBN
    9781032451909 hbk | ISBN 9781032451893 pbk | ISBN 9781003375821 ebk
Subjects: LCSH: Bayesian statistical decision theory | Meta-analysis |
    Quantitative research
Classification: LCC QA279.5 .G73 2025 (print) | LCC QA279.5 (ebook) | DDC
    519.5/42--dc23/eng/20250422
LC record available at https://lccn.loc.gov/2024059598
LC ebook record available at https://lccn.loc.gov/2024059599

ISBN: 978-1-032-45190-9 (hbk)
ISBN: 978-1-032-45189-3 (pbk)
ISBN: 978-1-003-37582-1 (ebk)

DOI: 10.1201/9781003375821

Typeset in Latin Modern font
by KnowledgeWorks Global Ltd.

Publisher's note: This book has been prepared from camera-ready copy provided by the authors.

For Marios

To Sara, Luna, and Joshua, my daily inspiration, and to Claudio, a brotherly friend who has always believed in me.

Contents

Foreword

Scientific studies should never be seen in isolation—they add to existing knowledge, enabling us to learn and progress. This is the essence of Bayesian thinking; on receipt of new evidence, basic probability theory is used to update our beliefs in a coherent way. Meta-analysis—where the evidence from multiple studies is combined—is, therefore, a natural area for Bayesian methods, and so this book is extremely timely.

But of course things are rarely simple. Numerous complexities arise in trying to have a consistent approach to combining multiple sources of evidence with our previous understanding. Studies can vary for unknown reasons, use different designs, have missing information, or be subject to publication bias. Fortunately, a Bayesian approach allows extraordinary flexibility to non-standard features, which can otherwise be very difficult to handle.

The authors of this book have faced up to this complexity with relish, and systematically worked through a wide range of challenges encountered by those wanting to combine evidence in the real world. And this is not just a technical exposition, but provides practical guidance about using different software platforms as well as valuable advice about extracting summary statistics, eliciting prior information and communicating results, visualisation, and many other issues they and others have had to deal with. There is a wealth of useful guidance, whether adopting a Bayesian approach or not.

Although Bayesian methods are a natural fit for meta-analysis, their adoption has been surprisingly slow. Many of the challenges this book addresses were highlighted in seminal works from the 1990s and discussed extensively in the 2000s. However, currently only a small fraction of meta-analyses employ Bayesian approaches to address these issues. In contrast, Bayesian software has advanced remarkably, offering several powerful tools that this book explores. There has never been a better time to embrace Bayesian methods in meta-analysis.

This book reflects years of thoughtful experience, and should be of huge value to anyone faced with pooling studies into a coherent whole.

Professor Sir David Spiegelhalter, FRS OBE

About the Authors

Robert Grant is a statistician who has worked throughout his career with evidence synthesis and Bayesian models. He is one of the developers of Stan software, and a chartered fellow of the Royal Statistical Society. He worked on health service quality indicators and clinical guidelines for the Royal College of Physicians and the National Institute for Health and Care Excellence from 1998–2010, as well as epidemiological and health services research, and he taught health care professionals statistics and research methods at St George's, University of London and Kingston University from 2010–2017. He provided freelance coaching, training and consultancy to clients from various sectors from 2017–2024.

Gian Luca Di Tanna is a biostatistician and health economist who has focused his career on applied statistical methodologies for randomized clinical trials and observational research, particularly Bayesian methods and evidence synthesis/meta-analysis. He has held academic positions at Sapienza University of Rome, the University of Birmingham, the London School of Hygiene and Tropical Medicine, and Queen Mary University of London. He worked at the George Institute for Global Health at the University of New South Wales, Australia, where he served as head of the Biostatistics Division and co-head of the Meta-Research and Evidence Synthesis Unit.

From 2020–2022, he chaired the Statistical Methods for Health Economics and Outcomes Research Special Interest Group of the International Society for Pharmacoeconomics and Outcomes Research (ISPOR). He contributes as a statistical editor for Cochrane Review Groups and serves on the editorial boards of *PharmacoEconomics* and *BMC Medical Research Methodology*. He was listed among the World's Top 2% of Scientists in both the 2023 and 2024 rankings published by Stanford University and Clarivate Analytics. He is a Chartered Statistician of the Royal Statistical Society.

He is currently a full professor of biostatistics and health economics and head of research and services in the Department of Business Economics, Health, and Social Care at the University of Applied Sciences and Arts of Southern Switzerland (SUPSI). Additionally, he is a member of the academic board of the Swiss School of Public Health.

Preface

Meta-analysis is a statistical tool to combine the results reported by a collection of similar studies. The aim is to bring clarity to decision-makers (including the public), instead of expecting them to find and reconcile multiple studies. Peter Morgan, then scientific editor of the *Canadian Medical Association*, put it like this in 1986:

> The medical literature can be compared to a jungle. It is fast growing, full of dead wood, sprinkled with hidden treasure and infested with spiders and snakes.
> [...]
> Review articles will become increasingly popular as the size of the jungle of medical literature doubles every 10 years. The number of review journals and books continues to increase as more authors learn how to use the computer to search the literature. Writing review articles will be more competitive, but it also will be more rewarding [...] [171]

This book aims to help you continue that trend toward making sense of the literature jungle, and to use computer power effectively for this.

Unfortunately, the studies that have been done on a particular topic (which we call the *evidence base*) are not always very similar, and not always very well done and/or reported. Little problems crop up that prevent us from comparing like with like, because they cannot be accommodated in the usual meta-analysis methods.

The researcher then has a difficult choice of whether to make some bold assumption to simplify the problem, or to discard potentially useful studies, just to keep the meta-analysis show on the road. This book introduces a third option: to use Bayesian methods instead, which can include many difficult features in the evidence base in a more tailored statistical model, and allow useful ways of presenting results.

We have written this book for the majority of people doing meta-analysis today: researchers who understand systematic reviews, and perhaps simple descriptive and inferential statistics, and who now need to combine statistics from other people's studies. The book is subtitled "A Practical Introduction", a task we take very seriously. We provide not just formulas, but code and examples, to get you started, and advice on how meta-analysis can get tricky when the theory meets a real evidence base. We are opinionated, but we tell you what the opposing views are, too.

We expect that most readers will be new to Bayesian methods, and so we present multiple software options, especially in Part 1 of the book. The purpose of this is to let the reader compare them and decide which they would prefer to use.

Our examples are mostly drawn from biomedical research, as that is our background and the subject of most meta-analysis today, but we also reflect on research and policy in economics and education, where meta-analysis is growing rapidly in popularity. We have tried to keep all case studies simple so that experience of the substantive topic is not required. As this book is both practical and an introduction, we do not devote any space to history and very little to the philosophy of probability; these are interesting subjects, but belong elsewhere.

We mostly consider meta-analysis of studies that compare "arms" or groups, principally randomised experimental studies, but there is some consideration given to studies that cannot count on random allocation. Meta-analysis of diagnostic or prognostic models is an important topic, but requires more space than we can accommodate here. We also do not attempt to include borrowing of external information in clinical trials, or adaptive trial designs. Research designs other than trials that lie outside our scope include pharmaco-kinetic and pharmaco-dynamic research, Bayesian belief networks, hidden Markov models, and differential equation methods such as in infectious disease modelling.

Part 1 of this book contains a primer on the foundations of statistical inference (Chapter 1). Readers already familiar with statistics and meta-analysis should skim, but not skip, this chapter, because it introduces our terminology and notation, as well as a way of conceptualising analyses not found in introductory statistics textbooks. Bayesian statistics and software is introduced in Chapter 2. We then introduce meta-analysis, including Bayesian equivalents to common effect models, in Chapter 3 (often called "fixed effect"), and random effects models in Chapter 4.

Part 2 considers the inputs that are essential for Bayesian meta-analysis—extracting statistics from published studies, and obtaining prior distributions, including the opinions of experts—as well as how to present outputs. Part 3 explores specific problems and how they can be modelled. Each Part 3 chapter is as short and specific as possible so that once readers have covered the basics they can use this as a practical reference guide.

Throughout, we aim to start each chapter with a motivating problem, consider simple models of the data-generating process, and show the readers enough code that they can explore the problems and get a deeper intuition. At this stage, we keep the terminology basic and the language intuitive and informal. Once the problem is understood, we propose more complicated models to deal with it. Formal definitions, if needed at all, come at the end when the reader has reached the deepest understanding*.

We introduce seven software options in Part 1: BUGS, JAGS, Stan, Stata, bayesmeta, brms, and JASP. BUGS is still the most widely used software for Bayesian meta-analyses, so we mostly present BUGS code for models in Parts 2 and 3, but the accompanying website at **https://bayesian-ma.net** provides translations where possible; we use base (not "tidyverse") R as a *lingua franca*. The website includes all data and code from the book. The computer symbol in the margin† is there to encourage readers to play with data and models to gain deeper understanding.

We emphasise the responsibility on the meta-analyst (and any Bayesian analyst) to make modelling choices and be prepared to explain and justify them. Readers may find themselves on a miniature version of the famous Dunning-Kruger curve of confidence when learning and practising statistics (see Figure 0.1). Arriving at the right-hand side of the curve requires mathematical mastery‡, a deep understanding of why you are doing meta-analysis, and perhaps most importantly, a critical and curious mindset.

Although our emphasis is on mastery rather than a statistical cookbook, or theorems and proofs, we have maintained the spirit of mathematical rigour in that a term or symbol only ever means one thing. We remember how small ambiguities in notation and coding can leave the novice confused and dispirited. This means that our mathematical notation can seem complicated at first, but pays dividends later.

---

*Michael Greenacre's books on correspondence analysis were the inspiration for short chapters, and Lara Alcock's on learning mathematics informed the structure within each chapter.

†Icon produced by Linux GNOME Project, CC-BY-SA-3.0.

‡This is a concept widely discussed in primary and secondary school mathematics, but we feel it also applies to adult professionals who are moving into unfamiliar mathematical concepts and who will need to continually adapt what they learn to new challenges.

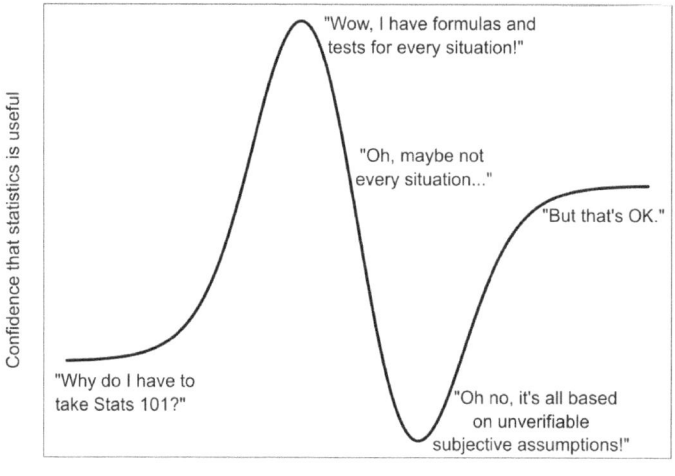

FIGURE 0.1

Our take on the Dunning-Kruger curve, based on our experience as students, then teachers of statistics. Learning Bayesian meta-analysis involves another roller-coaster ride.

Finally, we must warn readers that most people new to Bayesian methods encounter some frustrations in the early days. To have flexibility that allows tailored models, the software has to use simulation algorithms. Sometimes they will struggle, and it can be hard work to track down errors in your code or to set it up in the best way to get it running smoothly. We suspect that most new Bayesians at some point question whether it is worthwhile. We think it is. As John Tukey wrote more than 60 years ago:

> What of the future? The future of data analysis can involve great progress, the overcoming of real difficulties, and the provision of a great service to all fields of science and technology. Will it? That remains to us, to our willingness to take up the rocky road of real problems in preference to the smooth road of unreal assumptions, arbitrary criteria, and abstract results without real attachments. Who is for the challenge? [260]

We hope you will find Bayesian meta-analysis to be as useful as we have, and join us along the rocky road.

Robert & Gian Luca, Hampshire & Ticino, 2024

Acknowledgements

The development of this book has been profoundly shaped by our educational experiences, both as instructors and as perpetual learners.

We extend our sincere appreciation to the students who have participated in our various courses and seminars over the years. Their engagement, inquiries, and perspectives have significantly influenced our approach in this book. Thank you, for what we learnt from you.

Anonymous reviewers gave their time and expertise generously. Critical friends and experts helped refine the book, and suggested ideas and examples; thank you: Jay Brophy, Sylwia Bujkiewicz, Paul-Christian Bürkner, Meghan Cain, Giovanni Cerulli, Sofia Dias, Andrew Gelman, Nicholas Latimer, Rachael Meager, Emilia Riggi, Eric-Jan Wagenmakers, Ian White, and Vicki Yorke-Edwards.

We are deeply indebted to colleagues in research whose guidance and support have been invaluable in creating the time and opportunity to grow and refine our ideas. In particular, we want to thank: Luca Crivelli, Vari Drennan, Gary Globe, Mike Hurley, Derek Lowe, Jaime Miranda, Tom Quinn, Eva Segelov, Jill Stoddart, Armando Teixeira-Pinto, Giorgio Treglia, Maria Grazia Valsecchi, and Annarita Vestri.

We would also like to thank Kingston University, in particular Ann Ooms and James Denholm-Price, for hosting us during a productive writing week in June 2024.

Our profound appreciation extends to Joseph Alvin Ramos Santos, who transcends the role of researcher to that of a valued friend.

Notation

These tables set out all the algebraic notation used in this book so that you can refer back to it quickly if you are not sure what a particular symbol means. Unfortunately, different people prefer different forms of notation, and we have tried to be as simple and consistent as possible, except for where certain symbols are already widely used (for example, τ^2 for heterogeneity variance). We give priority to meta-analysis over other statistical claims on the same symbol (so τ does not mean precision). What appears complicated at first (for example, the $ijkt$ subscripts), will pay off later. Other textbooks on meta-analysis all differ somewhat in notation, so if you are taking a course on the subject, your instructor will probably have their own preferences too.

TABLE 0.1

Notation for data and statistics extracted from studies, part 1

Symbols	Meaning
y	Outcome variable
y_{ijkt}	The outcome reported for participant i in study j, arm k, at time t
$\bar{y}_{jkt}$	The mean outcome in study j, arm k, time t
$\bar{y}_{jk}$	The mean outcome reported in study j, arm k, where there is only one time point of interest
s_{jkt}	The observed standard deviation among participants in study j and arm k, at time t
r	An observed correlation coefficient (we mean the product-moment coefficient, unless we say otherwise); the details of what two variables are being compared depends on the circumstances, and is explained in each case
$\hat{\theta}_j$	The value estimated (the hat denotes an estimate) for some statistic that compares the arms in study j, such as a mean difference, log hazard ratio, and similar
$\hat{\theta}_{jk\ddot{k}}$	The statistic that compares arm k to a baseline arm $\ddot{k}$, in study j
$\widehat{\text{SE}}(\hat{\theta}_j)$	The estimated standard error of $\hat{\theta}_{jt}$; this can also apply to other statistics in studies, like $\widehat{\text{SE}}(\bar{y}_{jkt})$
n_{jkt}	The number of participants in study j, arm k and time t
m	The number of studies

TABLE 0.2

Notation for sample statistics extracted from studies, part 2

Symbols	Meaning
$\forall j$	for all values of j; a shorthand to say that a formula applies to all studies; we might also apply it to more than one subscript: $\forall(j,k)$
d_{jkt}	For a binary outcome, the number of *events* (however that is defined in the analysis)
p_{jkt}	For a binary outcome, the proportion of participants who were cases
w_{jkt}	The odds of a binary outcome in study j, arm j and time t
$\mathrm{LCI}(\hat{\theta}_j)$	The lower confidence interval (typically 95%) of $\hat{\theta}_j$ (or other estimates)
$\mathrm{UCI}(\hat{\theta}_j)$	The upper confidence interval (typically 95%) of $\hat{\theta}_j$ (or other estimates)

TABLE 0.3

Notation for unknown population statistics that we wish to estimate

Symbols	Meaning
μ	A population mean outcome value, defined in various ways as it is used
δ	An additive term, such as for a bias
u_j	The *random effect* or *fixed effect* of study j
θ_j	The causal effect of the intervention in study j
σ_{jkt}	The population standard deviation
τ	The standard deviation of the u_j random effects
ρ	A population correlation coefficient (typically, the product-moment coefficient)
π_{jkt}	The population proportion of cases
ν	Degrees of freedom, for the t and chi-squared distributions
β	A population regression coefficient, with subscripts determined by context as they are used
ω_{jkt}	The population odds for study j, arm k and time t
$\boldsymbol{\Sigma}$	A population covariance matrix; the subscripts will depend on the context; this is not the same as the summation operator $\sum$, and is smaller and bolder
$\mathrm{E}(\cdot), \mathrm{V}(\cdot)$	More generic notation for expectations and variances of any of these population or sample statistics

TABLE 0.4

Notation for probability distributions

Symbols	Meaning
$\sim$	The value on the left-hand side is distributed according to the probability distribution on the right-hand side
$N(\mu, \sigma)$	The normal distribution, with mean μ and standard deviation σ
$\phi(z)$	The "standard" normal distribution, that is, with mean 0 and standard deviation 1; z indicates such a standardised value
$\Phi(z)$	The cumulative density function $\int_{-\infty}^{z} \phi()$, in other words the probability of a standard normal distributed variable being z or lower
$\text{Binom}(\pi, n)$	The binomial distribution, with proportion π and sample size n
$\text{Poisson}(\mu)$	The Poisson distribution, with mean rate μ
$t(\mu, \sigma, \nu)$	The t distribution, with ν degrees of freedom, mean μ and dispersion (not the same as standard deviation) σ
$\chi^2(\nu)$	The chi-squared distribution with ν degrees of freedom
$\text{Beta}(\alpha, \beta)$	The beta distribution, with α and β defined the common way, so the mean is $\frac{\alpha}{\alpha+\beta}$
$\text{Cauchy}^+(0, \sigma)$	The half-Cauchy distribution, defined as 0 density for all negative values and $2 \times \text{Cauchy}(0, \sigma)$ otherwise, where σ is the dispersion
$f(\cdot)$	A generic symbol for a probability density function or probability mass function
$L(\cdot)$	A generic symbol for a likelihood function; $L(\theta \mid \boldsymbol{y}) = P(\boldsymbol{y} \mid \theta)$
$P(\cdot)$	The probability of some statement inside the brackets being true; this is used for prior and posterior densities

Part I

The Fundamentals

1

A Statistical Inference Primer

Learning objectives

After reading this chapter, you will be able to:

1. relate parameters to data and their distribution

2. explain the normal and binomial distributions for data

3. understand how the normal distribution is the sampling distribution for many statistics

4. appreciate the impact of the data distribution and sample size on the sampling distribution

5. consider data-generating processes

6. understand statistical inference as it relates to the sampling distribution

---

Inference means obtaining estimates of some unknown values from some known data, along with a measure of the uncertainty in those estimates. Most biomedical studies use data which are measurements from individual study participants and analyse these to report some summary statistics. Meta-analysis is rather different: the data are often the summary statistics reported by various studies, found by a systematic literature search, and included after critical appraisal [24].*

This chapter is intended for readers who have not studied statistical inference much, or not for a long time. Details of Bayesian statistics appear in Chapter 2, and meta-analysis is held back for Chapter 3, so if you are confident in your use of frequentist statistics (sometimes called "classical" statistics), including standard errors and confidence intervals, you can skip this chapter.

However, it also introduces the terminology we use in the rest of the book, the mathematical notation, and fundamentals of Bayesian programming code, and so we recommend looking through briefly even if you are a confident user of statistics.

Here, and throughout the book, we will write mostly about randomised controlled trials of healthcare interventions, but we will choose simple topics so that no specialist knowledge is required.

---

*Sometimes, meta-analyses can obtain and include individual participant data, which we consider in Chapter 10.

DOI: 10.1201/9781003375821-1

1.1 Thinking About Meta-Analysis

One example we will use repeatedly in this book is a meta-analysis of green tea extracts for weight loss. If you were the meta-analyst for that project, you would start with a collection of published studies found through a systematic review. You compile a list of each study's mean weight loss and standard deviation of weight loss—those are the knowns. Then, you want to *infer* the mean weight loss that we could expect from recommending people take green tea extracts—that is one of the unknowns.

There are a couple of steps that we just skipped over, and they can cause misunderstandings for meta-analysts. Let's consider them at the outset so that you can see how statistical inference will be used for challenging tasks, and how we need to be cautious at all times and to keep our judgements grounded in real-life experience and insight.

Firstly, the studies you have found do not necessarily represent the whole population: neither all *Homo sapiens* nor all people who might seek help for weight loss and start taking green tea extracts. Most of the studies were conducted in Asia, about half of them in Japan, and so the results they report might not be replicated elsewhere in the world, because of dietary, environmental or genetic differences. Extrapolating to other populations would be a leap of faith, more to do with clinical, behavioural, and biological judgement than evidence as such.

You don't need to know a reason why such a difference might happen; you should always be careful when extrapolating outside the kinds of people who were recruited into the studies. This is why you will often read this phrase in statistical inference: "...in the population from which the data were drawn". It acts as a handy reminder that inference is not magic and cannot tell you answers to things that you haven't even studied yet.

The second step that might cause you problems is that most modern randomised trials of interventions will allocate participants to interventions, and then compare their outcomes later, even if the individuals do not perfectly adhere to the recommended or prescribed intervention. Some people will not do exactly what they were told, for a wide variety of reasons. Studies which analyse everyone's data on the basis of what was recommended are called *intention to treat* analyses. These provide statistics which give insight into the *effectiveness* of the intervention: what results it will provide in the real world.

Not every study takes this approach. Studies sometimes monitor whether participants are adhering to the intervention and analyse only those that do so as expected. This is called a *per protocol* analysis, and it gives an estimate of the *efficacy* of the treatment: what its effect is when always applied as recommended. Most randomised trials now adopt intention to treat, but in practice, both insights have their use, and you are likely to find a mixture of the two in the evidence base—and sometimes, even within a single study[†].

So, we can see straight away, before even summarising what is involved in statistical inference, that the utility of what comes out depends on non-statistical considerations, especially when the data are actually summary statistics assembled by someone else for their own purposes.

For the rest of this chapter, we will step back from the specifics of meta-analysis and consider the basics. Our aim is to refresh your memory of the details of inference, to introduce our terminology and notation, and to lay the groundwork for thinking about meta-analysis as a statistical model that uses probability, not a fancy kind of weighted average.

[†]The topic of intention to treat and per protocol is dealt with further in Chapter 16.

1.2   Simple Inference for the Mean of Data

Imagine that you want to find out about the pulse rate of those recovering from a new viral infection. Is it different to the usual "healthy range"? You collect measurements from 100 patients at your clinic ($y_1, y_2, y_3, \ldots, y_{100}$; also, $n = 100$), and find that they are approximately normally distributed (Figure 1.1). Throughout this book, we will use notation for probability distributions like this:

$$y_i \sim \mathrm{N}(\mu, \sigma) \tag{1.1}$$

Here, the tilde symbol $\sim$ means that the variable on the left-hand side comes from a probability distribution, which is given on the right-hand side. In other words, there are some aspects to how specific values of y_i come about that we don't understand (nor do we need to; they might include whether participant i is feeling nervous or took a wrong turn coming into the clinic and had to climb up and back down a staircase), and added together, they produce that distributional shape (see Figure 1.1). For our purposes, y_i may as well be randomly generated from the distribution.

N() indicates the normal distribution, and it shows that every time you measure participant i's pulse, and get a value y_i, it will be just like a random number picked from this normal distribution. The Greek letter mu (μ) stands for the true mean pulse rate in the population from which the participants were drawn, and sigma (σ) for their true standard deviation. In some courses and textbooks, you will see the normal distribution written in terms of the mean μ and the *variance* σ^2, or even the *precision* $1/\sigma^2$, but we will use σ, because we find it is clearer for learners. Sometimes, you may see the normal distribution called the Gaussian distribution.

Later, we will start programming probability models like this. In the book, we mostly give extracts from code that can run in either the BUGS or JAGS software. We also give some indication of how this translates to other software, including Stan and Stata. In

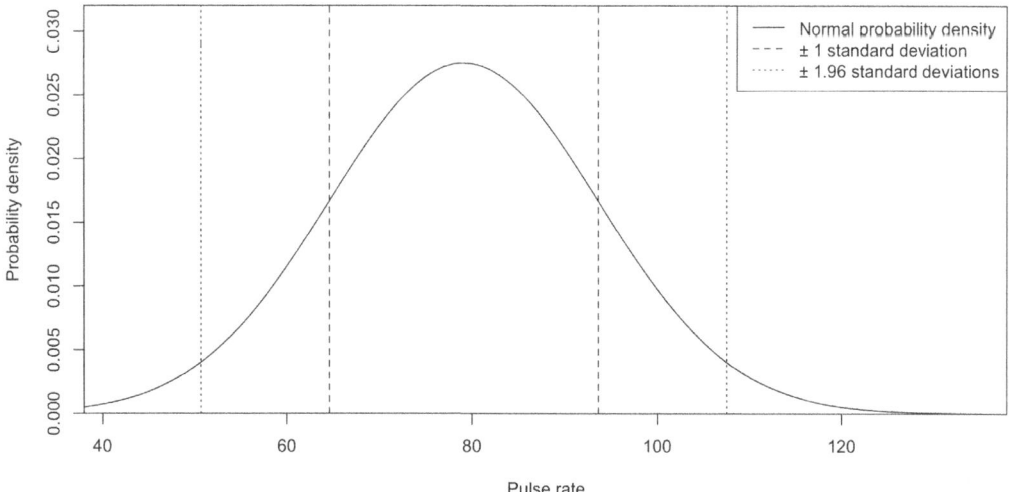

FIGURE 1.1
The normal distribution, with mean 79.1 and standard deviation 14.5. (From Ref. [136].)

BUGS/JAGS, we must provide the precision instead. We might write Equation 1.1 like this:

```
prec <- 1/(sigma*sigma)
pulse[i] ~ dnorm(mu, prec)
```

Some people find the mathematical notation easier to learn from, others prefer the code. You should pay attention to whichever version is best for you. In this chapter, there is more mathematics simply because the code that we use for Bayesian models will not appear until Chapter 2.

Now, you need to use statistical inference to estimate the mean pulse rate μ in the population of recovering patients, and also the uncertainty in your estimate. After all, it is only based on a sample of 100.

The estimate (statisticians often say *point estimate*) is simple enough—it is just the mean of your sample of 100:

$$\bar{y} = \frac{\sum_{i=1}^{n} y_i}{n} \tag{1.2}$$

Here, $\bar{y}$ indicates the mean of the sample: $y_1, y_2, y_3, \ldots, y_{100}$. This provides an estimate of the mean pulse rate in the population from which the data were drawn, but what about the uncertainty around that estimate? In frequentist statistics, probability is used for uncertainty, but only one kind of uncertainty: that arising from the fact that we have a sample of data and not the entire population. If we carried out another data collection process, recruiting and measuring participants, we would get a different sample, and therefore a different estimate of the mean.

Imagine all the possible samples and estimates that you might obtain from nearly identical data collection processes*. The estimates have their own distribution, the *sampling distribution*. It is often a normal distribution, and more likely to be so as the sample gets bigger, but it is not the same as the data's distribution.

Of course, this is just a theoretical point. We do not actually repeat the data collection process and directly assess the sampling distribution, but we do know that your study's estimated mean pulse rate is in the sampling distribution somewhere. Which one is it? Is it an over-estimate or an under-estimate of the true population mean? We will never know that for sure, but we can put bounds on the uncertainty around our estimate, using the shape and width of the sampling distribution, and that is a very valuable tool.

Suppose that in the population, there is no difference in mean pulse rate between infected and uninfected people. What are the chances of getting a very different mean in your data just by bad luck, as different as it could be? All of the data would have to bunch up at opposite ends of the distribution, and that is very unlikely, just like tossing a coin 100 times and getting 100 heads or 100 tails. So, the further away from our observed $\bar{y}$, the lower and lower the sampling distribution's probability must go. That should make you think of a shape like the normal distribution in Figure 1.1.

The standard deviation of the sampling distribution, which, confusingly, is in frequentist statistics called the *standard error* of the mean, gives us a measure of uncertainty, of how far away our estimate could be from the truth.

---

*These samples have to come from data collection processes which are similar enough to differ only in terms of the sample that they obtain. It would not be comparable to include a data collection which took place in a different country, for example.

Many learners find it helpful to play around with simulated data to understand how a statistical procedure really works. On this book's website, we include some suggested R code that you can run to see sampling from a known population in action.

When we want to learn about the sampling distribution of the mean, and the data distribution is neither too far from normal, nor too small, then we can estimate the sampling distribution's mean by just plugging in the sample mean, but the standard error (uncertainty in the estimate of the mean) is smaller than the standard deviation of the data. We can use this formula:

$$SE(\bar{y}) = \frac{SD(y)}{\sqrt{n}} = \frac{s}{\sqrt{n}} \tag{1.3}$$

SE stands for standard error and SD for standard deviation. Looking closely at Equation 1.3, you can see that $SE(\bar{y})$ applies to the sampling distribution of the mean, while $SD(y)$ applies to the data. s is our sample's observed standard deviation, which in practice we obtain directly from our software, for example by typing `sd(pulse)` in R. Inside the software, this is the calculation:

$$SD(y) = s = \sqrt{\frac{\sum_{i=1}^{n}(y_i - \bar{y})^2}{n-1}} \tag{1.4}$$

Beginners in inference are often tripped up by these similar terms, but the standard deviation is a statistic used to summarise the spread in the data distribution, while the standard error is a name for the same statistic when applied to the sampling distribution.

Armed with the standard error formula, we can now write down the sampling distribution of $\bar{y}$. It is not normal but a t-distribution instead, which is slightly more spread out for small values of n, allowing more uncertainty. This is because the formula for s relies on the estimate of $\bar{y}$, which is itself an estimate, so there is compounded uncertainty.

$$\bar{y} \sim t(\mu, \frac{s}{\sqrt{n}}, \nu) \tag{1.5}$$

We say that this follows a t-distribution with mean μ, *dispersion* (not the same as the standard deviation) $s/\sqrt{n}$, and ν *degrees of freedom* (ν is the Greek letter nu). The degrees of freedom control how much more the t-distribution is spread out than the normal: smaller degrees of freedom means extra uncertainty around s, and so wider spread. For the mean of one sample, $\nu = n - 1$. As n gets bigger, the sampling distribution becomes closer and closer to $N(\mu, \frac{\sigma}{\sqrt{n}})$.

The precision in the t-distribution is $\nu/s^2(\nu - 2)$, so the BUGS code equivalent would be:

```
nu <- n-1
prec <- nu / (s*s*(nu-2))
meanpulse ~ dt(mu, prec, nu)
```

Later (in Chapter 3 and Table 3.1), we will encounter an example of a meta-analysis where studies report means and standard deviations of change in body mass index [136]. The first of these studies, by Kozuma and colleagues, reports $n = 107$, $\bar{y} = -1.0$, and $s = 0.6$ in its intervention arm. Look through the calculation of the sampling distribution for the

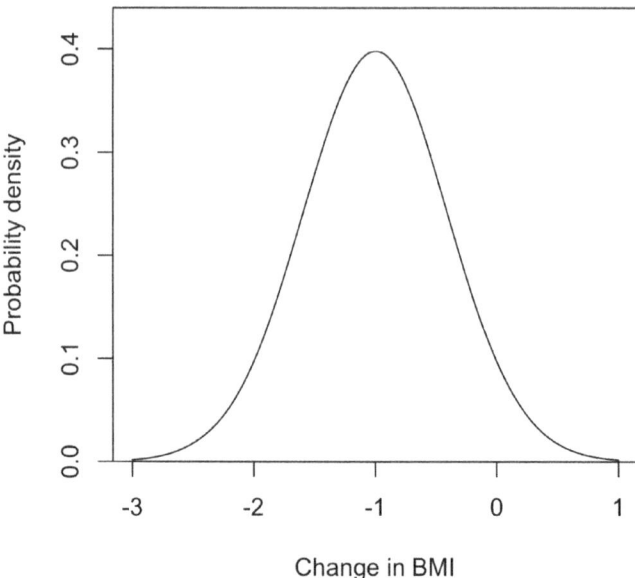

FIGURE 1.2

Sampling distribution for one study arm's mean. (Intervention arm of Kozuma. From Ref [134].)

(one-sample) mean below, referring to the formula above, to make sure that you can see how the values arise.

$$\text{Degrees of freedom: } 107 - 1 = 106$$

$$\text{Precision: } \frac{106}{(0.6)^2 \times (106 - 2)} = \frac{106}{37.44} = 2.83$$

This leads to a line of code:

```
change_bmi ~ dt(-1.0, 2.83, 106)
```

In practice, we do not have to do these calculations ourselves—the computer does them—but it is helpful to work through them at least once to understand what is happening. The t-distribution for Kozuma's intervention arm is shown in Figure 1.2.

In fact, regardless of the data distribution, as n grows, the sampling distribution of the sum of the data becomes normal. This is a statistical fact called the *Central Limit Theorem*. Properties like this, that apply as sample sizes get large, are called *asymptotic*. A lot of frequentist methods rely on shortcut formulas with known asymptotic properties.

A very common question that beginners ask is how they can tell when to use a normal sampling distribution, and when they should use the t-distribution. There is no universally reliable answer to this, as it depends not only on the sample size but also on how normal the distribution of the data is. Experimentation with the sampling code on the accompanying website will help you gain some intuition for this.

1.2.1 Confidence intervals and hypothesis tests

Having obtained the sampling distribution, we can find the pair of points that contain the central 95% of the area under the curve, and report these as the *95% confidence interval* for the mean. The 95% confidence interval around the mean—and most statistics as n grows— is the estimate ± 1.96 standard errors. In Bayesian statistics, we simply say that there is a 95% probability that the true population mean, μ, is in this interval.

In strict frequentist terms, the definition is more convoluted. This is a formula that produces an interval, and if we consider a collection of nearly identical data collection processes (with a shared μ), then each would have its own 95% confidence interval, and 95% of those confidence intervals would correctly capture the true μ.

We can also use the standard error to carry out a *hypothesis test* to assess the evidence that μ lies in a certain range or takes a certain value. These tests report *p-values* and might be divided into *statistically significant* or non-significant. This is a rather different paradigm to Bayesian statistics, and so we will not spend more time on it in this book. You might be concerned that your audience, accustomed to p-values in meta-analysis, will be disappointed by their absence from Bayesian meta-analyses. There are good alternatives, and we will return to them in Chapter 2, and other issues of reporting in Chapter 7.

1.3 Inference for the Proportion

So far, we have considered data $(y_1, y_2, \ldots, y_n)$ that could take any number, or perhaps any positive number. Often, however, research collects binary data on whether an event happened. In this book, we will encounter binary events such as: people on blood pressure lowering medication experiencing side effects, snow leopards having parasitic worms, and people surviving to 35 days after treatment for heart attack. Each study participant's outcome, y_i, must take a value of either zero or one. We typically summarise them by the proportion of events, p, which is actually just the mean of the zeros and ones:

$$p - \frac{\sum y_i}{n} \tag{1.6}$$

This formula also happens to be the ratio of two counts: the numerator $(\sum y_i)$ and the denominator (n).

With a binary outcome, p is the observed proportion in the study, and π is the proportion in the population. π can take any value between 0 and 1; it does not mean $3.14159\ldots$, the ratio between the circumference and diameter of a circle. Depending on the setting, you might also call π the population *risk*.

From now on, we will use the letter d for the observed numerator: $d = \sum y_i$. This is quite common in biostatistics (it probably started from counting **d**eaths) but can confuse learners because d refers to the **n**umerator and n to the **d**enominator!

The sampling distribution for d, given π and n, is *binomial*:

$$d \sim \text{Binom}(\pi, n) \tag{1.7}$$

The binomial distribution's probabilities are shown in Figure 1.3, for one example. This uses data from an example meta-analysis, which appears in Chapter 3 and Table 3.2. The first study, de Spoelstra 2006, reports that 1 out of 22 participants who received ACE inhibitors (a class of blood pressure medication) reported adverse events. You should note

Binomial distribution

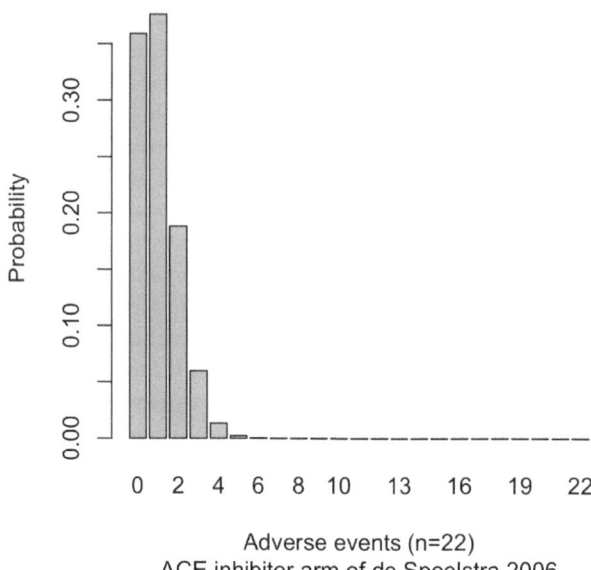

Adverse events (n=22)
ACE inhibitor arm of de Spoelstra 2006

FIGURE 1.3
Sampling distribution for one study arm's count of events.

that, in contrast to the t-distribution of Figure 1.2, the binomial is only defined for counts $0, 1, 2, \ldots$ (which mathematicians would call natural numbers).

In the case of de Spoelstra's ACE inhibitor arm, the estimate of π is $\frac{1}{22}$, and the code would be:

```
d ~ dbin(1/22, 22)
```

We can also apply this to each participant's binary data. The only difference to the formula is that $n = 1$:

$$y_i \sim \text{Binom}(\pi, 1) \tag{1.8}$$

The binomial distribution, with $n = 1$, is very often called the Bernoulli distribution, however, we prefer not to introduce new terminology if we can avoid it, so we will use the more general definition of the binomial distribution.

1.3.1 The odds of an event

A less intuitive but, as we will see, mathematically useful, statistic is the *odds*, which is the number of participants with the outcome, divided by the number without. We will use w

for the observed odds and ω (omega) for the population odds[†].

$$w = \frac{d}{n-d} = \frac{p}{1-p} \tag{1.9}$$

We will soon find ourselves working with its logarithm, or *log odds*. The function that takes p as input and produces $\log_e(w)$ as output is also called the *logistic function* or *logit*:

$$\begin{aligned} \operatorname{logit}(p) &= \log_e(w) \\ &= \log_e\left(\frac{p}{1-p}\right) \\ &= \log_e\left(\frac{d}{n-d}\right) \\ &= \log_e(d) - \log_e(n-d) \end{aligned} \tag{1.10}$$

The inverse logistic function reverses this, taking log odds as input and returning the probability of an event. Sometimes, it is called *expit*. To simplify the mathematics, let's define $z = \log(w)$.

$$\begin{aligned} p &= \operatorname{expit}(z) \\ &= \frac{e^z}{1+e^z} \\ &= \frac{1}{1+e^{-z}} \end{aligned} \tag{1.11}$$

For the rest of this book, we will only use logarithms to base e (sometimes called natural logarithms and written $\ln(\cdot)$), so they will just be denoted by $\log()$. In case you are wondering how we will handle situations where $d = 0$ and hence $\log(d) = -\infty$, in practice we do not compute these individual logarithms of d and n in Bayesian analysis.

1.4 Inference for Intervention or Treatment Effects

Studies usually do not just estimate one number, but instead some comparison between two groups, or the effect of one variable on another. These *contrasts* or *effects* manifest in slightly different ways for the statistics we have considered so far.

If there is a continuous outcome in the treatment arm of a study, and another in the control arm, then we will often focus our attention on the difference between the means. When there are binary outcomes, and two proportions, we often report a ratio of the risks, or a ratio of the odds.

1.4.1 Differences in means

Where a study reports a mean in a study arm receiving the intervention ($\bar{y}_{\mathbf{Int}}$) and a mean in the control arm ($\bar{y}_{\mathbf{Ctl}}$), we usually subtract them to estimate a *mean difference*, $\bar{y}_{\mathbf{Int}} - \bar{y}_{\mathbf{Ctl}}$. This provides an estimated effect of the intervention over and above that of the control.

[†]This is a strange choice, as ω (Greek omega) is not equivalent to the letter w at all, except that they *look* the same. But most papers and books use this, and we don't want to invent new notation if we can use a familiar one.

In general, we will use the Greek letter theta, θ, to denote any such contrast that might estimate a treatment/intervention effect.

The mean difference has a normal sampling distribution, just like the two means themselves. When we add two random variables, we obtain a new random variable with its own probability distribution. Its mean will be the sum of its components' means, and likewise for the variance if they are not correlated:

$$E(A + B) = E(A) + E(B),$$
$$V(A + B) = V(A) + V(B) \tag{1.12}$$

If we subtract them, which is the case for the difference of two means, then the resulting mean is the difference of means, but the variance is still the sum:

$$E(A - B) = E(A) - E(B),$$
$$V(A - B) = V(A) + V(B) \tag{1.13}$$

We can apply this to find the sampling distribution for the difference between two means:

$$E(\bar{y}_{\text{Int}} - \bar{y}_{\text{Ctl}}) = E(\bar{y}_{\text{Int}}) - E(\bar{y}_{\text{Ctl}}),$$
$$= \bar{y}_{\text{Int}} - \bar{y}_{\text{Ctl}},$$
$$V(\bar{y}_{\text{Int}} - \bar{y}_{\text{Ctl}}) = V(\bar{y}_{\text{Int}}) + V(\bar{y}_{\text{Ctl}})$$
$$= \left(\frac{\sigma_{\text{Int}}}{\sqrt{n_{\text{Int}}}}\right)^2 + \left(\frac{\sigma_{\text{Ctl}}}{\sqrt{n_{\text{Ctl}}}}\right)^2 \tag{1.14}$$

In a sampling distribution, the variance is the square of the standard error. This is a common source of confusion, which we think is worth summarising once more. The sampling distribution describes the uncertainty about the estimate of a statistic, and its spread is measured by the standard error. The data distribution describes the distribution of data values and its spread is measured by the standard deviation.

In the study we quoted above, Kozuma 2005, the intervention arm reported these statistics: $n_{\text{Int}} = 107, \bar{y}_{\text{Int}} = -1.0, s_{\text{Int}} = 0.6$.

The control arm reported: $n_{\text{Ctl}} = 119, \bar{y}_{\text{Ctl}} = 0.3, s_{\text{Ctl}} = 0.4$.

We can apply Equations 1.14 to this:

$$\text{Mean difference: } -1.0 - 0.3 = -1.3$$
$$\text{Variance of mean difference: } \left(\frac{0.6}{\sqrt{107}}\right)^2 + \left(\frac{0.4}{\sqrt{119}}\right)^2 = 0.0047$$
$$\text{Standard error: } \sqrt{0.0047} = 0.069$$

These formulas are useful in meta-analysis, so you should bear them in mind and know where to find them in this book. The accompanying website includes some suggested R code that you can use to simulate data from two groups, obtain their means and the mean difference, and repeat the process many times.

This lets you examine the sampling distributions in a way that we cannot do with real-life data. Many statistics students find that experimenting with simulations like this helps them to relate theory to practice and to remember what they have learnt for longer [82].

1.4.2 Differences in means from paired data

In parallel-arms randomised controlled trials, if everything has gone according to plan, $\bar{y}_{\mathbf{Int}}$ and $\bar{y}_{\mathbf{Ctl}}$ will not influence one another in any way. Their sampling distributions are *uncorrelated*. In some other study designs, they will be correlated, including pre-post comparisons, identical twins, family dyads, healthy and diseased organs from the same person, crossover trials and so on.

The effect on the difference of means is that a more complicated version of Equation 1.13 is needed. Suppose that two normally distributed random variables, A and B, are correlated with product-moment coefficient ρ:

$$E(A - B) = E(A) - E(B),$$
$$V(A - B) = V(A) + V(B) - 2\rho\sqrt{V(A)V(B)} \tag{1.15}$$

If some instances of paired data, for example pre- and post-treatment, we would expect there to be quite strong positive correlation, perhaps even up to $\rho = 0.9$.

What do you think it would indicate if a study had $\rho = 1$? Think about what would happen to the variance of $A - B$ as ρ gets closer and closer to 1. By looking at Equation 1.15, try to work out why this is the case. Then, you can try it out in the online simulation code.

1.4.3 Proportions, risks, and odds

In a two-arm trial with binary outcomes, all participants belong to one of the arms (intervention or control) and one of the outcomes (present or absent). We can split the total sample across a two-by-two table:

TABLE 1.1
Binary outcomes from a two group study

	Intervention	Control
Outcome present	$d_{\mathbf{Int}}$	$d_{\mathbf{Ctl}}$
Outcome absent	$n_{\mathbf{Int}} - d_{\mathbf{Int}}$	$n_{\mathbf{Ctl}} - d_{\mathbf{Ctl}}$
Total	$n_{\mathbf{Int}}$	$n_{\mathbf{Ctl}}$

From Table 1.1, the *risk* in the intervention group is $p_{\mathbf{Int}} = d_{\mathbf{Int}}/n_{\mathbf{Int}}$, which is just the observed proportion of participants who received the intervention and went on to have the outcome present.

The risk ratio or relative risk compares the two groups:

$$\frac{p_{\mathbf{Int}}}{p_{\mathbf{Ctl}}} = \frac{d_{\mathbf{Int}}/n_{\mathbf{Int}}}{d_{\mathbf{Ctl}}/n_{\mathbf{Ctl}}} \tag{1.16}$$

When a ratio is used to compare two groups and estimate treatment effect, rather than difference of means, the estimated effect is multiplicative, not additive. Using θ for the treatment effect (risk ratio, in this case), and $\hat{\theta}$ for our estimate of it, the risk in people receiving the intervention is $\hat{\theta}$ times the risk in those who receive the control. If $\hat{\theta} = 1$, there is no difference. If $\hat{\theta} > 1$, the risk is higher in the intervention group, and if $\hat{\theta} < 1$, the risk is lower in the intervention group.

Often, studies have to report odds and odds ratios instead. Referring again to Table 1.1, the odds of the outcome being present in the intervention group is $w_{\mathbf{Int}} = d_{\mathbf{Int}}/n_{\mathbf{Int}} - d_{\mathbf{Int}}$:

the number with the outcome, divided by the number without. The odds ratio is also a multiplicative treatment effect:

$$\frac{w_{\text{Int}}}{w_{\text{Ctl}}} = \frac{d_{\text{Int}}/(n_{\text{Int}} - d_{\text{Int}})}{d_{\text{Ctl}}/(n_{\text{Ctl}} - d_{\text{Ctl}})} \tag{1.17}$$

Some books, courses and websites rearrange the RR and OR formulas, for example,

$$\frac{w_{\text{Int}}}{w_{\text{Ctl}}} = \frac{d_{\text{Int}}(n_{\text{Ctl}} - d_{\text{Ctl}})}{d_{\text{Ctl}}(n_{\text{Int}} - d_{\text{Int}})}$$

In some epidemiology classes, students are taught that the odds ratio approximates the risk ratio, and can be interpreted as such. However, while this can be true if the outcome is rare, it is definitely not a universally reliable approximation and one should be converted into the other carefully, via a table like Table 1.1 if possible.

It is very useful to work with the logarithm of the odds ratio (you will often hear people say "log odds ratio") or risk ratio. There are three reasons for this:

1. If we take logarithms, the transformed effect becomes additive: $\log\left(\frac{w_{\text{Int}}}{w_{\text{Ctl}}}\right) = \log(w_{\text{Int}}) - \log(w_{\text{Ctl}})$

2. the logarithm of the odds ratio reaches a normal sampling distribution at smaller n than the odds ratio itself, and we may need to rely on known sampling distribution shapes in our meta-analysis models

3. it is used to predict the log odds for various situations, and the log odds can take any number from $-\infty$ to ∞, while alternatives are constrained in various ways that can cause problems*.

The asymptotic standard error of the log odds ratio (square root of the variance of its sampling distribution) has a surprisingly simple formula [138], related to Table 1.1:

$$SE\left(\log\left(\frac{w_{\text{Int}}}{w_{\text{Ctl}}}\right)\right) = \sqrt{V\left(\log\left(\frac{w_{\text{Int}}}{w_{\text{Ctl}}}\right)\right)}$$
$$= \sqrt{\frac{1}{d_{\text{Int}}} + \frac{1}{n_{\text{Int}} - d_{\text{Int}}} + \frac{1}{d_{\text{Ctl}}} + \frac{1}{n_{\text{Ctl}} - d_{\text{Ctl}}}} \tag{1.18}$$

Pause for a moment with this equation to think about what happens to the standard error as a study's sample size (n_{Int} and n_{Ctl}) gets larger.

The sampling distribution of the log risk ratio has the following asymptotic standard error [138]:

$$SE\left(\log\left(\frac{p_{\text{Int}}}{p_{\text{Ctl}}}\right)\right) = \sqrt{V\left(\log\left(\frac{p_{\text{Int}}}{p_{\text{Ctl}}}\right)\right)}$$
$$= \sqrt{\frac{n_{\text{Int}}}{d_{\text{Int}} n_{\text{Int}}} \frac{d_{\text{Int}}}{} + \frac{n_{\text{Ctl}} - d_{\text{Ctl}}}{d_{\text{Ctl}} n_{\text{Ctl}}}} \tag{1.19}$$

We worked through the binomial sampling distribution above for one study—de Spoelstra 2006—that reported the binary outcome of whether or not adverse events were reported, with participants allocated to either ACE inhibitors or angiotensin receptor blockers (ARBs)

---

*The odds must be positive, the risk must be between 0 and 1, therefore the log risk must be a negative number. The software we will use does not innately understand these constraints, so unless you are careful, it can propose impossible values, at the cost of computing problems or damage to the project's credibility.

to lower their blood pressure. In this study: $d_{\textbf{ACEI}} = 1, n_{\textbf{ACEI}} = 22, d_{\textbf{ARB}} = 3, n_{\textbf{ARB}} = 24$. We can work out the odds ratio (choosing to express it as $\frac{\textbf{ACEI}}{\textbf{ARB}}$), log odds ratio and standard error of the log odds ratio:

$$\text{Odds ratio: } \frac{1/(22-1)}{3/(24-3)} = 0.333$$

$$\text{Log odds ratio: } \log(0.333) = -1.099$$

$$\text{Standard error: } \sqrt{\frac{1}{1} + \frac{1}{21} + \frac{1}{3} + \frac{1}{21}} = 1.447$$

We describe, in more detail, how to convert one statistic into another when you are extracting data from published studies, in Chapter 5.

With the very small numbers in the de Spoelstra 2006 study, we should be cautious about the reliability of these formulas. Remember that they are asymptotic, which means that they apply as n grows large. With more than 100 in each group, Kozuma 2005 is likely to be well described above, but this smaller study is not. Later, we will examine more exact methods for small numbers, in the context of meta-analysis.

1.4.4 Survival or time-to-event data

It is common in biomedical research to look at the time until an event happens. If a study follows individuals, they will fall into four categories:

1. some will have the event of interest (such as attending hospital after a fall) first happen at some time,

2. others will reach the end of the study duration without it happening,

3. others will have some other event that disqualifies them from the rest of the study, and

4. the researchers may lose contact with others at some time during the study, and not know what happened after that.

This leads to time-to-event or survival analysis.

The likelihood is determined by the probability density of time at first event. This is a mathematical function showing how common first events are over time. It may have an off-the-shelf formula, such as the log-normal or Weibull distributions, in which case it is called parametric survival analysis. It may not have a formula but be learnt from the distribution of first events in the data; these are semi-parametric models such as Cox regression.

In either case, the probability density is potentially changed by the intervention arm or exposure to a risk factor. The combination of the intervention / risk factor effect, and the underlying distribution of first event times, together make the likelihood contribution. Semi-parametric methods do not explicitly quantify the underlying distribution's contribution.

Line charts with time on the horizontal axis and the proportion of "survivors" on the vertical axis are survival charts. If they are drawn based on the observed data, they will have a stepped appearance, dropping at each time that an event occurred, which is called a Kaplan-Meier plot.

The size of the vertical drop in the survival curve provides the probability of a first event in some period of time. An estimate of probability density at an instant in time, conditional on having survived up to that instant, is called the hazard. Two arms, or the presence and absence of a risk factor, can be compared by the hazard ratio.

The individuals in the fourth category above need to be treated differently in these calculations. They are *right-censored*: if the event did happen, it would be to the right of the censoring time on the survival curve. They still contribute to likelihood because we know that an event did not happen prior to censoring.

Hazard ratios are not the only output from survival analysis. They typically make an assumption that the ratio is constant over time, which is called *proportional hazards*. An increasingly popular alternative is the *restricted mean survival time* [207], which does not make this assumption.

There are more complications and innovations, and some statisticians devote their careers to survival analysis, particularly in clinical trials. Events may be interval-censored, in that we only know that they happened within some window of time. Parametric suvival curves may be made more flexible by the combination of multiple shapes. There may be more than one terminal event that removes the individual from the group of participants at risk, which leads to competing risks analysis.

1.4.5   A warning about interpretation

We have so far described randomised controlled trials, and in that study design, if everything is done properly, then the contrast between intervention and control should indeed give us an estimate of the intervention effect (as the section title promised). However, in non-randomised (observational) studies, in the presence of deviations from the study plan, or poor methodological practice, this interpretation cannot confidently be made. As the saying goes, correlation is not causation.

2

What is Bayesian Statistics?

Learning objectives

After reading this chapter, you will be able to:

1. differentiate Bayesian and frequentist analyses by the way they use probability distributions

2. explain the different meanings that prior and posterior probabilities can represent

3. summarise the posterior distribution for different needs

4. translate a data-generating process to a statistical model

5. use common probability distributions as sampling distributions of statistics, and as priors for their parameters

6. choose a preferred Bayesian software, based on its level of flexibility and ease of learning

7. use prior predictive distributions to check the compatibility of your prior distributions and data

8. use posterior predictive distributions to critically evaluate your model and identify areas for refinement

9. choose a summary of a posterior distribution that suits the question under investigation

Bayesian statistics differs from the more common frequentist and likelihood-based methods in how probability is used. Frequentist probability is only used to represent the way in which data might vary because of random sampling, given some data-generating process (DGP) and its parameters. Bayesian statistics applies probability to the parameters too, as well as other unknowns.

A simple way of explaining Bayesian probability is that it is a mathematical tool that represents how our data could have turned out differently. That would capture both aleatory unknowns (such as DGP parameters) and epistemic unknowns (such as missing data).

A nearly identical data collection process would give us another sample of data. No matter how many of these we might (at least in theory) collect, they would all be affected by the same DGP parameters, but each one would have its own unique missing data. Fundamentally, this is the reason why aleatory unknowns are amenable to frequentist analysis: the theory is centred on what would arise from a large collection of nearly identical data collection processes, and this would not allow epistemic unknowns.

DOI: 10.1201/9781003375821-2

Many people who adopt Bayesian methods for meta-analysis do so because there are epistemic unknowns that they need to estimate in order to get meaningful outputs from their work. For example, a common problem, which we return to in Chapter 11, is that studies sometimes do not report all the statistics that we need for meta-analysis. The means and sample sizes might be reported, for example, but not the standard deviations.

A Bayesian meta-analysis can include that study in the meta-analysis, representing the uncertainty in the unknown standard error with a probability distribution.

2.1   Likelihood

We can write down a formula for the probability of observing a certain outcome value for a study participant (i; people often say "the ith participant", rhyming with scythe), given the group they are in, such as the arm of a randomised controlled trial (RCT).

For a single normally distributed variable, we will need to know the mean and standard deviation: the *parameters* of the normal distribution. The normal probability density function allows us to combine the data y_i with the parameters and find the probability density for the ith participant. Although we might write this as $y_i \sim \mathrm{N}(\mu, \sigma)$, that's really a human-friendly shorthand for what's actually going on inside any calculation. The normal, or any other *probability density function*, takes both data and parameters as input, and returns a probability density as output.

If we have discrete-valued data, such as binary data or counts, we can use the binomial or other distributions in the same way, except that we obtain a probability and not a probability density[*].

The goal of likelihood-based statistical inference, in this example, is to find μ and σ so that they are the best possible match to the observed data. When they are a good match, the data get higher probabilities (densities). If we multiply all the data's probabilities (or densities) together, we get a summary measure of how well a given μ and σ match our dataset. That summary measure is called the *likelihood*. In machine learning, it would be called a form of *loss function*.

Because the likelihood can be an extremely small number, we usually work with its logarithm, the *log likelihood*. To calculate the log likelihood, we find the probability of each data point, given the model and the parameter values, we calculate their logarithms, and then *add* (not multiply) those together [†].

In Figure 2.1, we show points for the participants in an imaginary study of arthritis pain. Considering only one intervention, pre-treatment pain score is on the horizontal axis, and post-treatment is on the vertical axis. The two scores are correlated; someone who is

---

[*]We don't like to introduce technical complications, but we find that some learners rightly question this relaxed attitude to whether the function returns a probability or the probability density (which is really the derivative of the probability with respect to the parameter(s)). If this is you, think about it this way: any continuous variable, known or unknown, is measured only to some degree of precision (decimal places), so the probability $P(y_1 = 20.381)$ is really $P(20.3805 \leq y_1 < 20.3815)$, which is a narrow area under the curve of the PDF, so narrow it is well-approximated by a rectangle of area proportionate to the height of the curve (the PDF). In short, our work is made easier by the fact that we only need to obtain a value proportionate to the posterior density (explained in Section 2.2), so we do not have to suffer any integral calculus.

[†]This produces larger negative numbers that can be stored accurately. Digital computers have to represent numbers in a limited number of bits (0s and 1s), and so rounding error can creep in with extremely small (close to zero) values.

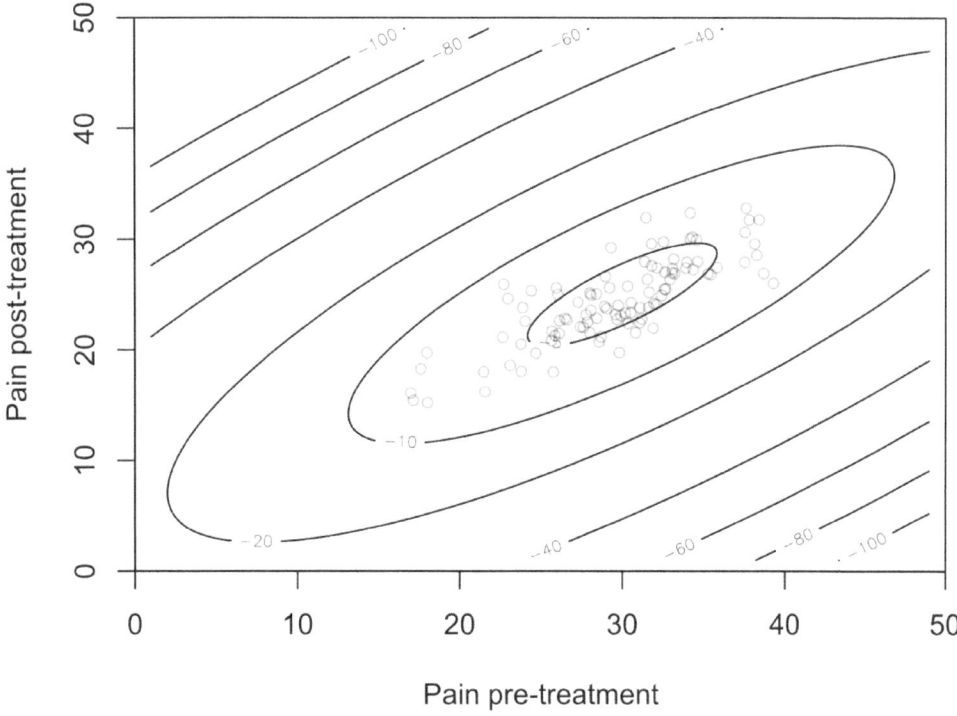

FIGURE 2.1

A normal probability model for pre- and post-treatment (correlated) data. The dots show 100 observations, while the concentric contour lines are an assumed *model*, in this case the log probability density from the bivariate normal distribution.

severely affected pre-treatment may be better afterwards but is likely still to be worse than most other participants.

The contour lines show the log probability density from the bivariate (two variables, on eon the horizontal axis, and one on the vertical) normal distribution that we encountered in Equation 1.15. A log probability density of -10 equates to a probability density of $e^{-10} = 0.000045$. A participant whose pre- and post-treatment outcomes led to a point lying on the -10 contour line would contribute -10 to the log likelihood. All the observed data are inside the -10 contour line.

Figure 2.1 shows the probability, and the axes are variables in our dataset. We call this *variable space*, and machine learning people use the term *feature space*. But because we are seeking to optimise the parameters, it is helpful to show *parameter space* too. In Figure 2.2, we only consider two of the parameters. Values of the pre-treatment mean are on the horizontal axis, and values of the pre-treatment standard deviation on the vertical.

We can estimate our parameters by finding values that maximise the log likelihood (the same values will also maximise the likelihood). This is called *maximum likelihood estimation* (MLE), and it is widely used in non-Bayesian statistics [189]. Considering the contours in Figure 2.2, this entails finding the "top of the hill" in parameter space: the point where log likelihood is highest.

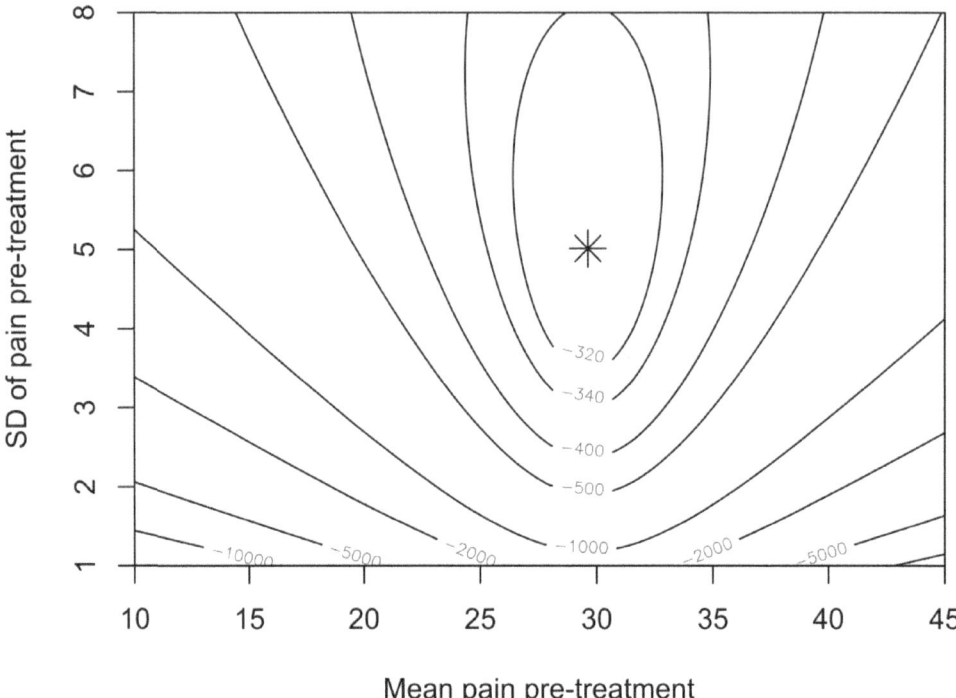

FIGURE 2.2
A normal likelihood in parameter space, for the pre-treatment pain data. The mean and standard deviation are the parameters. The contour lines show how the log likelihood changes with different values. The star indicates the observed mean and standard deviation of the data.

2.2   Bayes' Theorem: Likelihood and Prior

In all Bayesian work, we must supply some *prior distribution* for the unknowns, and then "update" that with the likelihood to obtain a *posterior distribution*. The likelihood, as we saw in Section 2.1, is the probability of obtaining the data, given the unknowns: in other words, the statistical model of the data-generating process.

The famous Bayes' theorem (Equation 2.1) was originally presented in 1763 in this context of updating prior information about the unknowns (θ) with new data (Y). Later, even among those who rejected this interpretation of probability, it remained an important part of the mathematics of probability, and was used in practice to reverse conditional probabilities.

For example, it often appears in health care professionals' courses to convert the probability of a positive test result, given the true presence of a disease, to the probability of having the disease, given a positive test result.

We will write the collection of values of unknowns as $\boldsymbol{\theta}$, using the bold typeface to indicate a vector*.

$$P(\boldsymbol{\theta}|\boldsymbol{Y}) \propto P(\boldsymbol{Y}|\boldsymbol{\theta})P(\boldsymbol{\theta}) \tag{2.1}$$

For our purposes, we can supply the prior, $P(\boldsymbol{\theta})$, and the likelihood, $P(\boldsymbol{Y}|\boldsymbol{\theta})$, for some combination of values making up $\boldsymbol{\theta}$, and by multiplying them together, obtain a value that is proportionate to the posterior density for that value of $\boldsymbol{\theta}$.

Bayesian analysis is implemented using simulation algorithms, and they generally do not need the exact posterior density, but just some value proportionate to it. This saves a lot of computer time.

2.2.1 Snow leopard parasites: a worked example

Let's consider a worked example that will make the concepts clearer. Suppose that you work for a conservation charity that runs a remote nature reserve in central Asia, where there are ten snow leopards. This is the population for which you want to infer results. Because of climate change, biologists are concerned about new parasitic worms entering the leopards' food chain [69, 185]. Expeditions have recently returned with three samples of snow leopard faeces, which you are able to screen for parasites. One of the three comes up positive for parasitic worms. This gives you the data, $Y = 1$.

Let's assume that you know that there are exactly ten snow leopards in the reserve, and that each sample is equally probable to have come from any of them; this is a statistics textbook, after all! Your task is to consider how many of the ten leopards are affected. This is your single unknown or parameter, θ, and it can take integer values $0, 1, 2, \ldots, 9, 10$.

We can use probability (binomial distribution) to consider the eleven possible scenarios, from $\theta = 0$, to $\theta = 10$. This gives us the likelihood:

$$Y \sim \text{Binom}(\frac{\theta}{10}, 3)$$

Suppose we wish to bring no prior opinion at all about how many snow leopards are affected. This means that our prior distribution will be equal for all eleven scenarios: $P(\theta) = 1/11$. That is a little contrived, but it keeps things simple for now.

For each possible value of θ and each possible value of Y, Table 2.1 shows the probability of obtaining Y, given θ. Each row contains the four possible outcomes given a value of θ, and so they add to one.

We saw in Section 2.1 that we can also use these probabilities as the likelihood of θ given Y. This involves looking down the columns rather than across the rows. In this case, we should look down the column for $Y = 1$.

Three things are worth noting:

1. we have not introduced our prior, which essentially means that the prior does not favour any value of θ: it is constant, or "flat", and a constant $P(\boldsymbol{\theta})$ can be dropped from Equation 2.1

2. $\theta = 0$ and $\theta = 10$ are impossible—they have likelihoods of zero—because there has to be a mix of some affected and some unaffected leopards, based on the data, $Y = 1$

3. the elements down the column do not add up to one

---

*In practice, your $\boldsymbol{\theta}$ might contain some unknowns which are themselves vectors or even matrices, so we just casually describe this as a collection of unknowns, to avoid being too esoteric in the terminology later.

TABLE 2.1
Probability of obtaining data Y given parameter θ, from the binomial distribution.

	$Y = 0$	$Y = 1$	$Y = 2$	$Y = 3$
$\theta = 0$	1.000	0.000	0.000	0.000
$\theta = 1$	0.729	0.243	0.027	0.001
$\theta = 2$	0.512	0.384	0.096	0.008
$\theta = 3$	0.343	0.441	0.189	0.027
$\theta = 4$	0.216	0.432	0.288	0.064
$\theta = 5$	0.125	0.375	0.375	0.125
$\theta = 6$	0.064	0.288	0.432	0.216
$\theta = 7$	0.027	0.189	0.441	0.343
$\theta = 8$	0.008	0.096	0.384	0.512
$\theta = 9$	0.001	0.027	0.243	0.729
$\theta = 10$	0.000	0.000	0.000	1.000

TABLE 2.2
Posterior probability of parameter θ, given data $Y = 1$, assuming a binomial likelihood and a flat prior.

$\theta = 0$	0.000
$\theta = 1$	0.098
$\theta = 2$	0.155
$\theta = 3$	0.178
$\theta = 4$	0.175
$\theta = 5$	0.152
$\theta = 6$	0.116
$\theta = 7$	0.076
$\theta = 8$	0.039
$\theta = 9$	0.011
$\theta = 10$	0.000

Because it does not add up to one, we cannot use this likelihood directly as a probability. But, if we rescale it so that it does add to one, then we can. The $Y = 1$ column adds up to 2.475, so if we divide all the values in the column by that (as in Table 2.2), we can use them as posterior probabilities.

From this we can make simple, probability-based statements, that are easy for everyone to understand. Looking at the row for $\theta = 1$, we see that there is a 9.8% chance that only one of the leopards is affected.

Suppose the team want to know the probability that 5 or more of the 10 leopards are affected. We can provide this by just adding together all the posterior probabilities from $\theta = 5$ to $\theta = 10$, to get 39.4%. Many real-life decisions in organisations are based on probabilities like this, so being able to provide them directly is an advantage of Bayesian analysis.

2.2.2 Continuous unknowns

The snow leopards example is simple to calculate because there is only one unknown and one known, and both are discrete-valued. Most often, we need to work with continuous-valued unknowns (and knowns), where we cannot simply add the probabilities up.

For discrete values, there is a probability, which we can imagine as a bar chart, and it must add up to one over all the possible values. For continuous values, there is a probability density, which is more like a smooth line chart, and it must *integrate* to one. Essentially, this means that the area under the curve must be one.

To deal with this, we use algorithms that provide a sample from the posterior distribution. To estimate the mean of the posterior density function, we can just calculate the mean of the sample. To estimate the probability of being over some threshold, we just find what proportion of the sample is over it. We can summarise the sample in other useful ways too. In Section 2.4, we expand on these algorithms a little more.

2.2.3   The possible meanings of prior & posterior

Frequentist statistics can only use probability for random sampling of data, but for the Bayesian, priors and posteriors can represent various concepts, such as previous evidence or expert opinion. These interpretations are philosophically justified, which is to say that various ideas have been proposed over the years, and you should consider them and decide which you are comfortable with. It is also reasonable for your views to change somewhat as you become more experienced in the practicalities of this kind of analysis.

Whatever interpretation you use to define your prior distribution will also be imposed on your posterior. Another important consideration is that mixing different interpretations within the same project or report is potentially misleading to your audience, and some would say that it cannot be justified at all. We think it is best practice to decide what interpretation is needed by your audience for effective decision-making and to accommodate any difficulties in the source data, and then stick with that. We are comfortable with choosing different interpretations for different projects; we don't believe (as some statisticians seemed to in the 20th century) that each of us should pick a side and stick to it for life.

In this section, we will describe a single unknown, θ. It is very common to specify priors for each unknown independently of the others. In fact, you should remember that the prior is really defined over all the unknowns jointly (a density in multi-dimensional parameter space). To specify each unknown independently implies that the joint prior density is uncorrelated.

2.2.3.1   Flat priors

We have already seen the choice of a flat prior, which just means that it takes the same value regardless of the unknown θ. For the discrete number of affected snow leopards, there are eleven possibilities (before we have seen the data), and so we can set the prior to $\frac{1}{11}$ throughout. This is so that they add up to one.

For continuous valued unknowns, the probability density function must integrate to one. This leads to a problem if θ can take any value over an infinitely long number line, because in this situation, there is no constant that would integrate to one. This is called an improper prior because it either does not integrate to one, or is zero everywhere.

Although it sounds like it is going to cause us a lot of trouble, the computational algorithms that we use in this day and age can effectively ignore it. In the snow leopard example, we worked with the likelihood alone, which is the same as setting a flat prior. Our algorithms only need to obtain some value proportionate to the posterior, so if the prior is constant, we can just leave it out of our calculation.

If we omit a prior from our calculations, or equivalently have a constant (flat) prior, we are basing our conclusions solely on the likelihood: the prior contributes no information. It is for this reason that flat (or nearly flat, as we'll see next) priors are sometimes called *uninformative*. To many beginners in Bayes, this sounds like a safe choice, but its implications are not always as straightforward as they seem.

Imagine an analysis where θ is the log odds ratio comparing two treatments. If we set a flat prior on this, we will not have a flat prior on the odds ratio, e^θ. The easiest way to understand this is to simulate some uniformly distributed numbers (representing the flat prior), draw a histogram of them, then exponentiate them and draw another histogram. For example, in R:

```
logOR <- runif(10000, -5, 5)
hist(logOR, breaks=30)
OR <- exp(logOR)
hist(OR, breaks=30)
```

The Jeffreys prior is an attempt to avoid this problem of uninformative priors becoming unexpectedly informative once the unknowns have been transformed [147]. It defines a prior in terms of the log likelihood, the details of which we will omit here.

Our preference, and suggestion to all new Bayesian meta-analysts, is not to try to sidestep the modelling choices contained in priors. All statistical analyses are somewhat subjective, in our experience. From the original hypothesis, to the choice of study design and setting, and the likelihood function, many choices have already been made which have shaped the results in one way or another. It is better to make choices, be transparent about them, and (try to) justify them, than it is to pretend that your analysis can be judgement-free and universally applicable.

In summary, we can impose flat priors if we so choose, but it may not be possible to use them as a way of avoiding responsibility for modelling preferences.

2.2.3.2 Diffuse or vague priors

An alternative to the totally flat prior is one that is just very wide, like a normal distribution with a very large standard deviation. These are often called *diffuse* or *vague*. Unfortunately, we have found that sometimes, analysts write words like those and then omit the specification of the actual distribution. So, we encourage you to always record the specific prior distribution.

Unknowns which could take any real value can be given normal distributions under this scheme. Those that must be positive can be given very wide gamma or inverse gamma distributions. Another distribution for positive unknowns is the half-normal, which is just equal to double the density of a normal distribution—with mean of zero—if the value is non-negative, and zero otherwise. We can double the value if we need it to integrate to one.

Unknown proportions must lie between zero and one, and we can give them beta distributions with parameters just a little above 1, to slightly prefer values away from the extremes[†]. We can also adapt these as rescaled betas for any unknown which has a minimum and maximum value. For $\theta_{min} \leq \theta \leq \theta_{max}$, we can instead estimate a transformed value $\phi = (\theta - \theta_{min})/(\theta_{max} - \theta_{min})$, which lies in the interval $0 \leq \phi \leq 1$.

 On the website, we provide some code to plot the densities of various common distributions used for priors. Experimenting with this will give you a better grasp of what prior to use in different circumstances.

You may wonder why we would bother with diffuse priors when we could just make them flat. There was a historical reason, because they simplify calculations of posteriors

---

[†] ... unless you feel that the extremes are feasible

using paper and pencil. A practical reason for contemporary, computer-intensive Bayesian statistics is that they include a slight gradient, which can help your software to find more likely values for the unknown θs, guiding it away from extreme values.

The characteristic of diffuse priors is that they are very wide. An obvious question is how wide is wide enough? You may find it annoying that we have not given you any formulas for a diffuse prior. In some contexts, $N(0, 100)$ might be very wide—if this prior estimates the mean change in body mass index (BMI) with green tea extracts, for example. In others, it would not, such as if we were estimating a change in annual income in Zimbabwean dollars. We expect the BMI change to be on the order of 0.1 or 1, while the income change might be on the order of 100,000 or 1,000,000.

This leads to a very important warning to budding Bayesians: **there is no such thing as a default prior distribution.** Every case must be considered on its merits. Just because someone else used a certain prior, and published their code online, does not mean that you can copy and paste it without changing the prior to your own circumstances.

Diffuse priors can be justified as representative of no opinion or prior evidence, and therefore stand in as a common frame of reference that all readers of your analyses can relate to. In his classic textbook on Bayesian theory, Peter Lee wrote "... it seems useful to have a reference prior to aid public discourse in situations where prior opinions differ or are not strong" (p.43 in [147]).

While we think that it is justifiable to present analyses with diffuse priors as approximations to the likelihood, we find the idea of a "reference" prior, and hence a "reference" posterior, hard to support logically. One cannot anticipate the opinions that all potential readers will hold, so it is far-fetched to claim to have found the common ground that will be informative to them all.

2.2.3.3 Weakly informative priors

We can set a prior that is quite diffuse, but actively guides our software away from completely implausible regions of parameter space. This aims to exclude the impossible (a subjective judgement), but not to impose much preference in terms of what we think is more probable. These are called *weakly informative priors* (WIPs).

In the example of green tea extracts for weight loss, with change in BMI as the outcome, we regarded $N(0, 100)$ as a diffuse prior, but a mean change of 100 or 200 in BMI would be ridiculous. Even a mean change of 10 or 20 seems highly implausible, especially for a lifestyle intervention that we would not expect to be enormously powerful.

A WIP would be something like $N(0, 3)$; we should consider whether it allocates a reasonable probability density to all the values that we think are possible. A change of 2 standard deviations would take us to the edge of the central 95% of probability, and that would be at a change of ± 6kg.m^{-2}, which seems implausible. The principal purpose of a WIP is as a computational aid: if the software tests out values much beyond ± 6kg.m^{-2}, it will be steered firmly back towards smaller values [87].

It is tempting to use bounded uniform distributions for WIPs, which are constant within a given range and zero outside it, but this carries some risk. Firstly, if your judgement about the bounds of possibility are wrong, the analysis will not even consider parameter values where the prior density is zero. Secondly, the lack of gradient provides no guidance in low-posterior regions.

2.2.3.4 Priors based on previous analysis results

The Bayesian concept of prior times likelihood can be interpreted as learning from data, updating the uncertainty with new insights from the data (plus the model assumptions).

This idea of updating is often mentioned in Bayesian courses and is one of the attractions that draws analysts to consider learning about Bayes.

In meta-analysis, there is a valuable application of this. If someone has previously carried out a painstaking literature search, systematic review and meta-analysis on your topic, then there is really little point in re-examining the same evidence base that they found (unless you disagree with the search or appraisal methods). Instead, you can take their results (even if they were not Bayesian) and use them as a prior. Then, you only need to consider the likelihood based on new studies published since the previous review was finished.

However, implementing this is not simple. We consider it further in Chapter 12.

2.2.3.5 Personal opinion priors

The interpretation of probability as a degree of belief is one of the oldest philosophical stances, and underpinned much early work on Bayesian statistics. It is a sound approach to take, mathematically the same as any other prior, and philosophically defended by many experts over the years. It has declined in popularity recently, at the same time as Bayesian methods have been more widely used for challenging real-world problems.

The process of eliciting opinion priors from individuals, and with a panel of experts, perhaps combining them or seeking consensus, is an interesting and important part of a Bayesian analyst's skills set. We discuss this in detail in Chapter 6.

2.2.3.6 Sensitivity analysis with priors

Whatever type of prior or interpretation of probability is chosen for a project, there should be some sensitivity analysis, re-running the analysis with somewhat different priors, to make sure that they are not having an unanticipated strong influence on the results.

Suppose that we chose the WIP $N(0,3)$ for the change in BMI attributable to green tea extracts. We should also run our analysis with an optimistic informative prior like $N(-1,1)$, and a pessimistic informative one like $N(0,0.4)$.

Priors on standard deviations or variances can be harder to imagine, but we can easily visualise them by generating random numbers from the distribution, and drawing a histogram or kernel density plot. For example, alternative priors of $Gamma(1,4)$ and a half-normal (defined only for non-negative values) $N^+(0,0.5)$ for a standard deviation can be shown in R using:

```
plot(density(rgamma(10000,1,4),bw="SJ"), main="")
lines(density(abs(rnorm(10000,0,0.5))),bw="SJ"),lty=2)
legend(x="topright",lty=c(1,2),
       legend=c("Gamma(1,4)","N+(0,0.5)"))
```

The gamma prior prefers very small standard deviations, below 0.3, while the half-normal prior is more lenient about those between 0.3 and 1.2. Above that, they are both equally dismissive.

If these priors lead to qualitatively different conclusions, or to notably different estimates and credible intervals, then our analysis must present the range of results and conclusions, describe the uncertainty which means that no firm conclusion can be made, and recommend caution when making decisions based on the analysis. It is of course disappointing to arrive at this level of uncertainty after a lot of work, but it is our duty to be honest with our audience, and to give them impartial information.

A set of posteriors may be rather similar in mean or median, yet quite different in the tails, or vice versa; the measure of whether they are sensitive to the prior or not depends on the question which we believe the audience will ask.

The priors that are used for sensitivity analysis should be chosen carefully, to represent all the alternative viewpoints that might have led to different priors. The sensitivity analysis is only as good as the set of priors you try out. Take care not to be influenced, consciously or unconsciously, to reverse-engineer the desired result.

2.3 Inference from a Posterior Sample

In practice, we do not calculate the distribution formulas for posterior distributions, but instead collect a sample of values for our unknowns, which follow that posterior distribution. Our *posterior sample* will contain many *draws* from the posterior, usually thousands. We can summarise those draws to obtain statistics that give us information about the posterior.

This helps because there might be no simple formula for the posterior, like the normal or other familiar distributions. If we can obtain a sample from it, there is no need to know its formula. We can instead summarise the sample and infer using that. Algorithms that generate simulated samples like this are in general called Monte Carlo methods (in reference to the casino and the randomness of processes like roulette wheels).

By *describing* the posterior sample, we are estimating the shape of the posterior. This works in exactly the same way as the simple statistical inference of Chapter 1, where a sample of observations provides an estimate of the shape of the distribution in the whole population from which the sample was drawn.

There are four common questions which our audience might ask of the data and model. These translate to tasks for the Bayesian analyst.

1. What is the most likely value? What is our best estimate?—*What is the centre of the posterior distribution?*

2. What is the range that the true value might be in?—*What interval contains 95% (or some other proportion) of the area under the curve?*

3. What is the chance that the true value is higher than this threshold?—*How much of the area under the curve is above that threshold?*

4. What is the weight of evidence for Hypothesis A, compared to Hypothesis B—*How much has the data (likelihood) increased the prior probability of A into the posterior probability of A? And how does that compare with the same for B?*

2.3.1 Centre of the posterior distribution

To describe the central location of the posterior, we can use the mean, median or mode of the sample. This gives us a best estimate of the unknown value that we want to investigate. The mean is the *expectation*, the value that we will expect on average, according to statistical theory. However, the median has a particularly clear interpretation in Bayesian statistics: there is a 50% chance of the true value being above it and 50% of being below it.

To estimate the posterior mean, we only have to calculate the mean of the posterior sample. The same applies to the median. Obtaining the mode is not so simple, because the point of highest density may lie between posterior draws. In Stan software, there is an optimisation function that will locate the value of θ with the highest posterior density, without running MCMC. Alternatively, you can use kernel density functions (such as `density()` in R or `kdensity` in Stata) to smooth out the distribution of draws for each unknown in turn, and find the interpolated value with the highest density.

2.3.2   Interval containing a certain probability

A range or interval of values that contain a high probability essentially tells us how far the true value might be from the best estimate. The most common form this takes is the 95% credible interval, analogous to the 95% confidence interval. In contrast, it does not require the complicated explanation required in frequentist statistics (see Section 1.2.1): we can simply say "there is a 95% chance that the true value lies in this interval," and that will likely be clearly understood by our audience.

Credible intervals can be calculated from the posterior sample in two ways. The simpler method involves finding the 2.5 and 97.5 centiles: the values define an interval so that 2.5% of the posterior draws lie below the 2.5 centile, and another 2.5% lie above the 97.5 centile. The advantage of the centile-based credible interval is that we can keep using the powerful communication based on probability that Bayesian methods allow us: we can say that there is a 95% chance that the true value lies in that interval, a 2.5% chance of being below, and a 2.5% chance of being above.

The other method finds an interval containing 95% of the area under the posterior density curve, but to maximise the height of the curve in that region. Rather than insisting on there being 2.5% probability on either side, this highest density interval (HDI) could slide down to the minimum and the 95th centile, or up to the 5th centile and the maximum, but is likely to be somewhere in the middle and not radically different to the centile-based credible interval. If you are interested in the 95% region, not the two 2.5% regions, then the HDI makes most sense.

There is nothing magical about 95%, and the same methods can be used to obtain other widths of credible interval, if they are appropriate to the needs of the audience. This should be decided in advance of analysis, and certainly should not be reverse-engineered in order to obtain a desired conclusion.

Stan software reports 90% credible intervals by default, based on a concern that Bayesian analyses often do not contain enough posterior draws to make reliable inference in the tails of the posterior distribution. Later in this book (page 41), we show you how to obtain any credible interval from Stan. In general, if you want to make statements about probability above and below some threshold, ensure there are enough draws on either side to locate the threshold precisely.

2.3.3   Probability of being above or below a certain threshold

The credible interval methods started with a pre-defined probability, and found thresholds to capture the correct probability. The opposite is also useful, and is a hallmark of Bayesian analysis. We can report the probability of the true unknown value lying above or below a pre-defined threshold, or of lying in a pre-defined interval.

This is especially useful to decision-makers who need to consider the risk of events. What if the new drug turns out to fall short of a minimum clinically important difference? What if the new public health intervention ends up making less of a difference than the established method? With Bayes, we can directly put probabilities onto these intervals, and report them. The decision-maker might accept a certain risk and reject others. It is certainly easier for them to absorb the information we provide in terms of probabilities and risks than it is with p-values and confidence intervals.

TABLE 2.3

Interpretation of Bayes factors [140].

Bayes factor	Evidence for Hypothesis A
1 to 3.2	"Not worth more than a bare mention"
3.2 to 10	"Positive"
10 to 100	"Strong"
> 100	"Very strong"

Source: Ref. [140].

2.3.4 Ratio of posterior to prior odds (Bayes factors)

This measure of evidence (or lack of evidence) has some similarities to a p-value in frequentist statistics. However, rather than simply assessing one null hypothesis, it can be used to compare two models, or two specific values of our unknowns $\boldsymbol{\theta}$. We will call them Hypothesis A and Hypothesis B, and they respectively fix $\boldsymbol{\theta}_A$ and $\boldsymbol{\theta}_B$. However, we should bear in mind that they can also compare two quite incompatible models with entirely different unknowns making up $\boldsymbol{\theta}$.

The straightforward implementation, as:

$$\frac{P(\boldsymbol{\theta}_A|\boldsymbol{Y})}{P(\boldsymbol{\theta}_A)} \bigg/ \frac{P(\boldsymbol{\theta}_B|\boldsymbol{Y})}{P(\boldsymbol{\theta}_B)} \tag{2.2}$$

is known as a Bayes factor. Among Bayesian ideas, it is relatively old, dating to a time of computation by pencil and paper, when Bayesian models had to be simple. In more challenging, 21st century settings, calculating it is more complicated. The details of this are beyond the scope of this book, but Bayes factors can be computed, regardless of the software choice you make, although it may have to be done as a second step after obtaining your posterior samples.

The connection to hypothesis testing has made it popular with some Bayesians [271], and simultaneously unpopular with others [249]. This is because of recent controversies around the use and abuse of hypothesis testing [163]. There are also concerns about how the prior odds can be unexpectedly large (or small) with diffuse priors, or those that align only slightly with the likelihood, leading to an unstable Bayes factor [90].

There have been some suggestions for interpretation of different values, such as the taxonomy in Table 2.3 [140].

In meta-analytic applications, we do not find it as useful as the other three outputs above, for just the same reasons that a p-value alone is not as useful for clinical decision-making as a best estimate of effect, a confidence interval for that effect, and comparison with the pre-specified minimum clinically important difference. We critique one such interpretation in Section 4.4.5.

2.4 Options for Software and Algorithms

2.4.1 Markov Chain Monte Carlo

The most widely used algorithms for sampling from a posterior distribution belong to a class called *Markov Chain Monte Carlo* (MCMC). They generate a sequence or *chain* of posterior draws. Each draw is a collection of values for each of the unknowns in $\boldsymbol{\theta}$. Together, lots of draws make up a sample. When MCMC works properly, the distribution of those draws in parameter space approximates the posterior distribution.

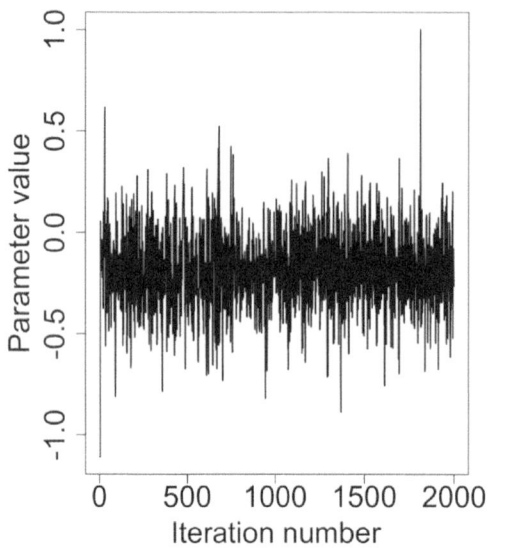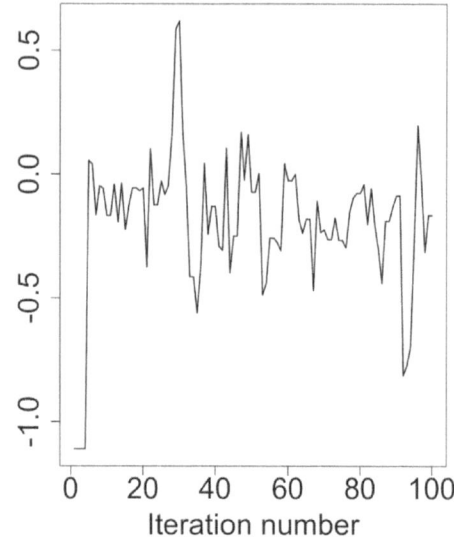

FIGURE 2.3

Traceplots from MCMC sampling. The first 2000 iterations on the left show the characteristic "hairy caterpillar" shape, discussed further in Section 2.5. On the right, zooming in on the first 100, we can see some iterations that rejected the proposed value and hence have a short flat line, for example at iterations 39 and 40. The initial value, at iteration 1, was -1.11, the next three iterations failed to improve log posterior and thus retained the initial value, and then the software (Stan, in this instance) rapidly moved to the posterior distribution. We can say it has converged after just a few iterations (not every model is so well-behaved).

The process can be summarised, for a model with one unknown θ:

1. Choose a starting value of θ

2. Calculate the log prior and the log likelihood given θ and the data

3. The sum of the log prior and the log likelihood is the log posterior, plus-minus some constant; we can ignore the missing constant

4. Move to a proposed new value of θ, and calculate the sum of the new log prior and the new log likelihood

5. If the sum of the new log prior and the new log likelihood is higher than the old one, probably stay at this new value

6. Otherwise, probably reject this new value and go back to the old one

Obviously, we are being deliberately vague about how the new value of θ is found, and about "probably" accepting or rejecting it; these are details that you do not need to know to get started with an intuitive appreciation of what is happening. After a few thousand steps, we can examine the chain of θ values and do the summary calculations described above. This is shown for the mean of normally distributed data in Figure 2.3.

The various versions of MCMC differ mainly in how the new proposed value is found. The Software appendix lists packages, their interfaces, algorithms, and other facts. The software we will consider here all uses the same criterion to accept or reject the proposed value, called the Metropolis-Hastings formula. We will not dig deeper into its computational details, as they do not impact on how you will work with this software.

We suggest to Bayesian newcomers that, once you have acquired some familiarity and confidence with the software, you read a little more about the computation, either in a review article [99] or a reference textbook [27, 87].

The earliest form of MCMC used a random walk to generate new proposed values of $\boldsymbol{\theta}$. This requires some function that generates random values, positive or negative, and adds them to the elements of $\boldsymbol{\theta}$. This is still used today as *random walk Metropolis-Hastings*. This is implemented in Stata as well as some R packages and functionality in JASP.

Algorithms that include some randomness will produce slightly different results each time they run, even if the specification of the model, and the data, are the same. In all the software examples that follow, we have tried to keep the code as simple as possible so that you can see what it might be like to work with it, and choose the software that best suits you. However, please bear in mind that Bayesian modelling should usually also involve specifying random number generator seeds. These ensure that exactly the same results appear each time*.

We should bear in mind that there is could be many unknowns in $\boldsymbol{\theta}$ that must be estimated, and together, they could have a complicated distribution. A variant of MCMC, called the Gibbs sampler, calculates the *conditional* distribution of one unknown (or a group of them) while holding the others constant. This allows for somewhat quicker movement through the posterior distribution than a random walk, and is implemented in BUGS, JAGS, Stata, and in some R packages and functionality in JASP.

Hamiltonian Monte Carlo is a more recent innovation, which uses calculations from physics to imitate physical objects moving while being pulled towards values of higher probability. This can move from one end of a posterior distribution to the opposite in a single proposal step, which is very advantageous if the posterior is correlated. This is implemented in Stan, which can be called through interfaces in R, Stata and other programming languages, and in turn is used by some higher-level R packages (including `brms`), and some of the functionality in JASP.

Below, we show various software options and how they can be used for two basic models:

1. 100 binary observations—30 events and 70 non-events—where we want to infer the population probability of an event

2. the 50 petal length measurements on *Iris versicolor* flowers, from Anderson's famous iris dataset [267]—which has sample mean 4.26cm and sample standard deviation 0.47cm—where we want to infer the population mean and standard deviation

The files needed to try these on each of the software options are available at this book's website.

Broadly speaking, the software options here exist on a spectrum from easier to learn, but restrictive, to harder to learn, but flexible. In our opinion, the order is: JASP, bayesmeta, brms, Stata, BUGS, JAGS, Stan. JASP in markedly simpler in interface (and more restricted) than the others, which all require a little programming. In some situations, programming can be avoided in Stata.

In the space of this book, we cannot provide more than a brief overview of each of the software options. We hope that this helps readers who are new to Bayesian statistics to

---

*This is not quite the whole truth! The version of software you are using, your operating system, and even your processor chips can affect the behaviour of the *pseudo*-random number generators. Your pseudo-random numbers will be stable if you set the seed, but may still differ between computers.

choose one that they are interested in, and in each case below, we give some direction to further reading. The versions we used are the most recent at the time of writing (2023-4).

2.4.2   BUGS

In this book, we will mainly show code from the popular software BUGS (Bayesian inference Using the Gibbs Sampler). BUGS is available as a standalone Windows application called WinBUGS, or as open-source software, OpenBUGS, which can be accessed from various interfaces in R, Python or Stata software. The best source for learning more is *The BUGS Book* [156].

In BUGS, we write our models as a short script, which defines the prior and likelihood. These are wrapped inside a "model block" like this:

```
model{
   ...YOUR MODEL CODE GOES HERE...
}
```

For simplicity, we omit the model block brackets in this book, along with BUGS code for the data and initial values. Details of these aspects can be found in print and online [156].

Below, we have some binary data and want to estimate the proportion of events (1s). We use a beta prior (flat within the range $[0, 1]$) and a binomial likelihood for single observations.

```
prop ~ dbeta(1, 1)
for(i in 1:n) {
  x[i] ~ dbin(prop, 1)
}
```

Below, we have continuous-valued data, and want to estimate a mean and standard deviation. In BUGS and JAGS, the normal probability density function takes mean and *precision* as input. The precision is the reciprocal of the variance. We use informative priors: a truncated $N^+(6, 1.5)$ prior for the mean (standard deviation of 1.5 implies precision of 0.444) and a gamma prior Gamma$(2, 4)$ for the standard deviation. The code `I(0,)`, which appears after the `dnorm` statement for the prior, truncates the distribution to the positive domain (which has a lower value of 0 but no upper value after the comma). We then convert the standard deviation to a precision for BUGS. The likelihood is normal.

```
mu ~ dnorm(6, 0.444)I(0,)
sigma ~ dgamma(2, 4)
prec <- 1/(sigma*sigma)
for(i in 1:n) {
  x[i] ~ dnorm(mu, prec)
}
```

BUGS has a wide range of probability distributions built-in, but if something really bespoke is needed, we have to trick it. The *ones trick* calculates the probability (either likelihood contribution $P(y_i|\theta)$ or prior $P(\theta)$), and supplies this as the probability of an event to a binomial (Bernoulli) distribution, where it so happens that every observation was an event. The name "ones trick" comes from the fact that this binomial distribution is supplied with phony data that is always 1. This has the effect of contributing the bespoke probability to the likelihood or prior as required.

There is also a *zeros trick*, where $-\log P(\cdot)$ is supplied as the parameter of a Poisson distribution, and we supply a phony variable which is always 0. These tricks are detailed in BUGS examples and literature [156].

2.4.2.1 WinBUGS

Historically, the most common software for Bayesian meta-analysts has been WinBUGS [94]. This is a Windows application which provides a graphical user interface for BUGS. It has not been maintained or updated since 2007, but still functions as intended, up to and including Windows 11. We will describe a simple walk-through example of its use, but we strongly recommend *The BUGS Book* [156] if you intend to use it. Installations also come with a large collection of well-documented examples.

After opening WinBUGS, we can click on `File / New` to open a document. The BUGS code is enclosed in curly braces and preceded with the word `model`, as shown in Figure 2.4. Data can be included here, or in a separate file, in R list format (there are other options [156]).

We click on the `Model` menu and choose `Specification...` to bring up the "Specification Tool" dialog box. Next, highlight the word `model`, at the beginning of the model code, and click on the `check model` button. If WinBUGS understands everything in our code, we will see a small message in the bottom left corner of the window: "model is syntactically correct" (see Figure 2.4).

Now we can load the data by highlighting the word `list` and clicking on `load data`. The message in the bottom left should be "data loaded".

Next, we choose to run two chains by changing the `num of chains` text box to 2, and click on `compile model`. Here, BUGS creates some internal code to be used for sampling, and may issue error messages if it cannot do so. If compilation happens without problems, the message "model compiled" is shown in the bottom left of the window.

Finally, we must set initial values for the unknowns. We can supply these in the same format as the data input, or we can ask WinBUGS to pick them at random (from the prior distributions). It is always a good idea to provide sensible initial values.

We highlight the word `list` at the beginning of the initial values input, and click on `set inits`. If you want to run more than one chain, there should be initial values input for each chain, and you will repeat the `set inits` on each of the inputs.

If some unknowns in the model are left uninitialised, the message at bottom left of the WinBUGS window will read "chain initialized but other chain(s) contain uninitialized variables". When initial values are loaded for more than one chain, this will appear until they are all loaded; it does not indicate an error.

The `gen inits` button asks WinBUGS to generate initial values for any remaining unknowns for the chain. However, this is not advisable because it draws at random from the prior and can take extreme values, affecting convergence of the chain.

Finally, the message in the bottom left reads "model is initialized" and we are ready to sample from the posterior. We click on the menu bar at `Inference`, then `Samples`. We can identify the unknowns for which we want to collect posterior draws. We type the name ("prop", in this example) into the `node` box and click on `set` for each one.

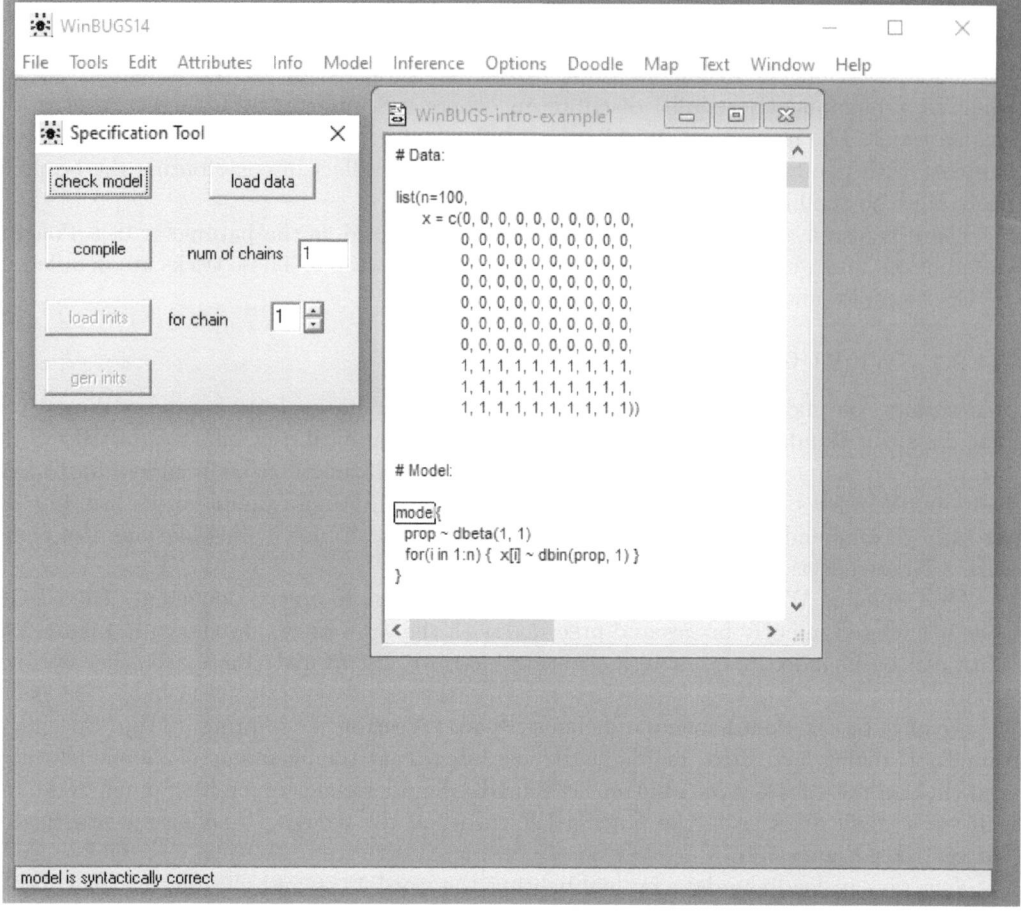

FIGURE 2.4
WinBUGS code providing data and model for the binary example.

Then, if we click on the `Model` menu, and choose `Update`, we will see a dialog box, where we can choose how many iterations to carry out (default 1000). When we click on `update`, the MCMC algorithm runs; "model is updating" appears briefly in the bottom left.

Returning to the "Sample Monitor Tool" dialog box, we can choose `prop` from the `node` drop-down list, and click on `history` to see a traceplot of the two chains of the unknown `prop`. The `density` button will produce a kernel density plot, and `stats` will produce a table of essential summary statistics. These outputs are all shown in Figure 2.5.

Following exactly the steps above, we have captured ("monitored") the draws of `prop` from the initial values to the 1000th iteration. This will show us whether the chains have converged, but then, we should discard some as burn-in or warm-up. To do this, we can change the iterations that will be used in outputs in the `beg` and `end` boxes. Suppose we decide to drop the first 100: set `beg` to 101 and `end` to 1000, then generate the statistics and plots as before; they will display iteration numbers 101 to 1000.

When we have `set` more than one unknown, we can get outputs for them all together by typing an asterisk into the `node` box.

WinBUGS provides further useful outputs: an autocorrelation plot from the `auto cor` button (and draws can be thinned in the "Sample Monitor Tool" dialog box), a "dynamic

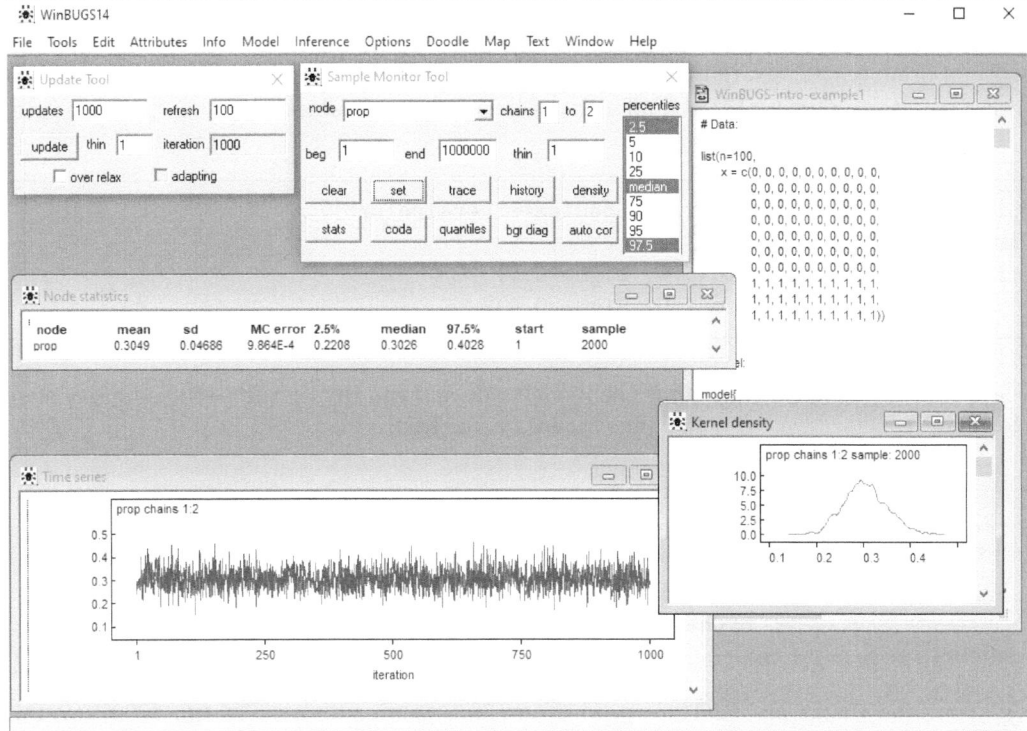

FIGURE 2.5
WinBUGS output with traceplot, density plot and statistics.

traceplot", which moves in real time as the algorithm runs, from the `trace` button, and a line chart of r-hat statistics from the `bgr diag` button.

Posterior draws can be exported using the `coda` button, and imported into R using the `coda` package.

2.4.2.2 Other interfaces to BUGS

There are other ways to link to WinBUGS or OpenBUGS, such as R packages `BRugs` and `R2WinBUGS`. Stata commands for interfacing with BUGS are described in Section 2.4.6.

2.4.3 JAGS

JAGS is an open-source alternative to BUGS, which uses an almost identical language for specifying your models. The main differences are:

1. truncation of distributions uses the `T(,)` syntax instead of BUGS' `I(,)`

2. some calculations can be applied to a vector in a single step, without looping over individual elements

3. it is possible to add a `data` block to JAGS code, which creates new variables, derived from the data, to be used inside the `model` block

JAGS must be installed as a standalone application, but the usual way to access it is through the R package `rjags`.

The first step to use JAGS is to write the model code in a text file. For the two examples used here, the JAGS code is identical to that given above for BUGS, except for the half-normal prior, which uses the T(0,) syntax. In R, this is the code to load the iris data, make a list of data to pass to JAGS, and a list of lists for initial values:

```
pl <- iris$Petal.Length[iris$Species=="versicolor"]
irdata <- list(n=50, x=pl)
irinits <- list(list(mu=3.0, sigma=0.5),
                list(mu=2.5, sigma=0.4))
```

Next, we get JAGS to compile the model code and run (by default) 1000 adaptive steps to tune the algorithm, with the jags.model() function:

```
irmod <- jags.model("JAGS-example-2.txt",
                    data=irdata,
                    inits=irinits,
                    n.chains=2)
```

Now, the chains are ready to produce useful posterior draws. We run 1000 warm-up iterations with the update() function, then sample 5000 iterations from each of two chains with the coda.samples() function.

```
update(irmod, n.iter=1000)
irdraws <- coda.samples(irmod,
                        variable.names=c("mu","sigma"),
                        n.iter=5000)
```

When this has run, we can print summary statistics with summary(irdraws), and draw traceplots and density plots with plot(irdraws), which are shown in Figure 2.6.

This is the summary output:

```
Iterations = 2001:7000
Thinning interval = 1
Number of chains = 2
Sample size per chain = 5000

1. Empirical mean and standard deviation for each
   variable, plus standard error of the mean:

        Mean      SD  Naive SE Time-series SE
mu    4.2649 0.06810 0.0006810      0.0006597
sigma 0.4776 0.04858 0.0004858      0.0006451
```

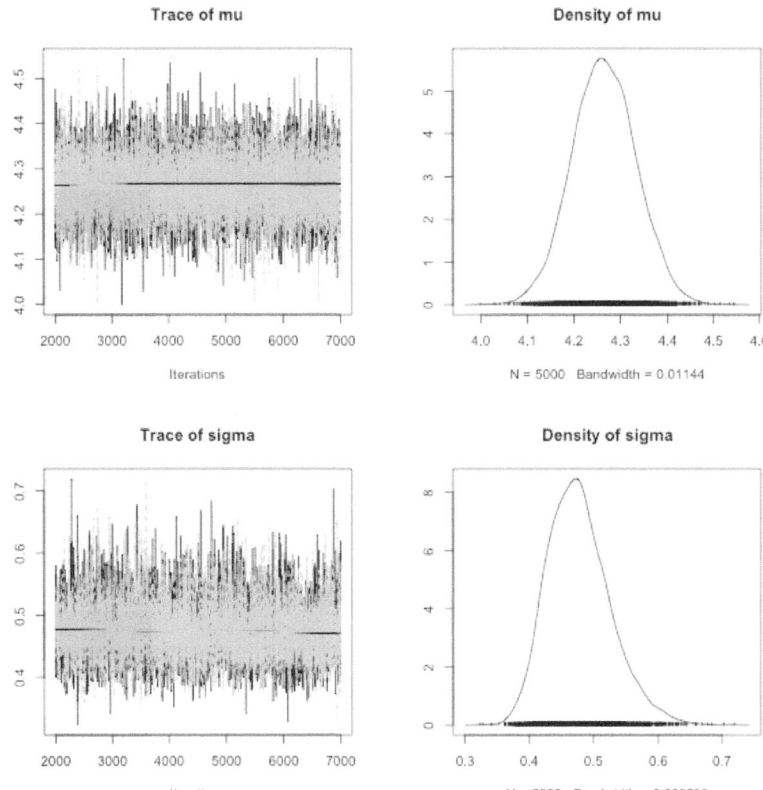

FIGURE 2.6
JAGS output with traceplots and density plots.

```
2. Quantiles for each variable:

         2.5%    25%     50%     75%   97.5%
mu     4.1313 4.2183 4.2641 4.3101 4.3979
sigma  0.3949 0.4429 0.4736 0.5074 0.5857
```

2.4.4 Stan

Stan is also open-source Bayesian software. Unlike BUGS and JAGS, it has a very active developer and user community, an online forum and conferences. Like BUGS and JAGS, Stan uses a script for the model, which specifies the prior and likelihood. After some experience of teaching Bayesian methods to beginners, we prefer to use Stan; although it is newer than BUGS, and therefore regarded as an advanced tool, its code is more explicit in exactly what is going in and out of the software, which helps to avoid misunderstandings.

There are two immediately apparent differences from BUGS/JAGS code. Firstly, any value that Stan deals with must be declared before it is used, like this:

```
real theta;
```

Each line in Stan code ends with a semicolon. When we declare it, we state a name which can then be used in deterministic and probabilistic lines of code. We also say what data type it will hold: `real` for real numbers (floating-point), `int` for integers. We might also declare an array with one dimension to hold a data variable, though we must declare N, the length of that array, first:

```
int N;
array[N] real x;
```

There are other data types available, all described in the Stan manuals [242].

Secondly, there are multiple blocks of code, each contained in curly braces. As a minimum, they include `data`, `parameters`, and `model`. The `data` block defines what will be sent to Stan, usually starting with the number of observations, N. The `parameters` block defines the unknowns that we want to infer, and the `model` relates the data and the parameters together.

This is the code for the simple binary proportion model:

```
data {
  int N;
  array[N] int x;
}
parameters {
  real<lower=0, upper=1> prop;
}
model {
  prop ~ beta(1,1);
  x ~ binomial(1, prop);
}
```

When we declare `data` or `parameters`, we can set lower and upper bounds on the values they can take, for example using `<lower=0, upper=1>`. In this case, it is merely a safety net, as the beta prior distribution on `prop` will apply the same constraint to lie between zero and one.

You might also notice that in the line for the likelihood (`x ~ binomial(1, prop);`), x is an array on the left-hand side. This implicitly means that every element of that array has the same formula for its likelihood. If you prefer, you can write it as a loop instead, applying it to each element of x:

```
model {
  prop ~ beta(1,1);
  for(i in 1:N) {
    x[i] ~ binomial(1, prop);
  }
}
```

This is the code for the iris model:

```
data {
  int N;
  array[N] real x;
}
parameters {
  real<lower=0> mu;
  real <lower=0> sigma;
}
model {
  mu ~ normal(6, 1.5);
  sigma ~ gamma(2,4);
  x ~ normal(mu, sigma);
}
```

The `normal()` distribution function takes the mean and standard deviation as input.

By constraining `mu` to be zero or positive, we have truncated the prior. There is no equivalent to the BUGS T(0,) syntax in Stan, which directly acts on the distribution[†].

The algorithm in Stan (Hamiltonian Monte Carlo) is less sensitive than the Gibbs sampler to the choice of prior distributions, so you could use a uniform or half-normal prior on the standard deviation without slowing down computation or risking non-convergence.

2.4.4.1 The R package `cmdstanr`

At the time of writing, the best way to interface from R to Stan is via the `cmdstanr` package. This sends your data and code to the standalone CmdStan application, which means that execution is as fast as possible, there are fewer ways in which integration between Stan, R and the operating system can go wrong, and CmdStan can easily be updated or rolled back to an old version, independently of R.

You can either write your Stan code in a separate text file, or type it inside your R code like this:

```
library(cmdstanr)

stancode <- "
data {
  int N;
  array[N] int x;
}
parameters {
  real<lower=0, upper=1> prop;
}
```

[†]If you want to use truncated distributions a lot, and prefer code that made the choice of distribution obvious, you could program a new density function in Stan with a name like `trunc_normal()`—but that is beyond the scope of this book. The Stan user guide shows how bespoke functions can be added.

```
model {
  prop ~ beta(1,1);
  x ~ binomial(1, prop);
}
"
```

The first task is to compile the Stan code into an executable application. It can take 10-30 seconds, and feels frustrating for beginners. However, as your data and the complexity of your models grow, compilation time remains fairly constant, and once compiled, sampling from the posterior happens very much faster than in BUGS or JAGS. The first example below compiles from a separate code file, the second from an inline R string of code.

```
stanmodel <- cmdstan_model("mycode.stan")
```

```
stanmodel <- cmdstan_model(write_stan_file(stancode))
```

Having compiled, we then sample from the posterior. This is the point at which the data are sent to Stan as an R list object. Assuming the binary data exists as a vector called x in R:

```
stansample <- stanmodel$sample(data = list(N=length(x),
                                            x=x),
                      iter_warmup = 500,
                      iter_sampling = 5000,
                      chains = 2
                      parallel_chains = 2,
                      seed=1234,
                      init=list(list(prop=0.5),
                                list(prop=0.4)))
```

The arguments of this function do the following:

1. define the list containing the data objects N and x; their names must match the names in Stan's `data` block

2. ask for 500 warmup iterations, which we will not store afterwards (although you can change this with another argument, `save_warmup=TRUE`)

3. ask for 5000 iterations (in each chain) that will be stored

4. run 2 chains

5. run them in parallel (this assumes you have enough CPU cores on your computer)

6. set a random number generator seed so that each time you run the sampling code, you get the same posterior sample

7. set initial values; this is a list with one sublist for each chain

The object that is returned in `stansample` can then be used to get graphics (we recommend the **bayesplot** package for this) and summary output. Below, we store the posterior draws first, then print the summary, then obtain traceplots and density plots.

```
standraws <- stansample$draws()
stansample$summary()

library(bayesplot)
mcmc_trace(standraws)
mcmc_density(standraws)
```

This is the output from `stansample$summary()`, showing the first seven columns:

```
# A tibble: 2 x 10
  variable    mean  median     sd     mad      q5     q95 ...
  <chr>      <num>   <num>  <num>   <num>   <num>   <num> ...
1 lp__       -63.2   -62.9  0.727   0.335   -64.6   -62.6 ...
2 prop       0.302   0.301 0.0459  0.0468   0.230   0.380 ...
```

In any Stan output, we obtain the unknowns in the model in addition to `lp__`, which is the evaluated log posterior density at each draw (plus-minus some constant).

`stansample$summary()` prints a 90% credible interval in line with the developers' scepticism about inference in the tails of the posterior. However, if you run enough draws to get reliable information that far out in the tails, you can use the **posterior** package, which `cmdstanr` uses in the background:

```
posterior::summarise_draws(standraws,
                           mean,
                           ~quantile(.x,
                                     probs=c(0.025,
                                             0.975)))
```

The final three columns of the summary table are useful for diagnosing problems in how the algorithm ran—the r-hat statistic and the effective sample size in the central 50% of the sample, and in the lower 25% and upper 25%:

```
# A tibble: 2 x 10
  variable    ...    rhat  ess_bulk ess_tail
  <chr>       ...   <num>     <num>    <num>
1 lp__        ...    1.00     4605.    5566.
2 prop        ...    1.00     3354.    4867.
```

We discuss these outputs and other diagnostics in Section 2.5.

2.4.4.2 The R package `rstan`

Before `cmdstanr`, the R interface to Stan was through the `rstan` package. It is actively maintained and very popular. It has the advantage that the Stan functionality is entirely contained in R, and you don't have to install CmdStan, but it also is a disadvantage that R, Stan and your operating system all have to fit together perfectly for it to work (and, for many users, RStudio as well). In recent years, `rstan` users have had difficulty updating and running it because of small changes to the Windows 11 operating system and the adoption of the Apple M-series chips. These have been fixed, but we anticipate more occasional problems like this in future.

This is the `rstan` code that corresponds to the `cmdstanr` steps above. First, we set two options, which allow parallel sampling and do not re-compile a model that is being run again, if nothing in the model code has changed:

```
options(mc.cores = parallel::detectCores())
rstan_options(auto_write = TRUE)
```

Supposing that we saved out Stan model script in a file called `mymodel.stan`, we can compile and sample from the model in one step:

```
stansample <- stan("mymodel.stan",
                data=list(N=length(x),
                        x=x),
                warmup=500,
                iter=5000,
                chains=2,
                cores=2,
                seed=1234,
                init=list(list(prop=0.5),
                        list(prop=0.4)))
```

Next, we extract the draws, print a summary table, and draw traceplots:

```
posterior_draws <- extract(stansample)
print(stansample)
traceplot(stansample)
```

As for `cmdstanr` above, additional summary statistics can be obtained from the `posterior::summarise_draws()` function. The `bayesplot` package provides a simple interface to many `ggplot2`-class graphics.

2.4.4.3 Other interfaces to Stan

Several other interfaces have been written for Stan, listed on the website `mc-stan.org`. Some are wrappers around CmdStan, like `cmdstanr`, and others bundle the C++ library like `rstan`. The former are generally preferable for stability and keeping up to date with new Stan versions. Python, Matlab and Julia are all included in the list. We describe the Stata interface to Stan in Section 2.4.6.1. The brms R package is an important alternative to writing Stan code directly, especially for regression models. We discuss it from Chapter 3 onward.

2.4.5 The R package bayesmeta

bayesmeta is a specialised R package for simple Bayesian meta-analyses. We introduce it in Chapters 3 and 4.

There are many other R packages which implement specific Bayesian models, including some for meta-analysis. We prefer to recommend that you learn a generic tool, which can be used in many different scenarios. This also has the advantage of reproducibility in that the model specification is all contained in your code.

2.4.6 Stata

Stata is proprietary, but relatively affordable, statistical software, which brings the advantage of customer support. There is also a very active user community with an online forum and meetings in many countries. Stata software, since version 14 (released in 2015), has included Bayesian functionality. Prior to version 14, it was possible to interface with Win-BUGS* through user-contributed commands by John Thompson [253]. There is also a Stata to Stan interface through a user-contributed command stan, described in Section 2.4.6.1. Since Stata 16, it has been possible to include blocks of Python code inside Stata scripts and pass data to and from Python, which raises the possibility of using CmdStanPy or PyMC (see Section 2.4.9).

In this book, we will only refer to the bayesmh command, introduced as part of Stata in version 14, which allows bespoke modelling. The point-and-click graphical user interface for this is shown in Figures 2.7 and 2.8.

However, bayesmh by default fits models into a regression framework, meaning that there is a dependent variable, which is predicted by a linear combination of independent variables. In meta-analysis (and many other problems), this requires either some rephrasing of the problem as one of regression, or some coding of bespoke likelihood and prior, as we will see below.

The normal functions in bayesmh take as their inputs means and variances, while all other built-in Stata functions for normal distributions take means and standard deviations. This difference in syntax is a common trap for beginners and regular users alike.

Stata uses curly braces to indicate unknowns, hence a population proportion called "prop" must be written as {prop}. The clear delineation between data (which is open in a Stata data frame) and "parameters" (which appear in curly braces) introduces some barriers for more complex models where the division is not so clear (such as missing data), but nevertheless, Stata allows considerable flexibility.

For the binomial model, if our binary data are in a variable called x, we can use this command:

```
bayesmh x, likelihood(dbinomial({prop}, 1)) ///
        prior({prop}, beta(2,2))
```

---

*Experimental commands exist for OpenBUGS and JAGS too. These are no longer actively maintained.

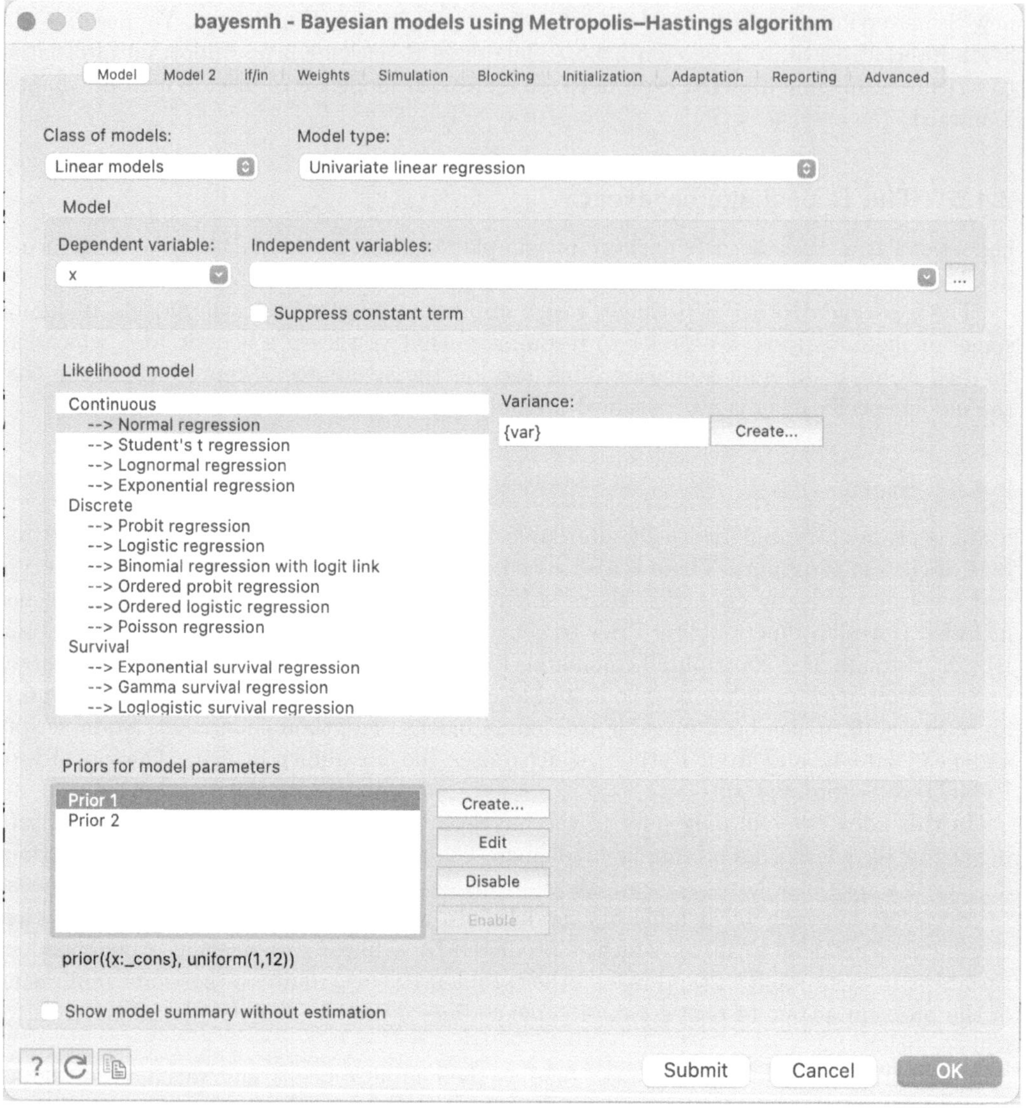

FIGURE 2.7
Stata `bayesmh` dialog box.

This will not simply estimate the probability of an event, because the binomial likelihood in `bayesmh`, by default, fits a logistic regression. In this case, there are no predictor or independent variables, only a constant, β_0. The implicit model is:

$$\beta_0 \sim \mathrm{N}(0, 10)$$
$$\log(\omega) = \beta_0$$
$$\pi = \frac{1}{1 + e^{-\beta_0}} \tag{2.3}$$
$$x \sim \mathrm{Binom}(\pi, 1)$$

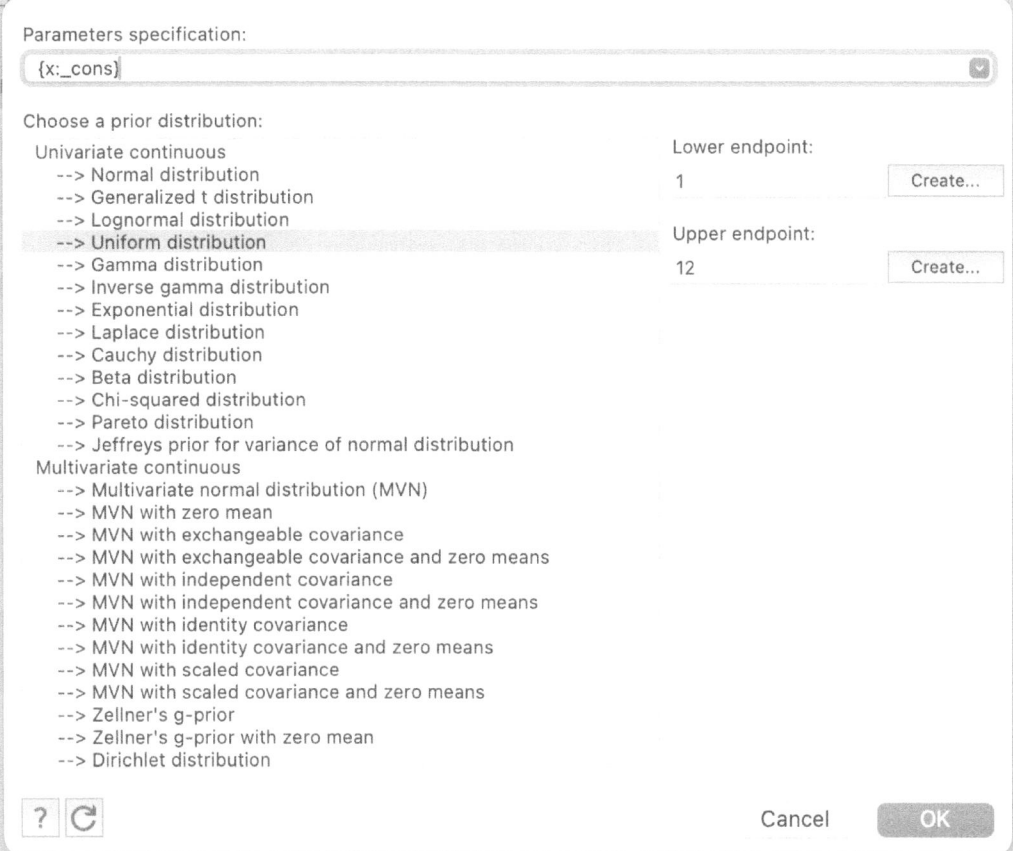

FIGURE 2.8
Stata `bayesmh` dialog box for priors.

The output provides posterior mean, standard deviation, Monte Carlo standard error, median and 95% centile credible interval. The default is to generate 2,500 burn-in (also known as warm-up) iterations, before storing the following 10,000. The iterations can be specified, and chains can be saved. Full detail is given in the help files and manual.

```
Burn-in ...
Simulation ...

Model summary
------------------------------------------------------------------------------
Likelihood:
  x ~ binomial({prop},1)

Prior:
  {prop} ~ beta(2,2)
------------------------------------------------------------------------------
```

```
Bayesian binomial model                          MCMC iterations    =      12,500
Random-walk Metropolis-Hastings sampling         Burn-in            =       2,500
                                                 MCMC sample size   =      10,000
                                                 Number of obs      =         100
                                                 Acceptance rate    =       .4423
Log marginal-likelihood = -63.042393             Efficiency         =        .242
```

	Mean	Std. dev.	MCSE	Median	Equal-tailed [95% cred. interval]	
prop	.3084663	.0446126	.000907	.3063096	.2247377	.3984222

The posterior mean of the probability (risk) is 0.308.

Additional commands `bayesstats` and `bayesgraph` then provide more statistics and graphics.

In the case of the normally distributed data, we estimate the mean (`{_cons}`) and the variance (`{var}`), which we can afterwards convert to the standard deviation. The reason why the mean is by default called `{_cons}` is that Stata's default interpretation of the "varlist" of variables before the comma is to treat them as a regression specification. With only one variable listed, there will be a constant term but no coefficients.

The sample variance in the *Iris versicolor* petal lengths is $(0.47)^2 = 0.22$. The truncated normal is not an off-the-shelf option in Stata, so first we substitute a uniform distribution, and later we will program it. We use Gamma$(1,4)$ for the variance so it prefers small numbers.

```
bayesmh x, likelihood(normal({var})) //
           prior({_cons}, uniform(1, 12)) //
           prior({var}, gamma(1, 4))
```

The equivalent action in the graphical user interface would be obtained by clicking on the Statistics menu, then Bayesian analysis, then General estimation and regression. The model setup is made in a multi-tab dialog box (Figure 2.7), and priors are defined in the further dialog box in Figure 2.8.

The output follows:

```
Burn-in ...
Simulation ...

Model summary
------------------------------------------------------------
Likelihood:
  x ~ normal({x:_cons},{var})

Priors:
  {x:_cons} ~ uniform(1,12)
      {var} ~ gamma(1,4)
```

```
Bayesian binomial regression
Random-walk Metropolis-Hastings
                                MCMC iterations  =      12,500
                                Burn-in          =       2,500
                                MCMC sample size =      10,000
                                Number of obs    =          50
                                Acceptance rate  =       .4815
                                Efficiency:  min =      .07829
                                             avg =      .09674
                                             max =       .1152
Log marginal-likelihood = -40.413152
```

	Mean	Std. dev.	MCSE	Median	Equal-tailed [95% CrI]	
x						
_cons	4.2558	.0672	.0019	4.2595	4.1194	4.3899
var	.2384	.0483	.0017	.2307	.1647	.3536

In order to use the truncated normal prior for the mean, we must create a bespoke prior in Stata. This needs a rather different syntax. We define a new **program** that will return a posterior log density in the scalar called `lnp`, and we supply the name of that program to the **evaluator()** option, instead of using `prior()` and `likelihood()`. Once we start writing a bespoke log posterior density program, we could adjust the model in any way we can imagine. For example, we might infer our preferred standard deviation, instead of the variance.

The truncated prior log density does not need to be adjusted so that the density integrates to one, because the algorithm only needs the log posterior plus-minus a constant.

```
program mylogdensity
  args lnp xb sigma
  // prediction (mu) is passed from Stata as variable xb

  tempvar lnfj // individual log likelihood contributions
  quietly generate double 'lnfj' = lnnormalden($MH_y, ///
                                               'xb', ///
                                               'sigma')
  // the dependent variable is passed as $MH_y

  tempname lnf // total log likelihood
  quietly summarize 'lnfj'
  scalar 'lnf' = r(sum)

  tempname lnpriormu // log prior for mu
  // the coefficients are passed as $MH_b
  scalar 'lnpriormu' = lnnormalden($MH_b[1,1] , 6, 1.5)
  if $MH_b[1,1] <0 {
```

```
   quietly replace 'lnfj' = -200 // proxy for zero prob.
}

tempname lnpriorsigma // log prior for sigma
scalar 'lnpriorsigma' = log(gammaden(1,4,0,'sigma'))

tempname lnprior // total log prior
scalar 'lnprior' = 'lnpriormu' + 'lnpriorsigma'

scalar 'lnp' = 'lnprior' + 'lnf' // total log posterior
end

bayesmh x,  evaluator(mylogdensity, parameters({sigma})) ///
        initial({x:_cons} 3.0 {sigma} 1.0)
```

Initial values, critically important with these priors, are set in `bayesmh`. The results, omitted here, are very similar to those obtained above.

In some simple settings, it may be possible to use an expression inside a `density()` sub-option for `prior()` and `likelihood()`; examples can be found in the Stata Bayesian manual. However, some of our more challenging meta-analytic applications will require the `evaluator` approach.

Stata can employ a method called *blocking* to aid convergence and thus reduce total computation time. Several elements of θ can be sampled simultaneously in one block, before turning to other elements or blocks. This works when the unknowns inside the block are correlated with one another and not much with those outside the block. Details of the `block` option are given in the Stata [BAYES] manual.

2.4.6.1   The StataStan interface

CmdStan, if installed, can be run from inside Stata using the user-written command `stan` [97]. Windows users will also have to install `windowsmonitor`. The simplest way to use this command is to have the Stan model code saved in a text file. Here, we will call it `mymodel.stan`.

The `stan` command gets CmdStan to compile the model code, and then sample from it. The data that can be sent includes: variables loaded in Stata, global macros, and matrices. The results are displayed inside the Stata console, and you can request the chains to be loaded, replacing the current data.

This is a basic example of its syntax, where data are stored in one variable, x:

```
// get number of observations
quietly count
global N = r(N)

stan x, modelfile("mymodel.stan") cmdstandir("/path/to/cmdstan") globals("N") load
```

The `modelfile` option identifies the file containing the Stan model, `cmdstandir` shows Stata the folder where it can find the executable CmdStan program, the `globals` option names the global macros that we wish to send to Stan, and `load` requests that the chains be brought back into Stata. The variable x (and any others required) is listed after the command name, in the usual Stata "varlist".

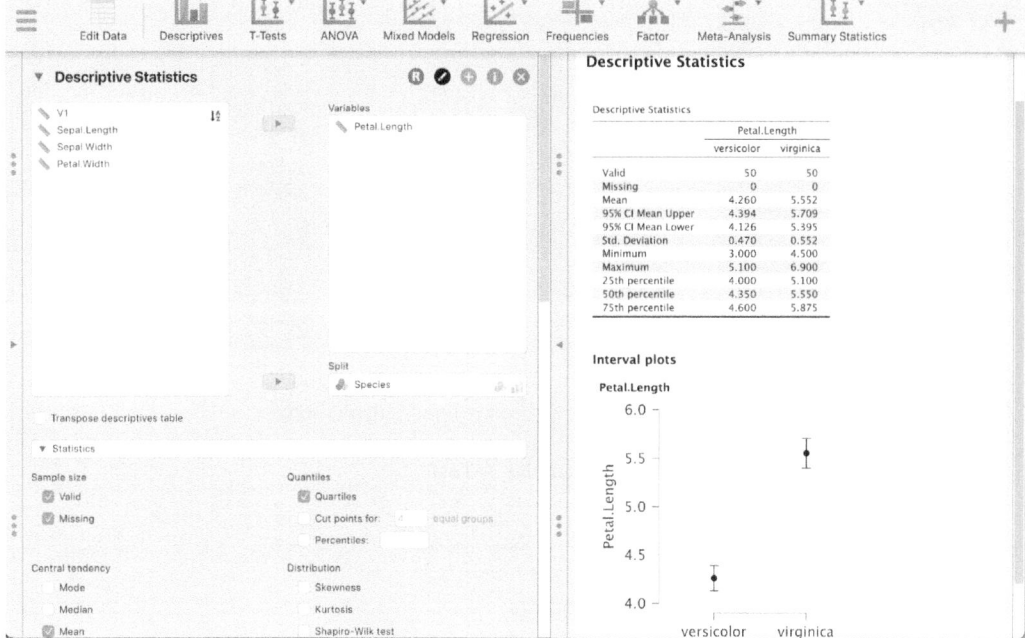

FIGURE 2.9
JASP interface for descriptive statistics. We are asking for comparison between petal lengths for different species in the iris dataset.

Diagnostic outputs are shown directly from CmdStan, further output can be requested with the `diagnose` option. There are no new commands for graphics, but traceplots, histograms, and density plots can be generated with standard Stata commands.

2.4.7 JASP

JASP is an open-source standalone application which runs various R programs in the background [133]. It provides a point-and-click interface (Figure 2.9) and offers Bayesian alternatives to a wide range of common frequentist inferential procedures.

The interface is likely to be the main attraction for beginners in Bayesian analysis, who are unfamiliar with a coding approach. The drawback is that your analysis needs to fit into one of the preset options in JASP. At the time of writing, these include some meta-analysis models but are rapidly expanding, making JASP a contender for many Bayesian meta-analyses in the near future. We cannot apply exactly the model for petal lengths or binary events that we used above in other software. Instead, we will compare mean petal lengths between two species (*Iris versicolor* and *Iris virginica*) with a Bayesian version of the t-test, which provides a more appropriate framework for this particular comparative analysis.

In JASP, we can select the "T-tests" menu, and click on "Bayesian independent samples t-test". The dialog box appears, similar to the one for descriptive statistics but also allowing specification of a prior for the effect size[†] (Figure 2.10). We set this prior to N(0, 0.8). Options are limited to Cauchy, normal and t-distributions.

[†]By clicking in the blue "i" information icon, we find that the effect size is defined as Cohen's d: the mean difference, divided by the pooled standard deviation of the groups.

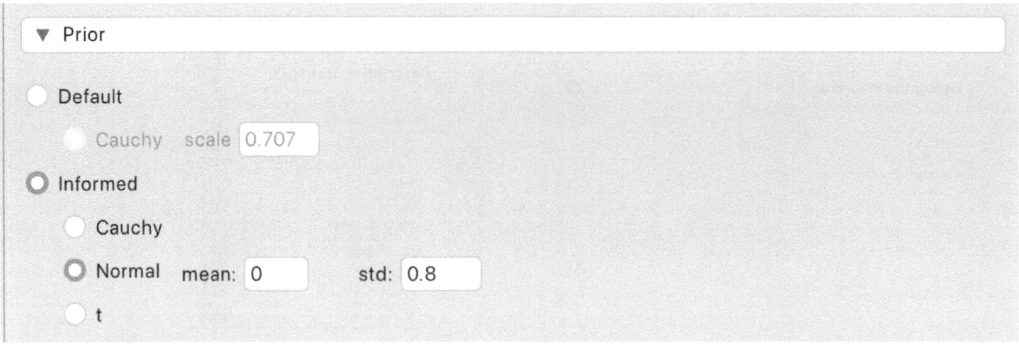

FIGURE 2.10
JASP interface to specify a prior for the independent-samples t-test.

Bayesian Independent Samples T-Test

Bayesian Independent Samples T-Test

	BF_{10}	error %
Petal.Length	$1.383\times10^{+18}$	

Note. No error estimate is available for normal priors.

Inferential Plots

Petal.Length

Prior and Posterior

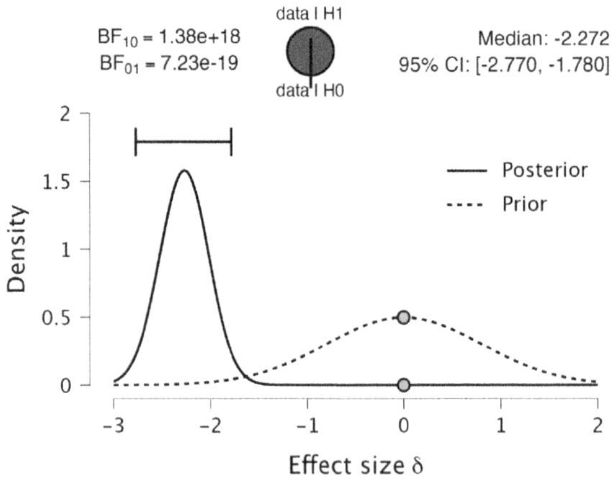

FIGURE 2.11
JASP output from the Bayesian independent-samples t-test.

Output includes a Bayes factor which is very large, showing extremely strong evidence that the two species do not have the sample mean petal length. We can also request graphics, including the density plots for the prior and posterior of the effect size (Figure 2.11).

If your model is not a novel one, and the Bayesian aspect is limited to applying priors, then you may be able to use JASP. It will provide a posterior median, and a 95% credible interval, but not the posterior sample. It includes some meta-analysis models, which we consider in Chapters 3 and 4.

2.4.8 A note on the Gibbs sampler

The Gibbs sampler, as described at the beginning of this chapter, is a potentially efficient algorithm because it divides the multi-dimensional joint posterior over all the elements of $\boldsymbol{\theta}$ into conditional distributions, one dimension at a time. These conditional distributions hold all the other unknowns fixed at their current values and then describe the posterior distribution of the one that is free to change, like a slice through the joint probability.

The details are beyond the scope of this book, but it is worth realising that, if you use the Gibbs sampler, its advantage over random walk Metropolis-Hastings depends on an assumption: that calculating each conditional posterior for θ_i in turn ($P(\theta_i|\boldsymbol{\theta}_{-i}, \boldsymbol{Y})$ is easier than calculating the joint distribution $P(\boldsymbol{\theta}_{-i}|\boldsymbol{Y})$. (Here, we use $\boldsymbol{\theta}_{-i}$ to mean all the elements of $\boldsymbol{\theta}$ except the ith.)

The computer has to calculate the shape of the conditional distribution at each step. This is quite simple if the priors and likelihood are *conjugate* [147, 156]. A simple example of conjugacy is using a beta distribution as prior for a proportion, along with the binomial likelihood. This will result in a beta posterior distribution, the same as the prior, but with different parameters. The definition of conjugacy is that the prior and posterior have the same distribution formula, but the parameters change as data are added via the likelihood.

If priors and likelihood are not conjugate, the computation may be slowed down very significantly, and there may be little or no advantage over random walk Metropolis-Hastings.

The Gibbs sampler is used all the time by BUGS and JAGS, and is available in Stata `bayesmh`, for certain combinations of prior and likelihood, if you add the `gibbs` option.

2.4.9 Other software

Bayesian functionality is available, with varying degrees of flexibility, in other software too. We will list and link here those that may be contenders for the sort of analyses in this book, which is to say that they provide more flexibility than mere presets.

SAS is proprietary software that includes MCMC functionality. At present, the part of the software that allows multilevel ("random effects") structure in models only allows random walk Metropolis-Hastings [219].

Multilevel models are the main focus of software written by the University of Bristol's Centre for Multilevel Modelling. This includes MLwiN, which is free to UK-based academics and students, and is inexpensive otherwise. MLwiN is available for Windows operating systems, has a unique graphical user interface where models are specified in mathematical notation, and implements an adaptive Metropolis-Hastings algorithm as well as maximum likelihood methods [150]. There are interfaces in packages for R and Stata. Other relevant software made by the same team can be found at their website [266].

PyMC3 and PyMC 4.0* are Python packages that implement a probabilistic programming language. Behind the scenes, they repurpose different powerful software for deep learning in order to sample from posterior distributions. PyMC 4.0 implements Hamiltonian Monte Carlo [199].

Julia is a programming language designed from the outset to be both fast and useful for scientific applications. There is a collection of Julia packages that can be used for Bayesian modelling, collectively called Turing, with a probabilistic programming language similar to Stan [245].

Most people call them PyMC3 and PyMC4. We decided not to feature them in depth in this book because, firstly, very few people we have met when teaching meta-analysis use Python, and secondly, the probabilistic programming language is quite unlike BUGS, JAGS and Stan, which closely mimic lines of mathematical notation. We intend to add PyMC translations of our examples to the book's website in due course.

There are many other cottage-industry probabilistic programming languages that can be found online, for example listed at Wikipedia [282]. Though we cannot vouch for their completeness or reliability, some may be of interest for didactic purposes.

2.4.10   Non-MCMC algorithms

MCMC is not the only way to get a posterior sample. Other approaches are an active area of methodological research, and hold promise for some of the most challenging problems, with extremely large datasets and extremely complicated models. However, meta-analysis is not in that category, and, in our experience, variants of MCMC are adequate for all meta-analytic tasks.

Some of the other algorithm names you might hear of include sequential Monte Carlo (also known as particle filters), sampling importance resampling, Metropolis-adjusted Langevin algorithm (MALA) and piecewise deterministic Markov processes (for example, the bouncy particle sampler or the zig-zag sampler) [99].

A quite different approach with some potential for meta-analysis is generically called simulation-based inference (SBI), where participant-level data are simulated to find out what values of θ lead to pseudo-data with study statistics that are similar to the real, reported statistics. We describe SBI in Chapter 17.

2.5   Checking Your Computation and Diagnosing Problems

2.5.1   Problems of convergence

For Bayesian sampling algorithms to work, they need to converge to the posterior distribution. Typically, the first iterations will move towards the posterior (see Figure 2.3), but until you can be confident that they have settled down there, they should be discarded. For random walk Metropolis-Hastings, this can take a thousand or more iterations; for Gibbs sampler it is faster and for Hamiltonian Monte Carlo faster still. More complex models with many unknowns, and correlated posteriors, will generally take longer. In each case you should discard the beginning of the iterations in each chain so that they do not bias your inferences about the shape of the posterior.

In BUGS and many other packages, this is referred to as burn-in, while in Stan it is referred to as warm-up. Most Bayesian analysts start by discarding the first 1000 iterations, and then examine the traceplot to see if it appears to be stable. A traceplot that has converged is characterised by random movement within the same distribution from left to right. Multiple chains' lines should overlap. This is the characteristic "hairy caterpillar" shape that indicates that all is well in the algorithm.

When the posterior cannot be trusted, we see one of three problems: slow mixing, convergence around one or more local maxima, or no convergence to any distribution.

In slow mixing, the traceplots move gradually around (they are autocorrelated), but seen in the longer run, they are within a distribution, but just moving slowly through it (Figure 2.12 shows an example from Chapter 9. This can be further assessed by looking at autocorrelation plots, which good Bayesian software will provide.

This might not be a problem, provided you have enough draws from the posterior. You might choose to *thin* the draws, keeping perhaps one in every hundred iterations. This helps with memory or disk space, but keeping all the autocorrelated draws is not necessarily a problem.

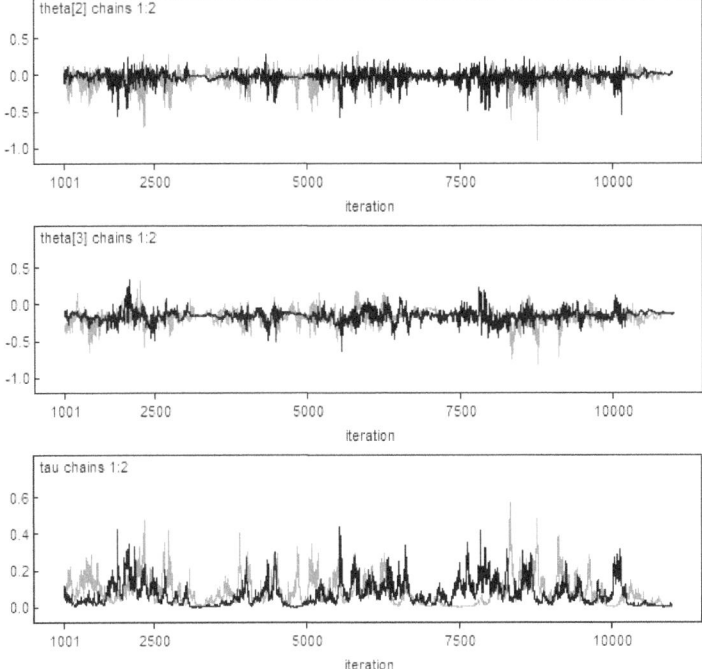

FIGURE 2.12
Traceplots indicative of slow mixing, from the "common heterogeneity" model in Section 9.1.4, implemented in WinBUGS.

In complex models, the posterior density might not have one hill (see Figure 2.2), but instead several local bumps (maxima). When chains settle on different maxima, each chain may look convincing, yet we see that they are not in agreement with each other. This is unlikely to arise in meta-analysis models, but if it does appear, it may indicate poor initial values or an incorrectly specified model.

When chains do not converge at all, it is typically because there is a flat region in the posterior density. Any direction is as good as any other in terms of the log posterior density, and so the algorithm moves entirely at random. Traceplots in this case will look more like snakes than hairy caterpillars (see Figure 2.13) and multiple chains may move to quite different values from each other.

One common mistake that can lead to non-convergence of some parameters is when we mistakenly make the model *under-identified*. A simple case of this is if we want to predict a dependent variable using a categorical predictor, and we include a coefficient for each of the categories, plus an intercept term[†]. Now, the intercept can be under- or over-estimated by any amount, so long as it is counter-balanced by the coefficients. In this case, traceplots will appear to be mirror images for some parameters, and this can give you a clue about how to correct the model.

Software will usually provide you with a simple statistic of convergence called r-hat or Gelman-Rubin, or Brooks-Gelman-Rubin. There are some slight differences in how these are calculated in different software, but the interpretation is the same. Ideally, the number should be close to 1 for all unknowns. If it exceeds 1.1 (as a rough rule of thumb), then

---

[†]Software using likelihood methods for regression will typically omit one of the categories automatically, so beginners in statistical analysis do not usually have to worry about this.

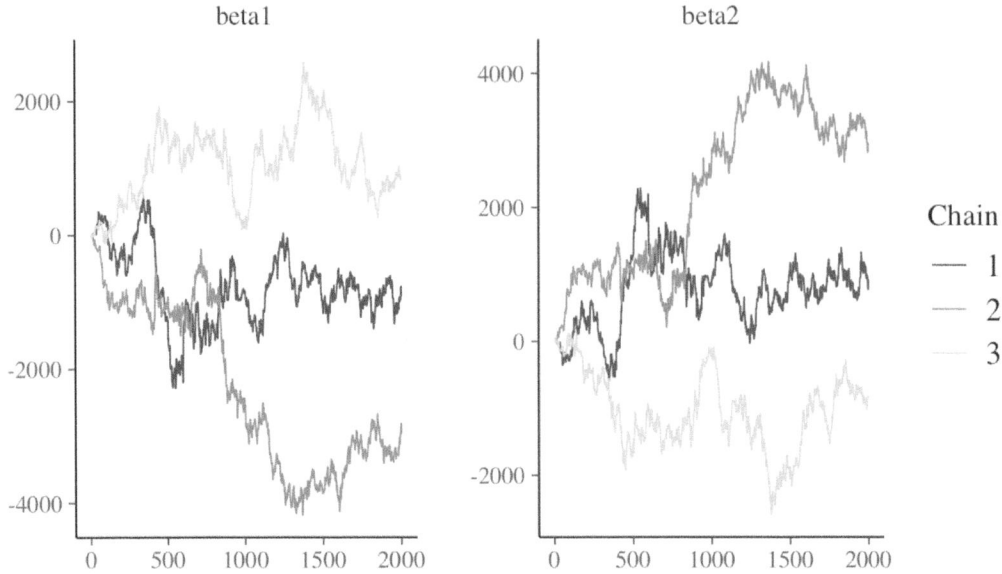

FIGURE 2.13
Snakes instead of a caterpillar: non-convergent traceplots from an under-identified model.
Note how the "beta1" traceplots are a vertical mirror image of those for "beta2". This is
because the mean of the data is estimated (a deliberate mistake) as beta1+beta2. Sampling
was done in Stan and the plot is from the `bayesplot` R package.

there is likely to be a problem with convergence, or perhaps the chains simply have to run
for more iterations.

2.5.2   How many posterior draws should be obtained?

In most meta-analysis settings, we expect the running of MCMC algorithms to be fast, and
so there should no need to compromise with small posterior samples. As a rough guide, if
you are interested in making decisions based on the tails of the posterior distribution, then
you will need more draws to provide certainty about those low densities.

Software output usually includes a Monte Carlo standard error (MC error) for the posterior mean. This is simply the standard error for the mean estimate, given that the posterior
sample is a random sample. The MC error of the mean or median will be smaller than the
MC error of values determined by the sparsely populated tails, such as limits of the 95%
credible interval.

MC error shrinks as the posterior sample grows, so one principled way to determine how
many iterations we need of our algorithms is to decide on a target MC error and increase
until this is achieved (or to estimate the sample size a priori from approximate formulas).

 The MC error can be estimated for quantiles, such as the credible interval limits, using
the bootstrap method. On the book's website, we provide code for this purpose.

We advise that you always begin by retaining 10,000 draws after warm-up, and examine
the effective sample size or autocorrelation. Strong autocorrelation means that the chains
move slowly through the posterior, and an even larger sample may be needed, particularly
if you are using software other than Stan. Thinning can be used to reduce autocorrelation,
while retaining a smaller posterior sample.

2.5.3   Initial values

Initial values can be critical to the success of MCMC algorithms. If you have problems with convergence, you should consider whether your initial values are going to be in the region of high posterior density, and if you are not sure, try some different values. There is no need to worry that you are hacking the algorithm until you get results you like: after autocorrelation has worn off, which is certainly within the warm-up, the initial values should have no influence.

2.5.4   Prior predictive and posterior predictive checks

A flexible and informative way of critiquing your models is to generate pseudo-data based on unknowns drawn only from the priors (a prior predictive check) or from the posterior (a posterior predictive check).

Generating these pseudo-data can be done inside BUGS, JAGS or Stan model code. Stata has a separate postestimation command for posterior predictive checks. Even if your software does not allow it, you can do it separately in a second step from your draws for $\boldsymbol{\theta}$.

In the prior predictive check, we expect to see pseudo-data that encompass the observed values (so the true data are not ruled out by the priors) and which have plausible and possible values (no negative counts, for example)—for example, Figure 2.14. The model code for this does not include the likelihood, only the priors. This is prior predictive WinBUGS code for the iris petals example:

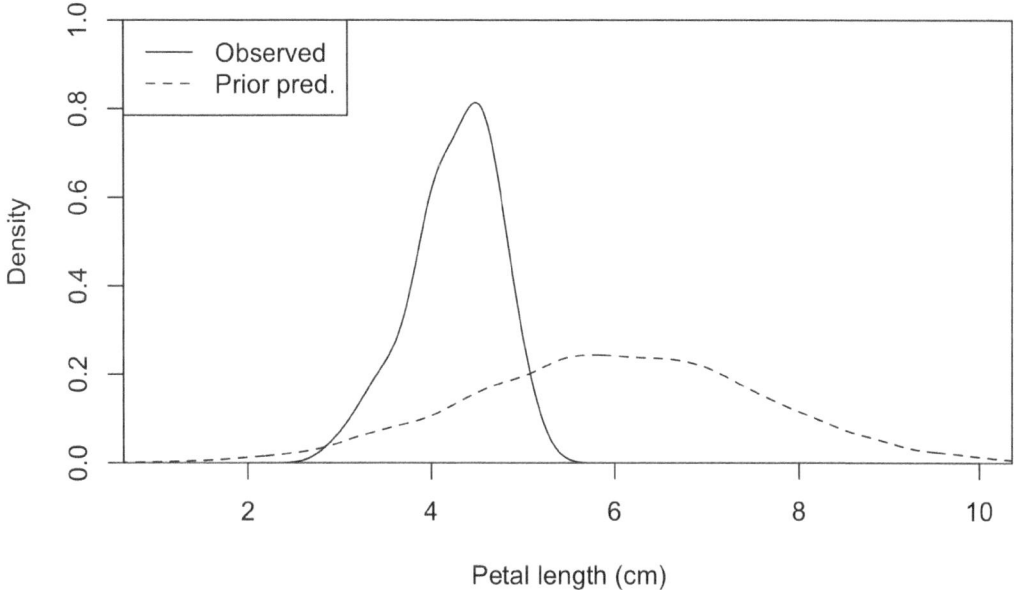

FIGURE 2.14
Comparison of observed data distribution and prior predictive distribution: in this case, the priors seem adequate because their predictive density encompasses the observed data with extra density on either side.

```
# model:
model{
  mu ~ dnorm(6, 0.444)I(0,)
  sigma ~ dgamma(2, 4)
  prec <- 1/(sigma*sigma)
  # constant (therefore negligible) likelihood
  x_pred ~ dnorm(mu, prec)
}

# initial values:
list(mu=3.0, sigma=0.5, x_pred=6.2)
list(mu=2.5, sigma=0.4, x_pred=5.8)
```

In this code, the unknowns are not affected by likelihood and simply follow the prior distribution. The predicted value is then drawn from the same distribution as the likelihood would have, taking the current μ and σ at each iteration as parameters.

Posterior predictive checks generate posterior draws as usual, from prior and likelihood, and then generate pseudo-data from those values of $\boldsymbol{\theta}$. We expect to see pseudo-data that look like the observed data, for example Figure 2.15. Ways in which they are not similar can provide us with ideas to refine the model further. This is posterior predictive BUGS code for the iris petals example:

```
# data:
list(n = 50,
     x = c(4.7, 4.5, 4.9, 4, 4.6, 4.5, 4.7, 3.3, 4.6, 3.9,
           3.5, 4.2, 4, 4.7, 3.6, 4.4, 4.5, 4.1, 4.5, 3.9,
           4.8, 4, 4.9, 4.7, 4.3, 4.4, 4.8, 5, 4.5, 3.5,
           3.8, 3.7, 3.9, 5.1, 4.5, 4.5, 4.7, 4.4, 4.1, 4,
           4.4, 4.6, 4, 3.3, 4.2, 4.2, 4.2, 4.3, 3, 4.1))

# model:
model{
  mu ~ dnorm(6, 0.444)I(0,)
  sigma ~ dgamma(2, 4)
  prec <- 1/(sigma*sigma)
  for(i in 1:n) {
    x[i] ~ dnorm(mu, prec)
  }
  x_pred ~ dnorm(mu, prec)
}

# initial values:
list(mu=3.0, sigma=0.5, x_pred=3.2)
list(mu=2.5, sigma=0.4, x_pred=2.2)
```

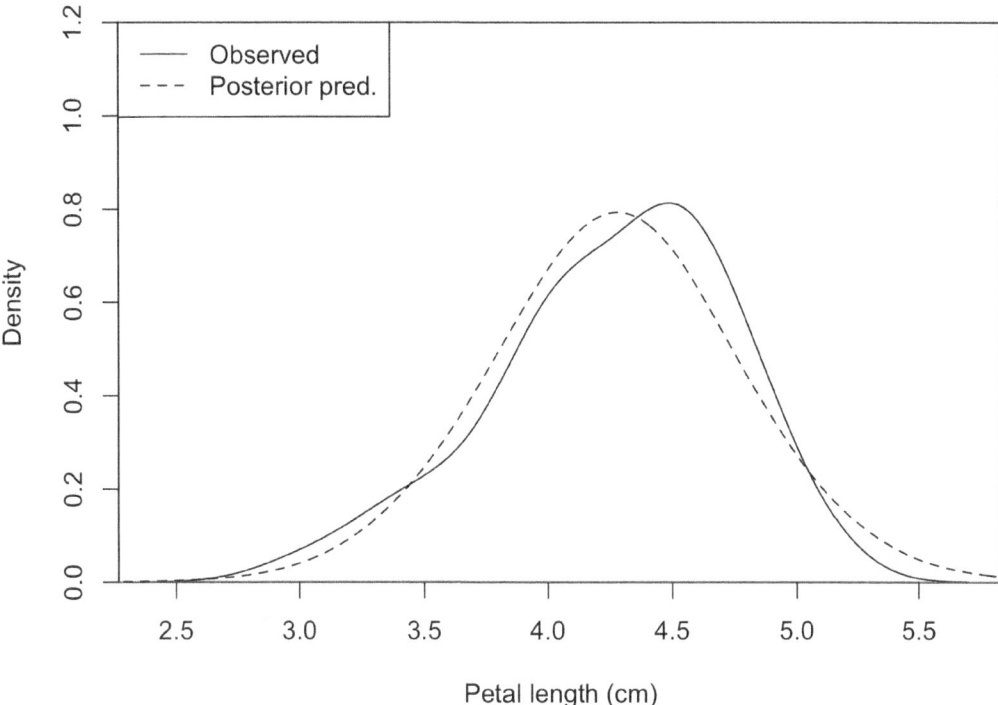

FIGURE 2.15
Comparison of observed data distribution and posterior predictive distribution: the normal model of the data (likelihood) assumes symmetry around the mean, while there is slight skew in the real data, though this is a small difference and unlikely to have introduced serious bias.

The difference is that the posterior predicted value (x_pred) is drawn from the likelihood distribution, given the parameters μ and σ, which are shaped by both prior and likelihood

Concepts of predictive checking as part of a modelling workflow are described clearly, but in a regression setting, in recent textbooks [88, 166]. In meta-analysis, the idea of predicting a future trial of a certain size is useful in itself, and is discussed in Section 3.7.

On this book's website, we supply examples of prior and posterior predictive checks in all the software packages where it is possible.

3

Common Effect Meta-Analysis

Learning objectives

After reading this chapter, you will be able to:

1. explain meta-analyses both as weighted averages and as statistical models

2. explain how likelihood and parameter space lead to an estimate and uncertainty around that estimate

3. use Bayesian software to conduct a common effects meta-analysis

4. recognise much of the notation used in this book

Meta-analysis is a collection of statistical methods to combine the results of multiple studies. Instead of starting with a file of data from individual observations, as we did in the previous chapter, we use published statistics from the studies* as our raw material.

We think it most likely that you, the reader, will have done some simple meta-analysis in the past, and that you have picked up this book because you need something more bespoke to deal with problems in the evidence base. You may be familiar with choosing meta-analysis options in software like RevMan, CMA or Stata.

This chapter will take you a little deeper, relating meta-analysis to the likelihood principles of Section 2.1. You will then have a framework on which you can build your own, more elaborate statistical models for specific projects. We will not give full details of non-Bayesian calculations in meta-analysis, as there are many textbooks on the subject [24, 248].

We focus on the meta-analytic calculations and assumptions that underpin them. Mostly, we do not explore the work of question definition, literature searching, and critical appraisal that precedes meta-analysis. These aspects are extremely important to the success of any effort to understand the evidence base and act on it, but are already explored very effectively in several textbooks [46, 64].

However, one important consideration for this chapter (and all that follow!) is that any meta-analysis seeks to answer a specific question, which should be defined as clearly as possible before modelling begins. This helps us humans to avoid the cognitive biases to which we are all prone: to see patterns that we would like to see, even where they do not really exist, and to be more critical of findings that go against our hopes and expectations than those that please us. In that way, it is like pre-registering the outcomes and analysis plan of a clinical trial.

---

*Sometimes, we have individual participant data (IPD) from one or more studies, and then the approach is a little different. This is discussed in Chapter 10.

3.1 How Does Meta-Analysis Work?

Our goal is to combine results from studies. So, we must be prepared to take statistics as our inputs, not individual observations.

Each study collected a sample of observations, drawn from a population. They then estimated some unknown population parameter. Because they have a sample, their estimates (statistics) might be over- or under-estimates, just by chance. Chapter 1 showed how summary statistics have *sampling distributions* which allow us to quantify the uncertainty arising from sampling.

If we average all the stats, we might reasonably expect the over-estimates to balance out the under-estimates, and give us a useful combined estimate. However, it needs to be a little more complicated: some studies will inherently have results that are less precise than others.

This is often simply because a study had fewer observations, and that enlarges the standard error of the statistic that they are reporting. As a result, their estimate could be further away from the true population value, and we should trust their results less. The simple way to do this is to use a weighted average, where the less precise studies get less weight.

In fact, many common calculations for non-Bayesian meta-analyses use exactly this weighted average approach, although they might differ on how to calculate the weights.

Next, we must have a way to calculate the extent of the uncertainty around our meta-analysis estimate. The most important consideration is whether we think that the outcome of interest had the same distribution in all the studies' populations.

It might be that the statistic of interest—typically, a summary of an outcome, or a contrast between two interventions' outcomes—differs between study populations. This is called heterogeneity, and is definitely important to capture in the meta-analysis.

In this chapter, we start with models where there is no heterogeneity, then we add it in Chapter 4.

Once we obtain a combined estimate by meta-analysis, and the size of the uncertainty around it (for example, a standard error, or the two ends of a confidence or credible interval), we need to interpret and present those results carefully. We must make sure that our audience understands it correctly, does not extend it into unsupported conclusions, and can use it for effective, data-driven decision-making.

We should contextualise our findings with reference to the studies that we were able to use as input. As an example with a continuous-valued outcome variable, we will take a Cochrane review of green tea extracts for weight loss[136], and in particular, a meta-analysis of randomised controlled trials (RCTs) where change in body mass index (BMI) was the outcome. For binary outcomes, we use a meta-analysis comparing two classes of blood pressure lowering drugs, and in particular, we compare them on the incidence of adverse events [149].

Suppose that a nurse in primary care picks up the green tea meta-analysis, with the intention of finding out whether they should recommend it to patients who are slightly overweight and want to control their weight with lifestyle interventions. The nurse will need to know whether the studies recruited participants that were similar to those that they see in their practice, and also, that the green tea preparations are similar to those that can be obtained locally, and that the control groups took steps to control their weight which are similar to the alternatives that local patients would consider.

To summarise this: are the studies representative of the sort of population, intervention, comparison and outcomes (PICO) that we want to make decisions about? If not, then we must be cautious about extrapolating the findings.

Some problems of limited evidence base are very common, yet hard to overcome, such as a lack of randomised controlled trials of health care interventions in children. Extrapolating from adult studies could be misleading, or perhaps even dangerous.

Perhaps the biggest challenge in effectively using meta-analyses to translate evidence into practice (and hopefully improved future outcomes) is this frank discussion of the limitations of the evidence base. We want the audience to understand the limitations of our work and use it within its capabilities, but we do not want them to give up all trust in our outputs and revert to prejudice. Finding this balance is a skill acquired over time, and has to be tailored to each situation.

3.2   Meta-Analysis of Mean Differences

Meta-analyses combine summary statistics of outcomes or contrasts of them. In a clinical trial, each arm will have some outcome statistic, and the principal focus of attention is likely to be the *contrast* between two arms. In this book, we mostly focus on randomised controlled trials, and in this setting, it is familiar to describe the intervention effect.

We will use $\hat{\theta}_j$ to indicate any intervention effect estimate from study j, and θ to indicate the true intervention effect in the population. (The hat indicates that $\hat{\theta}_j$ is an estimate.) The standard error of the intervention effect estimate is itself an estimate: $\widehat{SE}(\hat{\theta}_j)$.

In RCTs reporting means and standard deviations, this is usually just the difference between the means in the two arms: $\hat{\theta}_j = \bar{y}_{j\mathbf{Int}} - \bar{y}_{j\mathbf{Ctl}}$.

Taking the first green tea study in Table 3.1, Kozuma 2005, $j = 1$ and $\hat{\theta}_1 = -1.0 - 0.3 = -1.3$. Figure 3.1 shows the normal distributions for individual participants, implied by the statistics from each arm of this study.

TABLE 3.1

Study statistics from the green tea meta-analysis[136]. The outcome is change in body mass index, so a negative value is desirable.

Study	$n_{j\mathbf{Int}}$	$\bar{y}_{j\mathbf{Int}}$	$s_{j\mathbf{Int}}$	$n_{j\mathbf{Ctl}}$	$\bar{y}_{j\mathbf{Ctl}}$	$s_{j\mathbf{Ctl}}$
Kozuma 2005	107	-1.0	0.6	119	0.3	0.4
Takase 2008	44	-1.2	0.5	45	0.0	0.3
Nagao 2007	123	-0.6	0.6	117	0.0	0.6
Takeshita 2008	40	-0.5	0.4	41	-0.1	0.5
Kajimoto 2005	129	-0.2	0.5	66	0.2	0.8
Suzuki 2009	18	-0.2	0.5	20	0.0	0.6
Kataoka 2004	71	-0.4	0.8	71	-0.3	0.8
Takashima 2004	10	-0.5	0.6	9	-0.5	0.6
Auvichayapat 2008	30	-3.0	1.7	30	-1.9	1.8
Hill 2007	19	0.0	0.3	19	0.2	0.4
Hsu 2008	41	-0.1	2.8	37	0	0.8
Diepvens 2005	23	-1.5	0.7	23	-1.5	0.6

Source: Ref. [136].

Note: $k = \mathbf{Int}$ indicates the green tea extract arm (active treatment)

$\quad\quad k = \mathbf{Ctl}$ indicates the control arm.

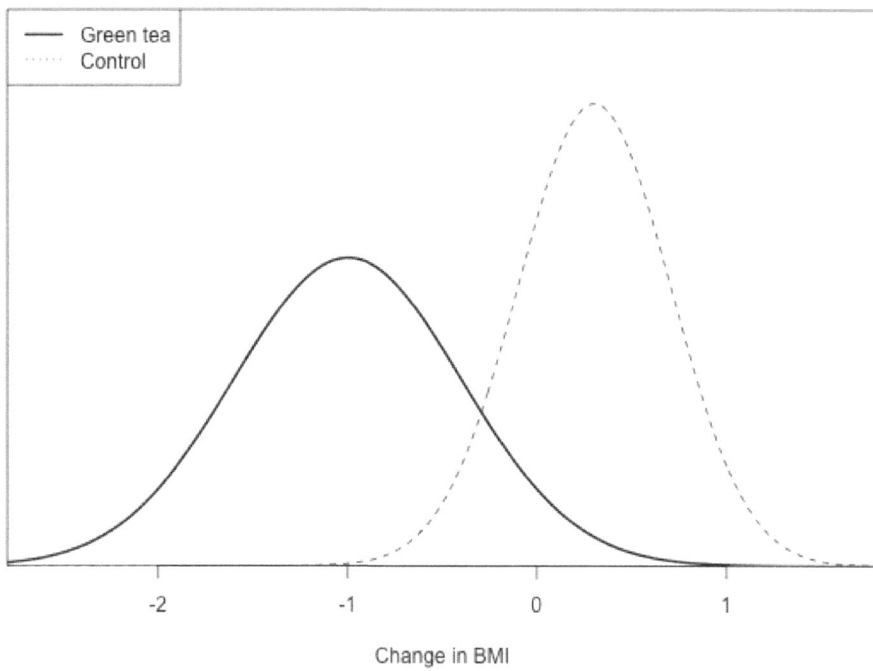

FIGURE 3.1
Normal distributions implied by the means and standard deviations reported in Kozuma 2005 (see Table 3.1).

We can also combine the variances (squared standard deviations) of outcomes in the two arms into a pooled estimate of variance, if we believe that they both drew from the same population (this should be the case in randomised studies). The *pooled variance* is an average of the arms' variances, weighted by the sample size minus one:

$$s_{j\bullet}^2 = \frac{(n_{j\mathbf{Int}} - 1)s_{j\mathbf{Int}}^2 + (n_{j\mathbf{Ctl}} - 1)s_{j\mathbf{Ctl}}^2}{(n_{j\mathbf{Int}} - 1) + (n_{j\mathbf{Ctl}} - 1)} \quad , \forall j \tag{3.1}$$

Equation 3.1 is applied to every study ($\forall j$ is read as "for all j"). It is an important part of the assumptions in our calculations when some formula is the same in all arms ($\forall k$) or studies ($\forall j$). From this point on, we will mostly omit the $\forall$ statements from our formulas, unless they help to clarify some point.

For example, in the paper "Kozuma 2005",

$$s_{1\bullet}^2 = \frac{106 \times 0.6^2 + 118 \times 0.4^2}{106 + 118} = 0.25$$

so:

$$s_{1\bullet} = \sqrt{0.25} = 0.50$$

Studies do not (we hope!) simply put all individual participant data from both arms into one big spreadsheet and calculate a single standard deviation, because if there is a difference in means, then one arm's data will be displaced above or below the other's values, which will falsely inflate the standard deviation estimate[†]. Instead, they use Equation 3.1.

Three differences from Chapter 1 are worth commenting on before we move on.

1. Our calculations will use study statistics as input instead of individual observations. We often hear study statistics referred to casually as "data", but strictly they are not. (We will introduce individual participant data (IPD) meta-analyses in Chapter 10.)

2. We are assuming, for now, that every study drew observations at random from the same population. This means that every $\hat{\theta}_j$ is an estimate of the same θ. This is called a *common-effect* model, and we will explore other options in Chapter 4.

3. We are going to start with models which include a mean (expected) outcome for each arm, but one shared standard deviation of the data for all arms of any studies, σ. That is an assumption in our model; we will look into how to change it later.

The sampling distribution of the study statistic around the true population value is at the core of all meta-analysis models. For means of outcomes, as long as the underlying data are not too few or too far from being normally distributed, that will be a normal sampling distribution:

$$\hat{\theta}_j \sim \mathrm{N}(\theta, \widehat{SE}(\hat{\theta}_j)) \tag{3.2}$$

Published studies generally provide us with $\hat{\theta}_j$ and $\widehat{SE}(\hat{\theta}_j)$. We might have to calculate $\widehat{SE}(\hat{\theta}_j)$ from a confidence interval (which is $\hat{\theta}_j \pm 1.96\widehat{SE}(\hat{\theta}_j)$), or from the pooled variance of Equation 3.1. Randomised controlled studies are designed so that data in one arm are independent of those in another arm, and this means that we can simply calculate:

$$\widehat{SE}(\hat{\theta}_j) = \sqrt{\hat{V}(\hat{\theta}_j)} = \sqrt{\frac{s_{j\bullet}^2}{n_{j\mathbf{Int}}} + \frac{s_{j\bullet}^2}{n_{j\mathbf{Ctl}}}} \tag{3.3}$$

You might notice that the mean difference in an RCT is the difference of two uncorrelated variables with normal sampling distributions, so the variance of the difference is the sum of the variances (see Equation 1.14). Other study designs, where the data are likely to be correlated, such as paired data or matched case-control studies, will not be so simple. We will return to them in Chapter 5.

The common-effect meta-analysis assumes that all studies drew their participants from the same population, at least in terms of the intervention effect θ, so we only need to estimate θ and σ. A weighted average of the $\hat{\theta}_j$s, where larger studies get more weight, is the most common method of non-Bayesian meta-analysis. There are a number of elaborations on it, but the simplest version produces a meta-analytic estimate of θ called the *weighted mean difference* (WMD). Just for this section, we will use the Greek letter lambda (λ_j) to indicate the weight given to study j.

In a common-effect meta-analysis, the usual weight is the precision of each study's estimate, which is the reciprocal of the variance of the sampling distribution: $\lambda_j = \frac{1}{V(\hat{\theta}_j)}$. A study with smaller variance of the estimate is a more precise one, and will get greater

---

[†]Try it yourself to get a deeper understanding: simulate 1000 random numbers from N(10, 1) and 1000 from N(5, 1). Combine them and calculate the standard deviation: you will find it is much bigger than 1. Plot a histogram to see what is going on. Then, find each group's observed standard deviation, and combine them with Equation 3.1.

weight in the meta-analytic estimate. This leads to the following weighted average estimate over all m studies:

$$\hat{\theta} = \frac{\lambda_1 \hat{\theta}_1 + \lambda_2 \hat{\theta}_2 + \ldots + \lambda_m \hat{\theta}_m}{\lambda_1 + \lambda_2 + \ldots + \lambda_m}$$

$$= \frac{\sum_{j=1}^{m} \lambda_j \hat{\theta}_j}{\sum_{j=1}^{m} \lambda_j} \tag{3.4}$$

with variance:

$$\hat{V}(\hat{\theta}) = \frac{1}{\sum_{j=1}^{m} \lambda_j} \tag{3.5}$$

In the case of the green tea studies, although a common-effect model seems implausible, we would obtain:

$$\hat{\theta} = -0.42$$

$$\widehat{SE}(\hat{\theta}) = \sqrt{\hat{V}(\hat{\theta})} = 0.22$$

You might like to check that you can obtain the same figures using a calculator, spreadsheet or statistics software. Another way to get a deep understanding of the calculations (and how they might not be appropriate for a particular evidence base) is to start with an assumed model, then generate simulated study data, obtain study statistics, and visualise them, to see what they would look like if the model were true. We take this approach in Section 3.5.

3.2.1 Combining different outcome scales: standardised mean differences

We might have to include studies in our meta-analysis which evaluate the same construct (underlying concept) but use different scales. For example, we might have a collection of studies looking at depression, but using different scales. Each scale has its own minimum, maximum, mean and standard deviation.

So far, we have been working with the *raw* or *unstandardised* mean differences, $\hat{\theta}_j$, but we obviously cannot try to average one study, with a scale from 0 to 10, and another, with a scale from 10 to 100. We need to convert the numbers first, to be comparable.

The most common approach is called the *standardised mean difference* (SMD). We divide each study's mean difference by the standard deviation of the outcome to put them all on the same scale, where 0 means no difference, and ±1 means a difference of one standard deviation on whatever scale. Then, they can be combined in a weighted average [41].

There are a few different proposed formulas for this standardisation. The most common are Cohen's d and Hedges' g[24]. Each has a formula for the standardisation, and a formula for the standard error of the standardised intervention effect.

We find these calculations too simplistic to cope with every case. In the example of depression scales, perhaps one gives a lot of its points for questions about social anxiety and low mood, while another might focus on self-harm and suicidal ideation. These are clearly going to give different distributions when applied to the same population of study participants, even if they have the same minimum and maximum values.

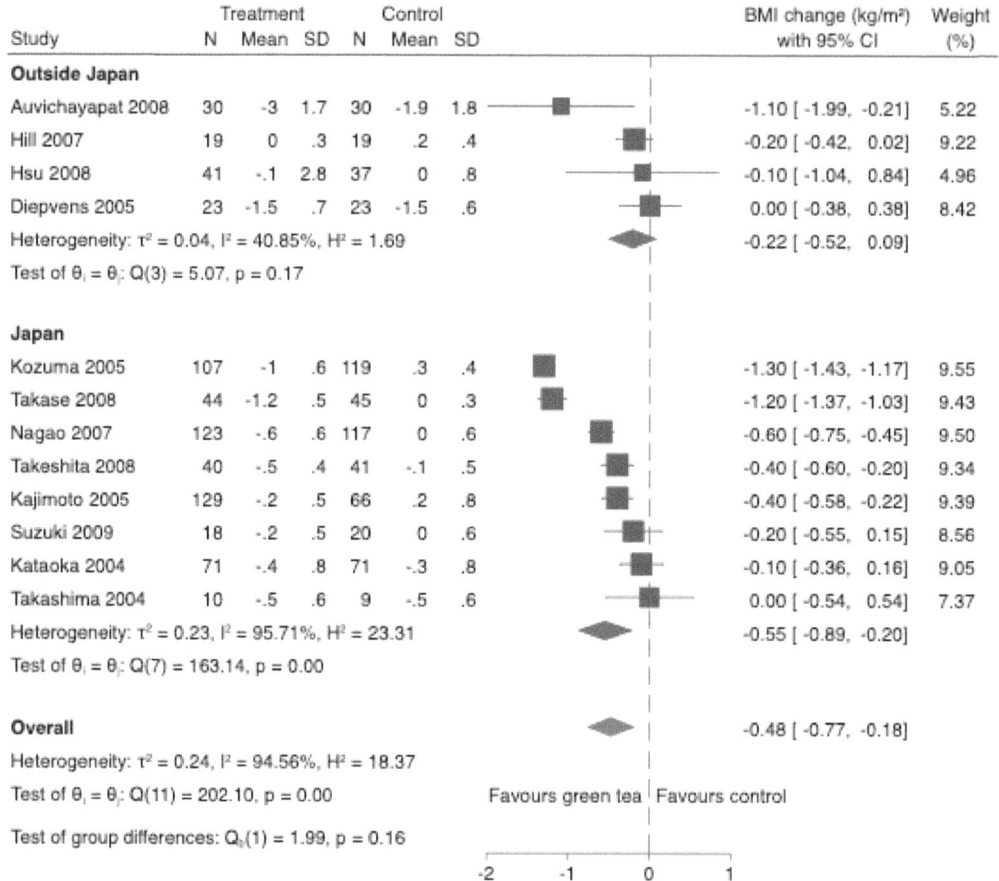

FIGURE 3.2

A typical forest plot, for the green tea meta-analysis, generated in Stata software using the DerSimonian-Laird random effects model with two subgroups (studies conducted in Japan, and elsewhere).

3.3   Forest Plots and Funnel Plots

The most common way to present meta-analyses graphically is the *forest plot* (Figure 3.2). This shows a shape, typically a square, for each study. Studies are arranged vertically at equal intervals, perhaps chronologically or alphabetically, and possibly in subgroups. The study effect (for example, the mean difference or log odds ratio) is encoded as the horizontal location of the square, and there is a vertical line for no effect. Often, the two sides of this line will be labelled as "Favours [intervention 1]" and "Favours [intervention 2]".

The weight given to each study is encoded as the size of the square*, and a horizontal line extends out of the square, showing the extent of the 95% confidence interval for each study's effect.

---

*whether area or length of a side differs depending on software

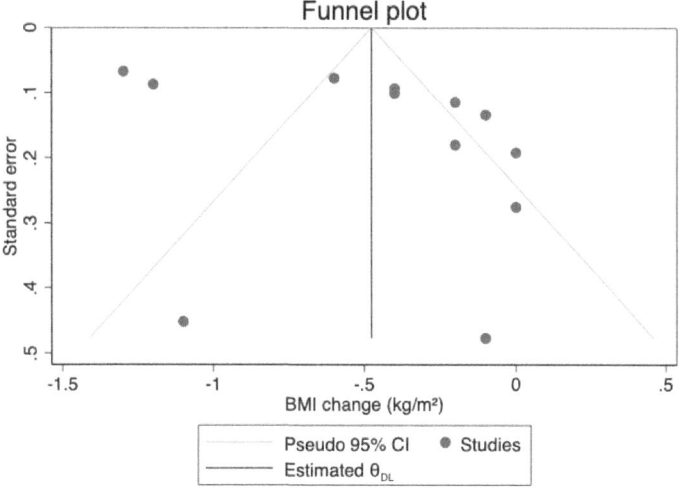

FIGURE 3.3
A typical funnel plot, for the green tea meta-analysis, generated in Stata software. There is some evidence of asymmetry.

At the bottom of the plot (and each subgroup, if they are present), a diamond shape shows the combined effect. The centre of the diamond is horizontally located at the chosen estimate, and its width shows the 95% confidence interval.

A common concern in meta-analysis is *publication bias*, the phenomenon where studies with striking, apparently definitive results[†] are more likely to be published than those that are inconclusive. We will investigate this further in Chapter 13, but it is worth introducing the *funnel plot* here (Figure 3.3), a chart that helps us consider whether there is evidence of publication bias.

Studies are again represented by markers, and study effects are again encoded as horizontal location. Some measure of study effect uncertainty, preferably the standard error, is encoded as vertical position. A vertical line is drawn at the combined effect estimate, and two diagonal lines are drawn along the estimate ± 1.96 standard errors (the 95% confidence interval for different standard errors). If our statistical model is accurate enough, and if there is no publication bias, we expect to see study markers symmetrically distributed around the vertical line and throughout the funnel. There may be 5% of them outside, but not too far from the diagonal lines.

3.4   Meta-Analysis of Log Odds Ratios

When the evidence base reports a binary outcome, then instead of means and standard deviations in each arm, we will find that studies report a proportion or percentage. Underlying this, there should be a numerator and denominator, which are both natural numbers $(0, 1, 2, 3, 4 \ldots)$. Sections 1.3 and 1.4.3 cover the basics of inference for proportions and odds respectively.

[†]often, this equates to statistical significance

To consider the comparison between arms, we usually work with the logarithm of the odds ratio, or log odds ratio. Each study has reported the numerator and denominator in each arm, and from that we can obtain the log odds ratio and its standard error or variance.

Take care over which way round the two arms appear: $\hat{\theta}_j = \log w_{j\text{Int}} - \log w_{j\text{Ctl}}$. We will use p for an observed proportion in a sample, and π for a population proportion; likewise, w for an observed odds and ω for a population odds.

$$\hat{\theta}_j = \log\left(\frac{w_{j\text{Int}}}{w_{j\text{Ctl}}}\right)$$
$$= \log w_{j\text{Int}} - \log w_{j\text{Ctl}}$$
$$= \log d_{j\text{Int}} + \log(n_{j\text{Ctl}} - d_{j\text{Ctl}}) -$$
$$\log d_{j\text{Ctl}} - \log(n_{j\text{Int}} - d_{j\text{Int}})$$
$$\widehat{SE}(\hat{\theta}_j) = \sqrt{V\left(\log\left(\frac{w_{j\text{Int}}}{w_{j\text{Ctl}}}\right)\right)}$$
$$= \sqrt{\frac{1}{d_{j\text{Int}}} + \frac{1}{n_{j\text{Int}} - d_{j\text{Int}}} + \frac{1}{d_{j\text{Ctl}}} + \frac{1}{n_{j\text{Ctl}} - d_{j\text{Ctl}}}}$$

(3.6)

For studies like this, we can take a weighted average of each study's log odds ratio, using the reciprocal of its variance (the standard error squared) as the weight. This is exactly the same as we saw for mean differences in Equations 3.4 and 3.5, and that is because the mean difference and the log odds ratio both have asymptotically normal sampling distributions.

In fact, for other statistics, we can also use this "inverse variance" approach, so long as we can coerce them, through some transformation, to have a normal sampling distribution. Log rate ratios and log hazard ratios, along with their standard errors, can be combined in this way.

3.5 Data-Generating Processes

Each model we will construct in this book is defined by a *data-generating process* (DGP). A common-effect meta-analysis is also a statistical model, even though when presented as an inverse-variance or other weighted average, it does not appear that way at first.

A DGP sets out some deterministic formulas and some probability distributions that together describe how the data came to have the values they do. It will necessarily be a simplification, or model, of reality, and we must use subject expertise and careful judgement in deciding how simple or complex to make it. When we make assumptions or simplifications, we should justify them.

Imagine a simple linear regression where x is the predictor and y is the outcome. The deterministic part of the DGP would be the line of the prediction: $\hat{y} = \beta_0 + \beta_1 x$. The presence of the equals sign shows us that it is deterministic. The probabilistic part is the scatter of the data above and below this line: $y \sim \text{N}(\hat{y}, \sigma^2)$. The tilde ($\sim$) shows that there is a probability distribution for the values of y, but they are not fixed.

3.5.1 DGP for continuous outcomes

Now we can set out a DGP for a collection of RCTs such as the green tea example. We will consider how the individual participant data comes into being, and then how they are then summarised to make the study statistics. We will be able to make simulated studies of various sizes, and see what their statistics look like.

The DGP modelled by a common effect meta-analysis assumes that all studies have randomly sampled participants from the same, normally distributed populations: one for the intervention arm and one for the control arm. The population has an unknown mean in the control group of μ_{Ctl}, and this is increased or decreased in the intervention group by adding θ. Note that, if we subtract the mean in the control group from the mean in the intervention group, we will obtain θ^*. To keep the DGP simple to start, let's assume that both populations have the same standard deviation, σ. Below, i is the participant number, j the study, k the arm.

$$\begin{aligned} y_{ij\text{Ctl}} &\sim \text{N}(\mu, \sigma) \\ y_{ij\text{Int}} &\sim \text{N}(\mu + \theta, \sigma) \end{aligned} \tag{3.7}$$

We can simulate a study like this ($j = 1$), with sample sizes `n_1Ctl` and `n_1Int` in R:

```
y_1Ctl <- rnorm(n_1Ctl, mu, sigma)
y_1Int <- rnorm(n_1Int, mu+theta, sigma)

mean(y_1Ctl)   # control group mean
mean(y_1Int)   # intervention group mean

mean(y_1Int) - mean(y_1Ctl)   # estimate of intervention effect
```

Next, we must consider how this is connected to the information that we typically have available, the sample mean and sample standard deviation. We will use the sampling distribution for the mean (Equation 1.5) and the formula for standard error of the mean (Equation 1.3). To keep it simple, we add an extra simplification: that the population standard deviation has been perfectly estimated by the sample standard deviation, so no inference is necessary for the standard deviation[†]

You might prefer to sketch out the DGP rather than use mathematical notation or code. Figure 3.4 summarises the essentials as a diagram, showing how the data in the control arms relate to the parameters via probability distributions.

Often in non-Bayesian meta-analysis, there is no attention paid to the control group mean (μ), and the participant-level standard deviation (σ) is merely a stepping stone to the standard error of the estimate $\hat{\theta}$. We include μ here so that we can simulate data for both arms, and fully explore the implications of our model.

Now, we can easily extend our code to summarise the simulated data and compare them with a t-test, if we input the three parameters, along with $n_{j\text{Int}}$ and $n_{j\text{Ctl}}$. For example, simulating one study in R:

---

[*]This all sounds like θ might be the *effect* of the intervention on the outcome, but that depends on what happens in the control arm (such as lifestyle advice and extended consultations with healthcare professionals), Hawthorne effect (of being knowingly observed), placebo or nocebo effects, and so on.

[†]In some situations, it is useful to consider the sampling distribution for the variance too, and this will appear in Chapter 11.

$$\theta$$

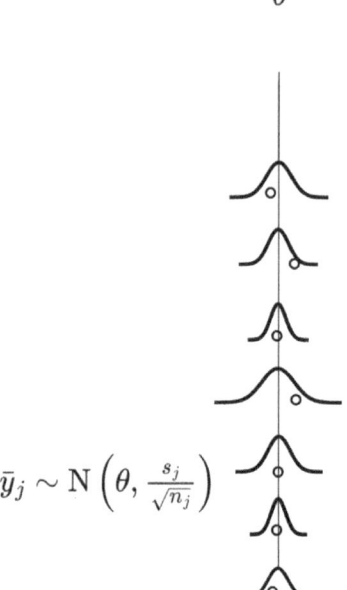

$$\bar{y}_j \sim \mathrm{N}\left(\theta, \frac{s_j}{\sqrt{n_j}}\right)$$

FIGURE 3.4

Data-generating process for a common effect meta-analysis. Observed statistics are scattered around a true and shared population value, θ, only by sampling error.

```
mu <- 0          # mean in control group
theta <- (-1)    # difference in means
sigma <- 2       # participant population SD

n_1Int <- 100
n_1Ctl <- 120

# data:
y_1Int <- rnorm(n_1Int, mu+theta, sigma)
y_1Ctl <- rnorm(n_1Ctl, mu, sigma)

# summary stats:
mean(y_1Int)
sd(y_1Int)
mean(y_1Ctl)
sd(y_1Ctl)
t.test(y_1Int, y_1Ctl)
```

On the website, we provide scripts that repeatedly do this simulation (for several studies), and then run a common effect meta-analysis on the resulting statistics. This allows you to see that this procedure works well if the assumptions are met. There, you will find equivalent code in Python and Stata.

Let's consider next the statistics that each study will provide, to complete our journey back to meta-analysis.

The observed mean in any arm ($\bar{y}_{jk}$) is drawn from a sampling distribution around the true arm-specific mean, μ_{jk}. As we have shown already, $\mu_{j\mathbf{Int}} = \mu_{j\mathbf{Ctl}} + \theta$.

$$\bar{y}_{jk} \sim \mathrm{N}\left(\mu_{jk}, \frac{\sigma}{\sqrt{n_{jk}}}\right) \quad, \forall (j, k) \tag{3.8}$$

$\hat{\theta}_j$ is the difference between the observed arm-specific means:

$$\hat{\theta}_j = \bar{y}_{j\mathbf{Int}} - \bar{y}_{j\mathbf{Ctl}} \tag{3.9}$$

Each study's estimate of the intervention effect is distributed about the true effect, θ, by a sampling distribution (Equation 3.10)*. In a randomised study, we know that the two arms' means are independent, so the variance (standard error squared) of the mean difference will be the sum of the arm means' variances (see Equation 1.14).

$$\hat{\theta}_j \sim \mathrm{N}\left(\theta, \sqrt{\frac{\sigma^2}{n_{j\mathbf{Int}}} + \frac{\sigma^2}{n_{j\mathbf{Ctl}}}}\right) \tag{3.10}$$

In practice, we must use the pooled observed standard deviation of the study, $s_{j\bullet}^2$, because we do not actually know σ. Our assumption here is that it is a perfect estimate, so there is no additional uncertainty that we are ignoring. This is not correct, but it may be close enough. The result is shown in Figure 3.4: each study has a sampling distribution for $\hat{\theta}_j$, and those have different standard deviations, but all share the same mean.

We expect that most readers will feel that this DGP approach is excessively complex for a meta-analysis, especially as we explained that non-Bayesian methods are elaborations on a weighted average. We have spelt out much more detail than you will need in order to perform a meta-analysis so that all the connections between data, parameters, and study statistics are clear at this early stage.

The DGP approach is not just a teacher's trick: it has two important benefits. In Bayesian analysis, we have to be explicit about all our assumptions, and we must not hide behind black box analyses. This helps us to question the evidence base, to be prepared to justify all our modelling choices, and to obtain approval from collaborators even when they are not statistical experts. Also, when we encounter problems in the evidence base, we have a framework ready. We can easily adapt the DGP to accommodate a wide range of problems.

3.5.2 DGP for binary outcomes

We consider a DGP for a binary outcome now, with an example of side effects from drugs for high blood pressure. We will use the evidence base from a Cochrane review [149] comparing two classes of drugs: ACE inhibitors (for example, lisinopril) and ARBs (for example, losartan). These studies do not have a control arm, so $k = \mathbf{ACEI}$ will indicate ACE inhibitors and $k = \mathbf{ARB}$ likewise for ARBs, and the odds ratio will be ACEI/ARB.

The studies had primary outcomes such as cardiovascular events, or reduction in blood pressure, and adverse events were only reported as secondary outcomes. The most common adverse events with ACE inhibitors is a dry cough, which can keep patients awake at night and seriously impact their quality of life. ACE inhibitors are cheaper, and so are often tried first.

---

*Some writers re-arrange the variance, $\frac{\sigma^2}{n_{j\mathbf{Int}}} + \frac{\sigma^2}{n_{j\mathbf{Ctl}}}$, into $\frac{(n_{j\mathbf{Int}} + n_{j\mathbf{Ctl}})\sigma^2}{n_{j\mathbf{Int}} n_{j\mathbf{Ctl}}}$, and replace σ^2 with its estimate, $s_{j\bullet}^2$.

TABLE 3.2

Study statistics from the meta-analysis of adverse events
with ACE inhibitors and ARBs[149]; log odds ratios can
be seen in the forest plot (Figure 3.5).

Study	$d_{j\mathbf{ACEI}}$	$n_{j\mathbf{ACEI}}$	$d_{j\mathbf{ARB}}$	$n_{j\mathbf{ARB}}$
de Spoelstra 2006	1	22	3	24
Lacourciere 2000	1	51	2	52
ONTARGET 2008	535	4687	465	4711
DETAIL 2004	24	102	16	100
Bremner 1997	30	167	37	334
Fogari 2012	7	103	3	102
Fogari 2011	7	130	3	132
Fogari 2008	5	124	1	122

Using the notation from Section 3.4, we can state the following basic DGP. The expit
function is the inverse logistic function, $\text{expit}(z) = 1/(1 + e^{-z})$, which converts log odds of
an event to risk (probability) of an event.

$$\text{Input parameters: } \mu, \theta$$
$$\text{Input sample sizes: } n_{jk}$$
$$\text{Data generation:}$$
$$\log \omega_{j\mathbf{ARB}} = \mu$$
$$\log \omega_{j\mathbf{ACEI}} = \mu + \theta$$
$$\pi_{jk} = \text{expit}(\log \omega_{jk})$$
$$d_{jk} \sim \text{Binom}(\pi_{jk}, n_{jk}) \qquad (3.11)$$

Study	Treatment Yes	Treatment No	Control Yes	Control No		Log odds-ratio with 95% CI	Weight (%)
deSpoelstra2006	1	21	3	21		-1.10 [-3.44, 1.24]	0.28
Lacourciere2000	1	50	2	50		-0.69 [-3.13, 1.74]	0.26
ONTARGET2008	535	4,152	465	4,246		0.16 [0.03, 0.29]	88.80
DETAIL2004	24	78	16	84		0.48 [-0.22, 1.18]	3.10
Bremner1997	30	137	37	297		0.56 [0.04, 1.09]	5.62
Fogari2012	7	96	3	99		0.88 [-0.50, 2.26]	0.80
Fogari2011	7	123	3	129		0.89 [-0.48, 2.27]	0.81
Fogari2008	5	119	1	121		1.63 [-0.54, 3.79]	0.33
Overall						0.21 [0.08, 0.33]	

Test of $\theta = 0$: z = 3.26, p = 0.00   Favours ACEI   Favours ARB

Common-effect inverse-variance model
Sorted by: _meta_es

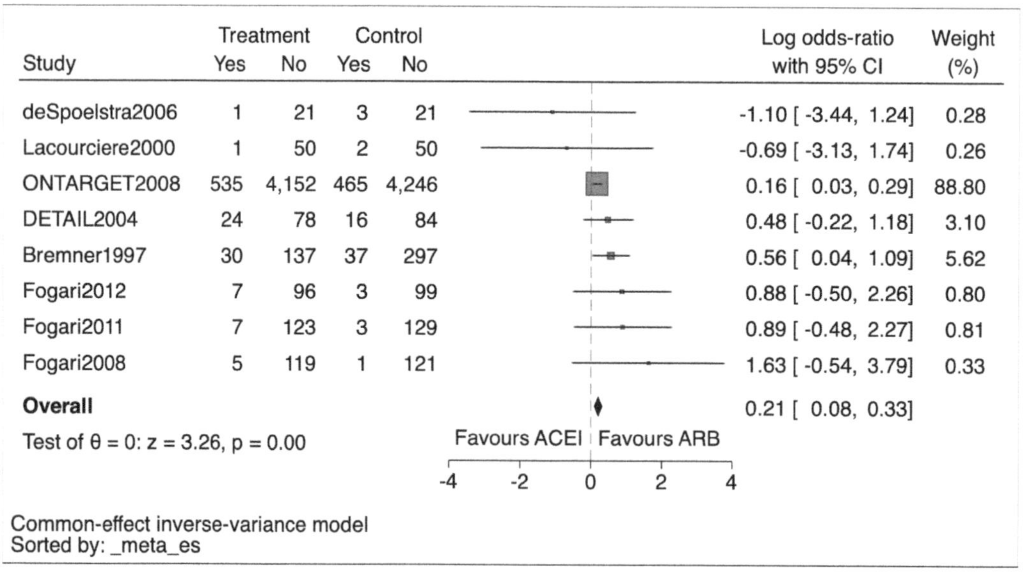

FIGURE 3.5

Non-Bayesian forest plot of common effect meta-analysis on the ACE inhibitor vs ARB
studies (produced in Stata).

You can see how the individual counts of participants with the outcome (d_{jk}) arise from the parameters in Equation 3.11, via a binomial distribution. Once d_{jk} is known, so is $n_{jk} - d_{jk}$.

We could equivalently have shown each participant's data (a 0 or a 1) arising from a Bernoulli distribution (which is just a binomial distribution with $n = 1$).

Studies probably report standard errors of the log odds ratio—or something that can be converted to them—and those would be used in a weighted average approach (as implemented in RevMan, Stata `meta`, R `meta`, and other software). However, they are not needed when taking the DGP approach to specify a likelihood. The uncertainty in the log odds ratio is determined entirely by the sample sizes, n_{jk}, and counts of participants, $n_{jk} - d_{jk}$, as seen in Equation 1.18. This is in contrast to continuous variables, where the standard deviation is an additional unknown which affects the standard error.

We can relate the log odds ratio and its standard deviation to this DGP and hence estimate the parameters using likelihood. If the studies are large enough, we could replace the exact binomial distribution with the asymptotically normal sampling distribution.

However, when studies are small, we might prefer to work directly with the counts of participants who had or did not have the outcome, to avoid the approximation error in the normal distribution. This cannot be processed through one of the weighted average meta-analysis calculations, but is amenable to maximum likelihood and Bayesian methods.

This is the R code to simulate one study's data:

```r
mu <- -2.4
# A log-odds of -2.4 is a proportion of 0.09
theta <- 0.4    # log odds ratio
n_1ACEI <- 36
n_1ARB <- 31


# arm-specific population odds and proportions:
log_omega_1ACEI <- mu + theta
log_omega_1ARB <- mu
pi_1ACEI <- 1/(1+exp(-log_omega_1ACEI)) # expit
pi_1ARB <- 1/(1+exp(-log_omega_1ARB))


# data:
d_j1 <- rbinom(1, n_1ACEI, pi_1ACEI)
d_j2 <- rbinom(1, n_1ARB, pi_1ARB)


# summary stats:
contingency_table <- as.table(rbind(c(d_1ACEI,
                                      n_1ACEI-d_1ACEI),
                                    c(d_1ARB,
                                      n_1ARB-d_1ARB)))
rownames(contingency_table) <- c("ACE Inhibitors",
                                 "ARBs")
colnames(contingency_table) <- c("Adverse event",
                                 "No event")


chisq.test(contingency_table)
```

(You should see a warning from R that, with small numbers like these, the chi-squared test is relying on an asymptotic assumption that may be unsound.)

On the website, we provide scripts that repeatedly do this simulation (for several studies), and then run a common effect meta-analysis on the resulting log odds ratios. You can experiment with the sample sizes and the scarcity of the events, to see what impact this has on the uncertainty in the meta-analysis, and the accuracy of the conclusion.

3.6   Software Implementation

Now that we have covered all the essential aspects of common effect meta-analyses, and have placed them in the framework of data-generating processes, we can proceed to the Bayesian form.

The unknown value that you are most likely interested in is θ, the population intervention effect. In the DGP for continuous outcomes in Section 3.5.1, if we assume that study standard errors are perfect estimates, then there is no other unknown. The DGP for binary outcomes in Section 3.5.2 do not require any other unknown anyway.

We start with code that will work in both BUGS and JAGS, giving a likelihood and a diffuse prior for these two DGPs. Then, in further sections, we show equivalent code for Stan, Stata bayesmh, and show how it is set up in the point-and-click interface of JASP. We encourage you to try running the code for yourself; the data files are available at the book's website. Please bear in mind, if you are running it, that Bayesian sampling algorithms are random processes and will differ slightly each time they run, unless you fix the random number generator seed (not shown here). BUGS is the exception, having a default seed preset each time it starts, unless you change it.

First, we can set up the variables we will need for most of the software options, in R, drawing on Equation 3.6:

```
ava <- read.csv("ARBvACEI.csv")

ava$ACEI_odds <- ava$ACEI_AE / (ava$ACEI_n-ava$ACEI_AE)
ava$ARB_odds <- ava$ARB_AE / (ava$ARB_n-ava$ARB_AE)

ava$logor <- log(ava$ACEI_odds / ava$ARB_odds)
ava$se <- sqrt((1 / ava$ACEI_AE) +
               (1 / (ava$ACEI_n - ava$ACEI_AE)) +
               (1 / ava$ARB_AE) +
               (1 / (ava$ARB_n - ava$ARB_AE)))

# drop one study that did not report adverse events
ava <- ava[!is.na(ava$logor),]
```

Note that we are dividing the ACE inhibitor odds by the ARB odds, so an odds ratio greater than one (equivalently, a log odds ratio greater than zero) means more chance of an adverse effect with ACE inhibitors than ARBs, which favours ARBs.

3.6.1 Prior and likelihood; BUGS / JAGS code

There is only one unknown in this model (θ). We give it a diffuse normal prior with a mean of 0 and a standard deviation of 100, which is a variance of 10,000 and a precision of 0.0001.

```
# data:
list(m = 8,
     logor = c(0.895, 0.163, 0.564, 0.48,
                1.626, 0.878, -0.693, -1.099),
     se_logor = c(0.701, 0.067, 0.267, 0.359,
                   1.103, 0.705, 1.241, 1.195))

# model:
model{
  theta ~ dnorm(0,0.0001)
  for(j in 1:m){
    prec_logor[j] <- 1/(se_logor[j]*se_logor[j])
    logor[j] ~ dnorm(theta, prec_logor[j])
  }
}

# initial values:
list(theta = -0.5)
list(theta = 0.5)
```

WinBUGS output is shown in Figure 3.6. The specifications that we entered are in the two dialog boxes at top and top left. The code is on the right. The traceplot is in the centre,

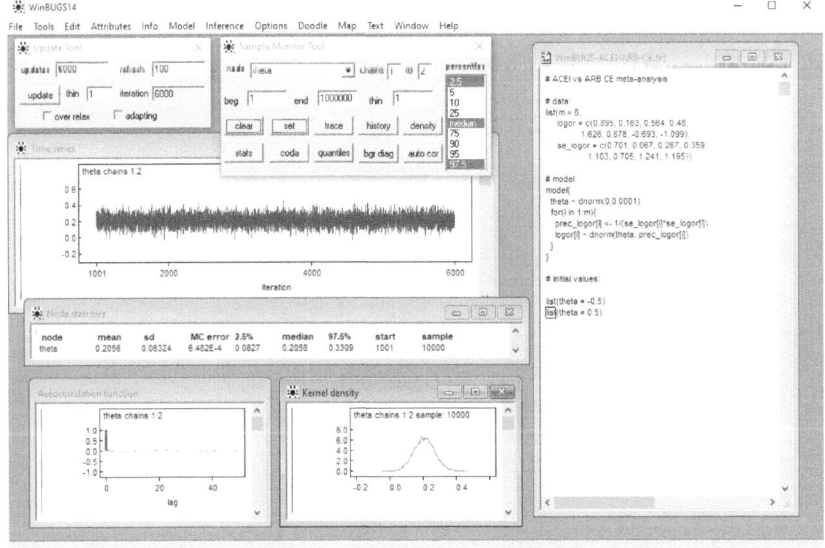

FIGURE 3.6
WinBUGS output for the common-effect meta-analysis of ACE inhibitors and ARBs.

the autocorrelation plot at bottom left, and the density plot for `theta` is bottom centre. We can see the hairy caterpillar shape indicating a healthy traceplot with convergence of chains. The autocorrelation plot shows only one spike at far left and no tail, so there is no autocorrelation. The density plot looks close to a normal distribution.

Comparing the Bayesian output with the inverse-variance weighted average in Section 3.5.2, we find negligible differences. The posterior mean (estimated population log odds ratio) is 0.2056, and the posterior standard deviation is 0.0632.

The very diffuse prior will not bias the Bayesian results relative to the weighted average results, but the fact that we are using a likelihood explicitly, rather than an approximate shortcut formula, will sometimes make a small difference later in this book, as models become more complicated (and approximations less adequate).

3.6.2   Stan code

In Stan, we specify the normal distribution in terms of the standard deviation. Here, the complete code is shown for using `cmdstanr`. The `stancode` object contains the code which can also be used in any other Stan interface.

```
stancode <- "
data {
  int m;
  array[m] real logor;
  array[m] real<lower=0> se;
}
parameters {
  real theta;
}
model {
  theta ~ normal(0, 100);
  for(j in 1:m) {
    logor[j] ~ normal(theta, se[j]);
  }
}
"

stanmod <- cmdstan_model(write_stan_file(stancode),
                         compile = TRUE)

stanfit <- stanmod$sample(data=list(m     = NROW(ava),
                                    logor = ava$logor,
                                    se    = ava$se),
                          iter_warmup=1000,
                          iter_sampling=5000,
                          chains = 2,
                          parallel_chains = 2)

stanfit$summary()

posterior_draws <- stanfit$draws()

mcmc_trace(posterior_draws, pars=c('theta'))
```

This is the output from `stanfit$summary()`, split into two parts for clarity:

```
  variable   mean median     sd    mad      q5     q95
  <chr>     <dbl>  <dbl>  <dbl>  <dbl>   <dbl>   <dbl>
1 lp__      -4.53  -4.26  0.708  0.320   -5.92   -4.03
2 theta      0.206  0.206 0.0633 0.0638  0.103   0.312

  variable   rhat ess_bulk ess_tail
  <chr>     <dbl>    <dbl>    <dbl>
1 lp__      1.00    4875.    5749.
2 theta     1.00    3830.    5166.
```

We see the same results as before, focusing on `mean` and `sd` columns, and the unknown `theta`. Recall that the `lp__` line refers to the log posterior density (plus-minus some constant), and can be ignored in this instance.

3.6.3 Stata code

In Stata (versions 16 and up), you can use `meta esize` to create variables with study estimates of intervention effect and its standard error.

```
import delimited "ARBvACEI.csv", clear

generate acei_no_ae = acei_n - acei_ae
generate arb_no_ae = arb_n - arb_ae

meta esize acei_ae acei_no_ae arb_ae arb_no_ae, ///
        studylabel(study) common(ivariance)
```

`meta esize` will create a variable `_meta_es` which contains the log odds ratios, and another `_meta_se` with the standard errors. Otherwise, if you already have those variables, `meta set` prepares the data. Then, `meta summarize` shows the results. The common effect meta-analysis for comparison is:

```
meta summarize
meta forestplot, nullrefline(lcolor(gray) ///
                            lpattern(dash) ///
                favorsleft("Favours ACEI") ///
                favorsright("Favours ARB"))
meta funnelplot
```

This is the `meta summarize` output:

```
     Effect-size label: Log odds-ratio
           Effect size: _meta_es
             Std. err.: _meta_se
           Study label: study

Meta-analysis summary                      Number of studies = 8
Common-effect model
Method: Inverse-variance

     -------------------------------------------------------------
            Study |     Log OR   [95% conf. interval]   % weight
     ---------------+-----------------------------------------------
        Fogari2011 |     0.895     -0.480      2.270       0.81
      ONTARGET2008 |     0.163      0.031      0.294      88.80
       Bremner1997 |     0.564      0.042      1.086       5.62
         DETAIL2004 |     0.480     -0.224      1.183       3.10
        Fogari2008 |     1.626     -0.536      3.788       0.33
        Fogari2012 |     0.878     -0.503      2.259       0.80
   Lacourciere2000 |    -0.693     -3.125      1.739       0.26
   deSpoelstra2006 |    -1.099     -3.441      1.244       0.28
     ---------------+-----------------------------------------------
             theta |     0.206      0.082      0.330
     -------------------------------------------------------------
Test of theta = 0: z = 3.26                  Prob > |z| = 0.0011
```

For clarity in the Bayesian version, we make a copy of the `_meta_es` variable and call it `logor`, and create a new `se2` because Stata `bayesmh` expects the variance (standard error squared):

```
gen logor = _meta_es
gen se2 = _meta_se^2
```

The `bayesmh` code anticipates a regression model. In this case, there is no predictor variable, just a constant, which Stata labels {_cons}.

```
bayesmh logor, likelihood(normal(se2)) ///
            prior({logor:_cons}, normal(0,10000)) ///
                        nchains(3)
bayesstats grubin
bayesgraph diagnostics {_cons}, title("Log OR")
```

This runs three chains with the default of 2500 burn-in iterations and 10,000 sampling iterations each. We generate the r-hat (Gelman-Rubin) statistic and obtain the usual graphics. This is the `bayesmh` output:

```
Chain 1
  Burn-in ...
  Simulation ...

Chain 2
  Burn-in ...
  Simulation ...

Chain 3
  Burn-in ...
  Simulation ...

Model summary
------------------------------------------------------------------
Likelihood:
  logor ~ normal({logor:_cons},se2)

Prior:
  {logor:_cons} ~ normal(0,10000)
------------------------------------------------------------------
Bayesian normal regression
Random-walk Metropolis-Hastings sampling

                              Number of chains    =          3
                              Per MCMC chain:
                                  Iterations      =     12,500
                                  Burn-in         =      2,500
                                  Sample size     =     10,000
                              Number of obs       =          8
                              Avg acceptance rate =      .4254
                              Avg efficiency      =      .2269
                              Max Gelman-Rubin Rc =          1

Avg log marginal-likelihood = -13.487

------------------------------------------------------------------
         |                                   Equal-tailed
  logor  |  Mean   Std. dev. MCSE   Median  [95% cred. interval]
---------+--------------------------------------------------------
  _cons  |  .2053   .0629    .0008   .2054   .0832        .3294
------------------------------------------------------------------
Note: Default initial values are used for multiple chains.
```

In Section 4.4.3, we will add options to control the number of iterations, thinning, and initial values.

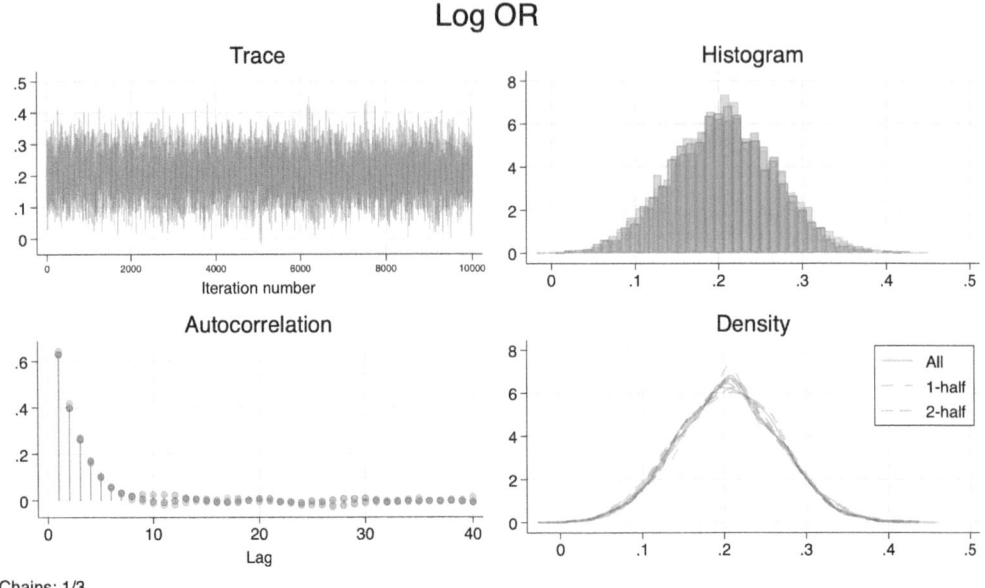

FIGURE 3.7
Graphical output from Stata `bayesgraph diagnostics`.

This is the output from the r-hat statistic:

```
Gelman-Rubin convergence diagnostic

Number of chains     =            3
MCMC size, per chain =       10,000
Max Gelman-Rubin Rc  =     1.000933


-----------------------
             |        Rc
-------------+----------
logor        |
       _cons |  1.000933
-----------------------
Convergence rule: Rc < 1.1
```

The r-hat statistic is 1.001, indicating chains that have converged and are mixing efficiently.

3.6.4   R `bayesmeta` packages

In this section, we consider the R package `bayesmeta` package, which provides higher-level, simple interfaces but in R code. `bayesmeta` can fit a Bayesian meta-analysis with normal sampling distribution (likelihood) and normal heterogeneity. Instead of sampling by

MCMC, it uses quasi-analytical posterior distributions [210], using the DIRECT algorithm [211], which avoids the burden of model checking and post-processing that accompanies general purpose MCMC. However, DIRECT can only accommodate certain preset models. bayesmeta also uses the metafor package, as it is required to calculate, for each study, the effect size and its standard error.

bayesmeta always includes a heterogeneity standard deviation, tau, which we explain in Chapter 4. However, in this setting of a common effect meta-analysis, we force tau to be very small, which is equivalent to a common effect meta-analysis, as we will show below.

We import the ARB v ACEI dataset, and create additional variables (the number of participants with no adverse events in each arm) necessary for the analysis:

```
library(metafor)
library(bayesmeta)

dataset <- read.csv("ARBvACEI.csv")

dataset$ACEI_no_AE <- dataset$ACEI_n - dataset$ACEI_AE
dataset$ARB_no_AE <- dataset$ARB_n - dataset$ARB_AE

# Define the dataset for analysis, specifying
#   effect size calculations for odds ratio.

dat <- escalc(measure="OR",
              ai=ACEI_AE,
              bi=ACEI_no_AE,
              ci=ARB_AE,
              di=ARB_no_AE,
              data=dataset,
              slab=Study)
```

We could have calculated the effect sizes and standard errors by using the standard formulas but it is easier to call the escalc() function of the metafor package. The ai input is the number of participants who experience the event in the intervention group, bi the number of participants who did not experience the event in the intervention group, ci and di the same numbers, respectively, in the control group. Alternative syntax would allow us to use n1i and n2i to consider the total number of participants in each group, if we prefer. The escalc() function will add to the dataset two new variables, yi and vi containing the effect sizes and the squared standard error respectively.

The dataset that we have prepared with the metafor package is ready for a common effect meta-analysis. We need to specify the data and the priors for the unknowns: the pooled effect size (mu) and the heterogeneity variance (tau). We define vague priors using a unit information prior for the log odds ratio with zero mean and a standard deviation of 4, corresponding to odds ratios roughly within a range from 1/2500 to 2500. We also provide a half-normal distribution for the heterogeneity variance, suggesting we expect positive values only for that parameter: as we are now considering a common effect model, tau is constrained to zero using a very small scale parameter of the dhalfnormal() function.

We also pass the study labels through the `bayesmeta()` function. Importantly, this function requires a vector of standard errors, therefore we need to apply a square-root transformation of `vi`, obtained with the metafor package:

```
metaCE <- bayesmeta(y=dat[,"yi"], sigma=sqrt(dat[,"vi"]),
                labels=dat[,"Study"],
                mu.prior.mean=0, mu.prior.sd=4,
                tau.prior=function(t){dhalfnormal(t, scale=0.0005)})
```

We can easily get the summary statistics of the main parameters, the additional "theta" column refers to the predictive distribution (for a "$(m+1)$th" estimate of an additional study). It is also possible to call a simple `print()` function to get a comprehensive summary.

```
# Generate exploratory plots and summaries to interpret the Bayesian
  meta-analysis

# heterogeneity (tau is the first column):
metaCE$summary[,1]
                tau
mode       0.000000
median     0.000337
mean       0.000399
sd         0.000301
95% lower  0.000000
95% upper  0.000980


# Exponentiate the summary to interpret effect sizes on the original scale

exp(metaCE$summary[,2:3])
                  mu     theta
mode       1.228383 1.228383
median     1.228383 1.228383
mean       1.228383 1.228383
sd         1.065217 1.065217
95% lower  1.085327 1.085327
95% upper  1.390322 1.390322
```

In bayesmeta summaries, mu is the overall, combined intervention effect. In this case, because we force the `tau` to be very small, `mu` and `theta` are identical. An estimate of I^2 can be calculated at the median value of `tau`:

```
# Calculate the I-squared statistic for evidence of heterogeneity

metaCE$I2(tau=metaCE$summary["median","tau"])
[1] 8.432043e-07
```

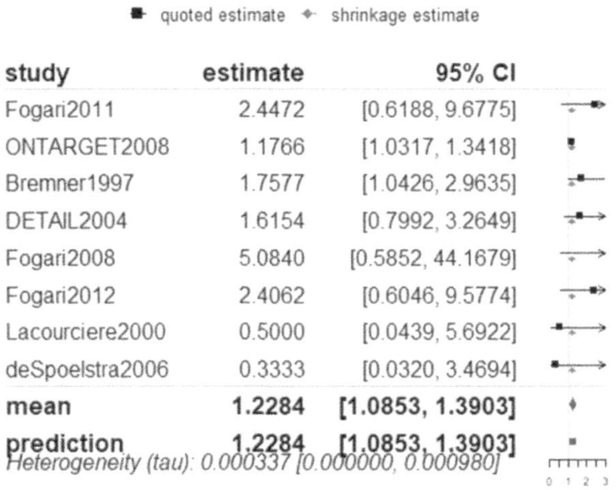

quoted estimate   shrinkage estimate

study	estimate	95% CI	
Fogari2011	2.4472	[0.6188, 9.6775]	
ONTARGET2008	1.1766	[1.0317, 1.3418]	
Bremner1997	1.7577	[1.0426, 2.9635]	
DETAIL2004	1.6154	[0.7992, 3.2649]	
Fogari2008	5.0840	[0.5852, 44.1679]	
Fogari2012	2.4062	[0.6046, 9.5774]	
Lacourciere2000	0.5000	[0.0439, 5.6922]	
deSpoelstra2006	0.3333	[0.0320, 3.4694]	
mean	**1.2284**	**[1.0853, 1.3903]**	
prediction	**1.2284**	**[1.0853, 1.3903]**	

Heterogeneity (tau): 0.000337 [0.000000, 0.000980]

0 1 2 3

FIGURE 3.8
Forest plot of Bayesian common effect meta-analysis via `bayesmeta`.

To graphically illustrate individual and pooled results, including an estimate of tau along with credible and prediction intervals, we can use the `forestplot()` function (see Figure 3.8). The forest plot includes all individual estimates `yi` with 95% intervals based on the provided standard errors, and also the intervals for each specific effect (based on the posterior of each individual study's true effect). The `tau` is practically equal to a fixed constant, 0. We can also visualize a series of accompanying graphs by calling the `plot()` function.

```
# Forest plot which include reported estimates and shrinkage ones,
#   pooled result, 95% Credible and Prediction intervals
#   It also reports the tau and its confidence interval

forestplot(metaCE, exponentiate=TRUE, zero=1, clip=c(0, 3))
plot(metaCE, prior=TRUE)
```

In Figure 3.9, the first plot (top left) is a simple forest plot with the individual point estimates of the pooled effect size with 95% credible interval, and the prediction interval for the effect size of a future study. The second plot (top right) shows the joint posterior density of the tau and effect size, with darker shading showing to higher probability density. The elliptical lines indicate 2-dimensional credible regions. Not easily visible, there are two cross symbols (+ and ×) at the far left of this plot, showing the posterior mode and the maximum likelihood estimate, almost identical (because of uninformative priors). The two other plots show the marginal posterior densities for the pooled effect and heterogeneity, with 95% credible intervals shown with a darker shading, and posterior medians indicated by the vertical lines.

The posterior density and probability can be accessed by the functions `dposterior()` and `pposterior()` respectively (the latter provides us with the cumulative distribution function). They have both a `mu=` or a `tau=` argument. For example, we can calculate the

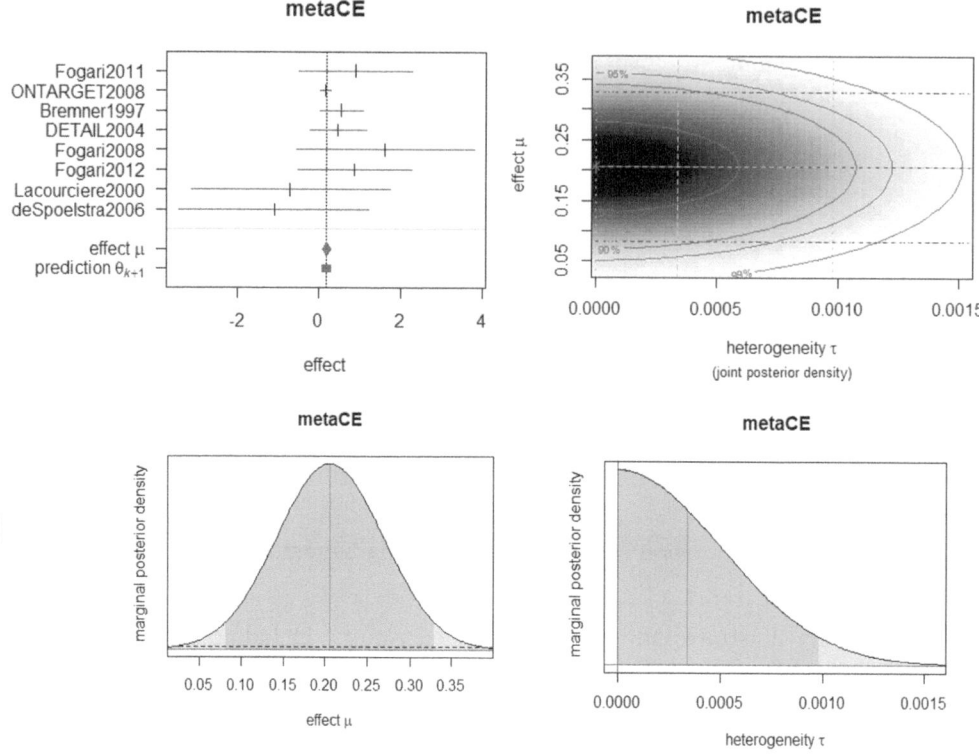

FIGURE 3.9
Exploratory plots of Bayesian common effect meta-analysis via `bayesmeta`.

posterior probability of `mu<=0` (that is, ACE inhibitors having lower risk of adverse events than ARBs) using the `pposterior()` function at `mu=0` as:

```
metaCE$pposterior(mu=0)
[1] 0.0005652734
```

3.6.5   JASP

The common effect meta-analysis is available in JASP, under the Meta-Analysis menu (which must be added from the blue + symbol of modules), at "Bayesian Meta-analysis".

Data must contain one variable with the studies' intervention effects ($\hat{\theta}_j$), and another with the standard errors ($\widehat{SE}(\hat{\theta}_j)$). Note that the JASP dialog box (Figure 3.10) refers to the intervention effect as "effect size", while in the output and the priors for the Bayesian t-test we showed in Section 2.4.7, that term is used to mean a standardised effect size, such as Cohen's d. Also, JASP uses the term "fixed effects" for what we call common effect.

We can choose priors from some preset options for the intervention effect (θ). In Figure 3.11, we use our weakly informative prior, $N(0, 3)$.

Output includes the posterior mean, standard deviation and 95% credible interval. Plots of the prior and posterior, and a basic forest plot, are available too (Figure 3.12).

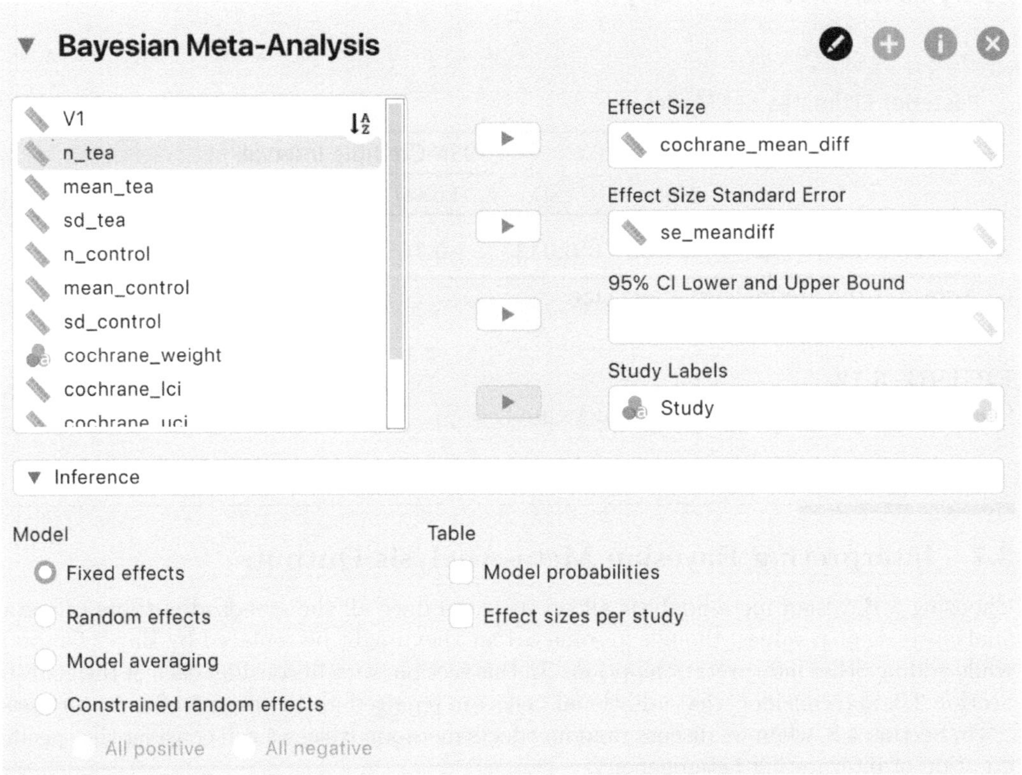

FIGURE 3.10
Input for JASP common effect meta-analysis.

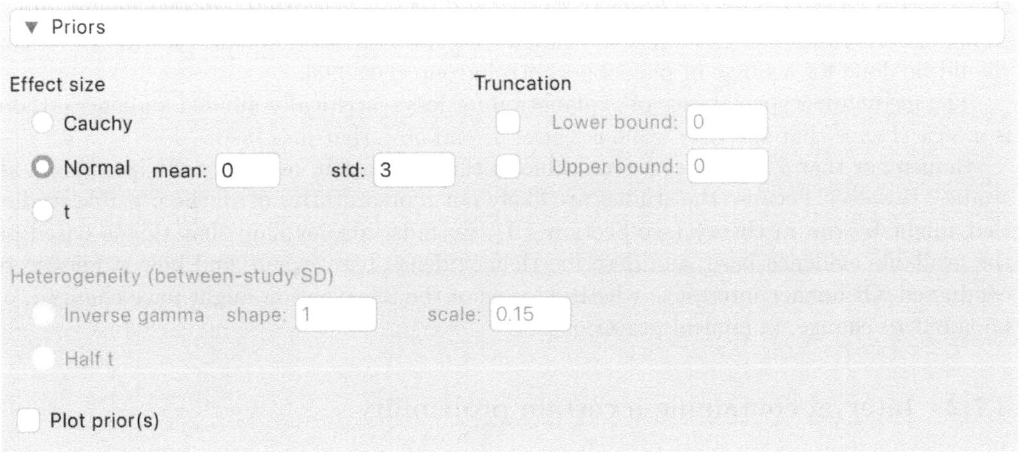

FIGURE 3.11
Prior for JASP common effect meta-analysis.

Bayesian Meta–Analysis ▾

Posterior Estimates per Model

		Mean	SD	95% Credible Interval		BF_{10}
				Lower	Upper	
Fixed effects	μ	−0.700	0.033	−0.765	−0.636	$2.719 \times 10^{+98}$

Note. μ is the group–level effect size.

FIGURE 3.12
Output from JASP common effect meta-analysis.

3.7   Interpreting Bayesian Meta-Analysis Outputs

Choosing a Bayesian meta-analysis allows us to produce all the standard outputs of meta-analysis (except p-values, though to some extent they might be replaced by Bayes factors), while adding other interpretation options. In this section, we will consider each of the goals in Section 2.3, and consider what additional tasks are required in the context of meta-analysis.

In Section 4.8, when we discuss random effects meta-analysis, we will consider the specific question of interpreting heterogeneity.

3.7.1   Centre of the posterior distribution

The mean (or median) of the posterior draws for θ, the intervention effect, is the point estimate of principal interest. Mean differences (such as in the green tea study) can be interpreted directly, as a mean reduction in BMI of θ. If it is a log odds ratio, then it is wise to convert it to the risk of the event in the control group, and in the intervention group. A common odds ratio does not imply a common risk ratio or risk difference, so the conversion should be done for a range of plausible control group risks [93].

The median has special ease of explanation for less statistically minded audiences: there is a 50% chance that the true value is above θ, and 50% that it is below.

Remember that θ estimates a true value in the population, over all participants and all studies. However, because the studies are likely not representative of all the possible studies that might be run in theory (see Section 1.1), we must also explain that this is based on the available evidence base, and describe that evidence base: where and how studies were conducted. Of further interest is whether forms of the intervention might have changed, or be about to change, in clinical practice.

3.7.2   Interval containing a certain probability

The 95% credible interval is obtained from most software, and with a little work, other credible intervals can be obtained too. This is literally an interval within which there is a 95% chance that the true θ lies.

In the absence of p-values and significance, clinical attention may focus on whether this interval crosses zero (or one, in the case of ratios). It is always a good idea to advise against reducing a complex and nuanced synthesis of studies to a binary decision[†]. A sensitivity analysis with different priors, likelihoods, or inclusion and exclusion of different papers, can help to remind the audience that evidence synthesis is not an automatic process.

3.7.3   Probability of being above or below a certain threshold

The most important threshold to use is the minimal clinical important difference. You might find that there are others that can be expressed too, such as the intervention effect of some other, well-known alternative (in the absence of head-to-head studies).

3.7.4   Ratio of posterior to prior odds (Bayes factors)

The Bayes factor can quantify whether the evidence base has shifted probability (whatever that may mean in the context, see Section 2.2.3) in favour of a particular hypothesised value of intervention effect. We could also consider whether it has favoured one hypothesised value over another. What we cannot do with Bayes factors is to falsify a null hypothesis, as a p-value might. Some argue that a Bayesian workflow can attempt this in a more holistic fashion [88], while others feel that this is too subjective a process to be satisfactory [163].

Most of the software that we have reviewed in this chapter, which allow flexible implementation of meta-analytic and other models, do not directly allow estimation of Bayes factors. JASP is a notable exception, though its modelling options are limited at present.

3.7.5   Predictive inference for a future trial

Prior and posterior predictive distributions were suggested in Chapter 2 to validate priors and likelihoods (or at least to invalidate bad ones). We can also create a posterior predictive distribution for a new study.

Such a hypothetical study will have a predicted intervention effect, $\hat{\theta}_{m+1}$, for a given sample size. Because our Bayesian sampling algorithm will be iterative, we will obtain a different $\hat{\theta}_{m+1}$ at each iteration, and their distribution will represent the uncertainty in what we would find if we conducted a new study of that sample size.

To determine the standard error, $\widehat{SE}(\hat{\theta}_{m+1})$, we can assume a particular standard error, based on an estimate of observed standard deviations from the existing evidence base. In Section 4.8, we will see how the participant-level standard deviation can alternatively be estimated as part of one combined model.

The steps that are taken are as follows:

1. take the current iteration's value of θ

2. take the assumed value of $\widehat{SE}(\hat{\theta}_{m+1})$, or simulate the participant-level standard deviation and compute it for a given sample size

3. draw the simulated new study's observed intervention effect as
   $\hat{\theta}_j \sim N(\theta, \widehat{SE}(\hat{\theta}_{m+1}))$

In the example code below, adapted from the green tea analysis, which has a point estimate of some modest weight loss, but a 95% credible interval crossing zero, we try to predict whether another study, similar to the larger ones already included, might clarify the issue with a credible interval on the side of weight loss[*]. To this end, we draw a new

---

[†]To see how this binary thinking is prevalent even in the presence of statistical uncertainty, search online for the name of any highly regarded medical journal, with the phrase `"is superior to"`. You will find plenty of papers that sound like the final word on their subject.

[*]...notwithstanding the warning we just gave about over-simplified binary interpretation ...

study from a distribution with mean θ and standard error of 0.11. This standard error arises from an assumed standard deviation of 0.8, which is typical of most of the studies in the meta-analysis, and a sample size of 100 in each arm, via the pooled variance.

```
theta ~ dnorm(0,0.0001)
for(j in 1:m){
  prec_logor[j] <- 1/(se_logor[j]*se_logor[j])
  logor[j] ~ dnorm(theta, prec_logor[j])
}
new_study_prec <- 1/(0.11 * 0.11)
new_study_logor ~ dnorm(theta, new_study_prec)
```

We can simulate multiple new studies, with various sample sizes, simultaneously, to explore the curve relating sample size to information.

This in turn allows us to re-run the predictive meta-analysis with one more study of a given size, to see what impact it might have on the conclusions. This *value of information* approach is widely used in health economics, and can help to justify funding for another study on a subject. We explore this and other economic outputs in Chapter 16.

3.7.6   Sensitivity analysis with priors

The goal of sensitivity analysis is not to choose one of the alternatives, but to describe how sensitive the results are to our modelling decisions. To help communicate this, we should present all the alternatives side by side. It is also important to see the shape of the priors, and perhaps to describe the probability they would give to unknowns lying in certain regions. This helps to make the alternatives more real and concrete to the audience.

Again, the goal is understanding sensitivity. If, for example, four out of five alternatives provide credible intervals that do not cross zero, that should not be interpreted as evidence for an effect. There should be one preferred model *a priori*, providing a "best guess", while the alternatives show us how much trust to put in it.

4

Random Effects Meta-Analysis and Heterogeneity

Learning objectives

After reading this chapter, you will be able to:

1. justify a choice of common effect or random effects models

2. interpret random effects meta-analysis as a form of hierarchical (multilevel) regression model

3. choose, and justify, prior distributions on the unknown quantities in the model

4. use Bayesian software to conduct a random effects meta-analysis

5. write Bayesian meta-analysis models that are close matches to the DerSimonian-Laird and Sidik-Jonkman methods

6. critically consider the shape of heterogeneity in the evidence base, comparing different distributions, and justify your choice in a model

7. critically investigate heterogeneity and justify your choice of modelling subgroups in the evidence base, or meta-regression

---

Each study in a meta-analysis will have collected data from a "population". The population might be people with the relevant health condition in the local hospital, or on some national register. It might not be people but instead care homes or schools, or even individual blood samples.

We saw in Chapter 3 how studies are performed in different parts of the world, at different times, and they are likely to have slightly different inclusion and exclusion criteria. This means that they are each drawing data from a somewhat different population, even before any intervention or follow-up. Then, there can be slight differences in how interventions are implemented and how outcomes are defined and measured, which can alter the intervention effect.

It is reasonable to expect such studies to arrive at somewhat different results. This inter-study variation, which is called *heterogeneity*, applies in addition to the sampling distribution.

In the early days of meta-analysis, this was a source of much concern: that we should not inform clinical decisions by averaging studies when we are not comparing like with like. "Comparing apples and oranges", people often say. The controversial psychologist Hans Eysenck was an early sceptic of meta-analysis, and called such combinations of studies not meta-analysis but "mega-silliness"[70].

Although we think he was wrong to condemn the majority of meta-analyses, based on early experiences in the questionably reproducible field of personality and intelligence scales,

DOI: 10.1201/9781003375821-4

we do think that he highlighted several problems that continue to trouble meta-analysts [71]. Bayesian approaches offer a solution to most of these.

In everyday practice, we have to consider the size of the heterogeneity, compared to the sampling distributions. We cannot simply refuse to meta-analyse any evidence base that exhibits even a small degree of heterogeneity, or we will be failing to help our audience. On the other hand, we cannot put a mismatched collection of statistics into one melting pot and expect it to be helpful.

We also have to think about what might be causing studies to arrive at heterogeneous results. If we can understand that, we should describe it, and if we can go further and quantify it, then we should at least consider whether we can adjust for it. This is the focus of later chapters, but for now, we will simply set out how we can assess the size and shape of heterogeneity and thus arrive at an estimate of the underlying effect and its uncertainty.

There are two approaches in widespread use to this question of how comparable the studies are, and a third that is much rarer. We will now show how they are defined and what the impact is on the meta-analysis.

1. *Common effect* meta-analysis works on the basis that all studies have drawn participants at random from the same shared population. The objective is to estimate the intervention effect (or other relevant statistic) in that population. This was covered in detail in Chapter 3.

2. *Random effects* meta-analysis assumes that the studies are themselves drawn from a population of possible studies, and then their participants' data are in turn drawn from a study-specific population. The random effects meta-analysis allows for heterogeneity, including it as a prior distribution of the study-specific intervention effects.

3. *Fixed effects* meta-analysis is rarer, and allows for differences between studies, but estimates a intervention effect in each study's population. The overall intervention effect from the meta-analysis is then a weighted average of these, without any claim to represent a population of potential studies.

Unfortunately, many researchers that we have met have some misunderstandings about what these different approaches entail. Often, it is said—incorrectly—that a common effect meta-analysis is appropriate when there is little or no heterogeneity, and a random effects should be used instead when heterogeneity is present. Worse yet, you might encounter the suggestion that the type of meta-analysis is chosen on the basis of some measure of heterogeneity. A clear description of these options, along with debunking other myths, is given by Borenstein [23].

You might feel that the notion of study designs and populations being drawn at random from a distribution of possible studies is far-fetched. We sympathise with this intuition, but experience has shown us that anything worth doing in statistics probably needs to be done because the answer is far from obvious. This means that we must make assumptions and simplifications—a model—that are not entirely realistic but are close enough to give us useful insights. Stangl and Berry expand on this point ([243], p.6).

The names given to these options are also not consistently used. You may see common effect described as "fixed effect (singular)" or as "equal effect".

In a Bayesian context, some of these distinctions become irrelevant, because of the flexible way in which we use probability. In particular, fixed effects and random effects models will lead to different results, but the choice between them is a philosophical one. In practical terms, a Bayesian fixed effects model is simply a Bayesian random effects model with a flat (or wide and uniform) heterogeneity prior distribution. For this reason, we do not consider fixed effects as a distinct class of meta-analysis in this book.

4.1 Heterogeneity in the Data-Generating Process

Meta-analysis often combines different studies, done in slightly different ways, in different places and times. Naturally, this causes some differences in the statistics that they report. Sometimes, we can understand the reason for such a difference, but sometimes we can't, and the best we can do is to model it statistically. It is called *heterogeneity*, from Greek meaning "coming from different sources".

In the previous section, we presented common-effect meta-analyses, which assume that all the variance between studies can be attributed to sampling.

The alternative, called *random effects models*, include heterogeneity as an additional variance, which has scattered the studies' populations' intervention effects (θ_j) around an underlying* intervention effect (θ), and then each study has sampled from their own populations to obtain their reported statistics ($\hat{\theta}_j$).

This means that the observed variance has two components: the sampling within each study (which the reported standard errors estimate), and the differences between the studies (which we meta-analysts must estimate).

$$\theta_j \sim N(\theta, \tau) \quad , \forall j$$
$$\hat{\theta}_j \sim N(\theta_j, \widehat{SE}(\hat{\theta}_j)) \quad , \forall j \tag{4.1}$$

There are a few aspects that you should pause to consider:

1. In every study ($\forall j$), participants were drawn from a population where the mean intervention effect is θ_j.

2. The study-specific (or local) populations' mean intervention effects are scattered around an underlying (or global) intervention effect, θ. We assume a normal distribution for this with standard deviation τ. This is the heterogeneity distribution.

3. Equivalently, we could instead represent heterogeneity as adding or subtracting some value u_j from the underlying intervention effect θ. This replaces θ_j with $\theta + u_j$, and then $u_j \sim N(0, \tau)$. Because the u_js are centred on 0, some are positive and others negative: some study populations have higher mean intervention effects than the underlying θ, other are lower.

4. This heterogeneity is treated as a purely random process. In other words, we are acting as though we understand nothing about why the studies differ.

5. The individual studies' estimates of their populations' mean intervention effects, $\hat{\theta}_j$, are in turn drawn from the sampling distribution around their respective θ_js.

6. The mean has a normal sampling distribution, as long as the samples are not too small and the data not too far from normality.

7. The standard error of the mean intervention effect is itself an estimate—hence the large hat on $\widehat{SE}(\hat{\theta}_j)$—though in the first models that follow, we ignore this.

Heterogeneity adds an inter-study variance, $\tau^2 = V(\theta_j)$ to the intra-study variance (standard error squared) of the sampling distribution, $\widehat{SE}(\hat{\theta}_j)^2 = \hat{V}(\hat{\theta}_j)$. Because the two are uncorrelated, the total variance is just the sum of the two component variances (see Equation 1.15). In fact, this is not a practical formula because there are multiple values of

---

*Names for this are all tricky. Sometimes people say "global" effect, but that implies validity for all people everywhere.

$\widehat{SE}(\hat{\theta}_j)$, one for each study. In the next section, we will show how this concept translates to a statistical model that leads to estimates and inference.

The challenge here is that differences between studies manifest as a sum of two variances: if we observe some estimate of the total variance, and wish to partition this, but know neither of the components, then we cannot proceed.

The DerSimonian-Laird method [53] tackles this in the simplest way, by providing a formula to estimate τ^2, which assumes that the standard errors reported by the studies are correct. (That is to say, $\widehat{SE}(\hat{\theta}_j) = SE(\hat{\theta}_j), \forall j$.) Other methods have been proposed too[24, 220], which take different approaches to including the uncertainty in the standard errors. We will create Bayesian models in this chapter that mirror the principles of the DerSimonian-Laird and another method, the Sidik-Jonkman.

If τ^2 is large, then a more complex model that accounts for heterogeneity is required. This typically means a random effects meta-analysis. Various measures have been proposed to assess the size of τ^2 relative to the total variance. The most common are a chi-squared statistic called Cochran's Q, with accompanying hypothesis test, and Higgins' I^2, which estimates the percentage of total variance arising from heterogeneity.

A common misunderstanding is that one should fit either common effect or random effects, depending on which fits the data best. In fact, the decision should be based on information outside the statistics, about the study populations, interventions, controls and outcomes, and other aspects of study design. Some people contend that heterogeneity should always be included, as studies are not (usually) intended as direct replications of one another, and always have some differences.

You should also be wary of over-optimism about what can be learnt from heterogeneity. Popular ideas such as "personalised medicine", in the Bayesian context, draw on the idea that we can make inferences about individual narrow zones of the posterior distribution pertaining to particular patients. The combined intervention effect θ is informed by all studies in your evidence base, but to make inferences in the tails of the heterogeneity distribution will draw on perhaps only one study, and also have relatively few posterior draws to inform it [28].

4.1.1   DGP for continuous outcomes

We will now amend the data-generating process (DGP) for continuous outcomes, seen for common effects meta-analysis in Section 3.5.1. We will consider only the difference between arms, the mean difference, and in Chapter 8, we look into the possibility of extending this to the individual arms.

As before, participants (i) are randomly drawn from normally distributed populations, but now, the studies (j) do not all draw from the same population. We simplify this by assuming that the studies are themselves drawn from a distribution (of potential studies that might be done). Further, we assume that studies draw from populations with different means, but all have one common population standard deviation, σ. There are only two arms: the intervention ($k = \mathbf{Int}$) and the control ($k = \mathbf{Ctl}$).

$$\text{Input parameters: } \mu, \theta, \sigma, \tau \tag{4.2}$$
$$\text{Data generation:}$$
$$\theta_j \sim \mathrm{N}(\theta, \tau) \tag{4.3}$$
$$\mu_{j\mathbf{Ctl}} = \mu \tag{4.4}$$
$$\mu_{j\mathbf{Int}} = \mu + \theta_j \tag{4.5}$$
$$y_{ijk} \sim \mathrm{N}(\mu_{jk}, \sigma) \quad , \forall (i, j, k) \tag{4.6}$$

Taking each line in turn, we can relate them to what we have already covered so far.

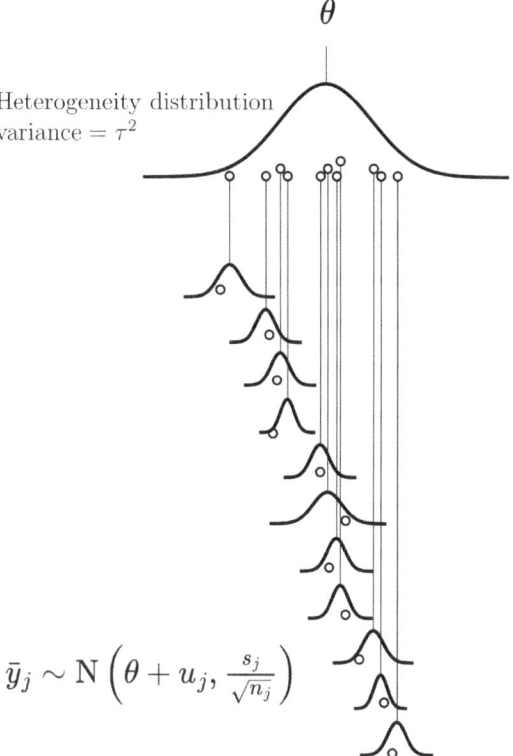

Heterogeneity distribution
variance $= \tau^2$

$$\bar{y}_j \sim \mathrm{N}\left(\theta + u_j, \frac{s_j}{\sqrt{n_j}}\right)$$

FIGURE 4.1

A continuous outcome data-generating process with heterogeneity. Each study has an observed mean drawn from the relevant normal distribution on the left. We assume the standard errors are perfectly known.

Equation 4.2: there are four parameters, whose values are not known to us, but we will estimate them and the uncertainty around our estimates: the mean outcome in control groups, which we assume is shared by all studies (μ), the population difference between intervention and control arms (θ), the common population standard deviation (σ), and the inter-study standard deviation of heterogeneity (τ).

Equation 4.3: each study has its own population (we will call it *study-specific*) intervention effect, θ_j. This can also be written as:

$$u_j \sim \mathrm{N}(0, \tau)$$
$$\theta_j = \theta + u_j$$
$$\therefore \theta_j \sim \mathrm{N}(\theta, \tau)$$
$$\theta_j = \mu_{j\mathrm{Int}} - \mu_{j\mathrm{Ctl}}$$

This is the difference between the arm-specific means ($\mu_{j\mathrm{Int}}$ and $\mu_{j\mathrm{Ctl}}$). As a linear combination of two normally distributed variables, we can use Equation 1.15 to find its distribution. Here, the heterogeneity distribution is derived; can you see why its standard deviation, τ, is the same as the standard deviation of the u_js?

Note that the heterogeneity models the scatter of studies' θ_js, not the μ_{jk}s; that is to say, heterogeneity affects the intervention effect (difference between arm means), not the arm means themselves.

Equation 4.4: the study populations for all control arms ($k = 2$) have means equal to μ.

Equation 4.5: the study populations in the green tea arms ($k = 1$) have means equal to $\mu + \theta_j$, so each study will differ somewhat.

Equation 4.6: the individual data in each study and arm come from a normally distributed population with the relevant arm-specific mean and common standard deviation σ.

Now, we can easily simulate data from this, if we input the four parameters, along with n_{j1} and n_{j2}. For example, simulating one study in R:

```
mu <- 0
theta <- (-1)
sigma <- 2
tau <- 0.5

n_1Int <- 100
n_1Ctl <- 120

# heterogeneity:
theta_1 <- rnorm(1, theta, tau)

# arm-specific population means:
mu_1Int <- mu + theta_1
mu_1Ctl <- mu

# data:
y_1Int <- rnorm(n_1Int, mu_1Int, sigma)
y_1Ctl <- rnorm(n_1Ctl, mu_1Ctl, sigma)

# summary stats:
mean(y_1Int)
sd(y_1Int)
mean(y_1Ctl)
sd(y_1Ctl)
t.test(y_1Int, y_1Ctl)
```

 On the website, we provide scripts that repeatedly do this simulation (for several studies), and then run a DerSimonian-Laird meta-analysis on the resulting statistics. This allows you to see that DerSimonian-Laird works well if the assumptions are met.

Let's consider next the statistics that each study will provide, to complete our journey back to meta-analysis. Equations 4.7 to 4.10 present the same ideas of sampling that we have already covered.

The observed mean in any arm is drawn from a sampling distribution around the true arm-specific mean:

$$\bar{y}_{jk} \sim \mathrm{N}\left(\mu_{jk}, \frac{\sigma}{\sqrt{n_{jk}}}\right) \quad, \forall(j, k) \tag{4.7}$$

The variances of each arm's mean can be added together because, as a randomised study, they are uncorrelated. Each study's estimate of the intervention effect is the difference between the observed arm-specific means:

$$\hat{\theta}_j = \bar{y}_{j1} - \bar{y}_{j2} \tag{4.8}$$

Each study's estimate of the intervention effect is distributed about the study-specific mean intervention effect θ_j by a sampling distribution:

$$\hat{\theta}_j \sim N\left(\theta_j, \sqrt{\frac{\sigma^2}{n_{j1}} + \frac{\sigma^2}{n_{j2}}}\right) \tag{4.9}$$

This is not very useful, because we have no idea what the values of θ_j are, so in Equation 4.10, we link this back further to θ, combining the heterogeneity and sampling distributions (because they too are uncorrelated):

$$\therefore \hat{\theta}_j \sim N\left(\theta, \sqrt{\frac{\sigma^2}{n_{j1}} + \frac{\sigma^2}{n_{j2}} + \tau^2}\right)$$
$$\hat{\theta}_j \sim N\left(\theta, \widehat{SE}(\hat{\theta}_j)\right) \tag{4.10}$$

We can write Equation 4.10 in a different way, by introducing u_j, which can be positive or negative with mean 0:

$$u_j \sim N(0, \tau)$$
$$\hat{\theta}_j \sim N(\theta + u_j, \widehat{SE}(\hat{\theta}_j)) \tag{4.11}$$

In BUGS, it will look something like this:

```
u[j] ~ dnorm(0, tau_precision)
theta[j] <- theta + u[j]
theta_hat[j] ~ dnorm(theta[j], se_precision[j])
```

We can easily simulate some study statistics that will look like these, and play with some different values of τ, to get a closer understanding of the model. On the website, we provide code where you supply τ and obtain a forest plot representing simulated study results. This will help you to acquire an instinctive recognition of what different levels of heterogeneity look like, and when the various statistics might be misleading.

This brings us full circle to Equation 4.1. We have started from the data-generating process for individual participant data and seen how this leads to the heterogeneity variance and the sampling error. This two-level scattering is captured in a random effects meta-analysis. It is also an example of what statisticians call a *hierarchical* or *multilevel model*. Hierarchical models are very widely used, for example in cluster-randomised clinical trials, or data from electronic health records, where patients attend one of a range of local health care providers, and we would expect the patients at one location to be somehow different to those at another location.

Now, consider the likelihood methods in Section 2.1, and how they could be applied here—just at an informal level of detail. If we have been given $\hat{\theta}_j$ and $s_{j\bullet}$ or something else that allows you to calculate $\widehat{SE}(\hat{\theta}_j)$, can you apply the equations above to evaluate the likelihood for various values of θ and σ? How might you also estimate τ? Do you need μ for this?

You might feel that this DGP approach is excessively complex for a meta-analysis, especially as we explained that non-Bayesian methods are elaborations on a weighted average. We have spelt out much more detail than you will need in order to perform a meta-analysis so that all the connections between participant data, population parameters and study statistics are clear at this early stage.

The DGP approach has two important benefits. We have to be explicit about all our assumptions, and can no longer hide behind black box analyses. This helps us to question the evidence base and to be prepared to justify all our modelling choices. Also, when we move to Bayesian analyses, we have the framework ready. We can easily adapt the DGP, for example, to allow for non-normal heterogeneity.

4.2   Bayesian Models and Priors

Like we did for common effect meta-analysis in Section 3.6, we will now show the corresponding models, and later the code, to implement a simple random effects meta-analysis. We will use a variety of priors here and in the code that follows, to illustrate options; they are not recommended in general.

4.2.1   Priors

To fit a Bayesian meta-analysis to our data, we need to supply prior distributions for the unknown parameters of the model: $f(\theta)$, $f(\tau)$, $f(u_j)$ in the case of the model in Equation 4.11. Noting the various approaches to prior distributions in Chapter 2, we will use weakly informative priors in this section, to focus attention on the construction of the model.

In experimental studies, it is typical to appeal to equipoise when designing the recruitment and seeking ethical approval. On this basis, a meta-analysis of these experimental studies (such as randomised controlled trials (RCTs)), with weakly informative or diffuse $f(\theta)$, can reasonably use priors with a median of 0: there is equal probability of the intervention effect being on either side.

We have been dealing with mean differences so far, and these can take both negative and positive values, so $f(\theta)$ should be defined for all real numbers from $\theta = -\infty$ to $\theta = +\infty$.

The normal distribution is the usual starting point. t and Cauchy distributions allow higher probability of being further from the mean—and in so doing, allow the computer to get into potentially troublesome territory, where posterior densities are extremely low and it takes a very long time to return to the high density region.

Remember that there is no safe "default" prior that can be applied to all instances of a certain statistic. Prior predictive checking, as described in Chapter 2, will help you detect mis-matches between your priors and your evidence base.

As with any standard deviation, τ can only take positive values, so its priors should do so too. It has been common practice for many years to use inverse-gamma distributions for variances (see Section 2.2.3.2), though this has been criticised in recent years in favour of normal, Cauchy or t-distributions, truncated to only the part above zero[85]. These are often called "half-normal", "half-Cauchy", and so on. We will write them like this: $\tau \sim \mathrm{N}^+(0, 2)$. Examples appear in the software-specific sections below. Several alternatives have been suggested in the past[247].

Some people use uniform priors for standard deviations or precisions, as there is usually no prior information or opinion to shape them other than ruling out completely unbelievable values. However, there is a risk in providing a flat region in the priors or likelihood for some sampling algorithms, and until you are a confident Bayesian modeller, we recommend something like a half-normal so that there is always a gradient[†] to guide the sampling algorithm back from extreme values.

The prior for each of the u_j parameters is the same, and is the heterogeneity distribution. If you make this normal, with standard deviation τ, then that is the prior: $u_j \sim N(0, \tau)$.

Note that u_j has a prior, the standard deviation of which (τ) has its own prior! Some people use the term "hyperprior" in this setting, but we prefer not to single it out as acting in any different way to other probabilistic statements in our model (also to avoid the need for hyperhyperpriors further down the line). It simply reflects the probability of finding different values of τ. It also functions to pool information (people often say "borrow information") across all the studies, because they all tell us something about τ.

4.2.2 Empirical priors to update a previous meta-analysis

The main unknown that you will seek to estimate is likely something that serves as an intervention effect between two arms. For this, whether it is a mean difference, a log odds ratio, or log rate ratio, the prior and posterior are going to be approximately normal. Take the green tea meta-analysis as an example ("Analysis 1.4", p.61 [136]). They reported a mean difference of -0.47 units of body mass index (kg/m^2), favouring green tea, and a 95% confidence interval from -0.77 to -0.17. Bearing in mind that the normal 95% confidence interval extends 1.96 standard errors on either side of the mean, that implies that the standard error was $0.3/1.96 = 0.15$. So we can set a prior as $N(-0.47, 0.15)$, and update it with just the latest studies.

There are some complications to this though. Firstly, our model should be comparable to the one that we are adopting from the previous meta-analysis. If we include heterogeneity, so should they. Inclusion / exclusion criteria should be the same for studies too, and if there is a marked change in the population or study designs and conduct between the old and new studies, then we should not take the old results as a prior for the new.

Secondly, there are other unknowns, notably the heterogeneity standard deviation. We should choose whether to impose a prior on those that is also based on previous results [264], or some kind of diffuse or weakly informative prior. If the posterior is correlated between our intervention effect and some of those other unknowns, then we will perhaps bias our results somewhat by having a more diffuse prior on the other unknown, and allowing it to accommodate less likely values.

This problematic correlation should not occur for simple meta-analyses, but there is no guarantee of that for more complicated models, such as we will construct in Part 3 of this book. In those models, a better idea would be to adopt the study statistics from the old evidence base and include them in your meta-analysis, effectively analysing all the data together from scratch. Unfortunately, as we will see, this can extend well beyond the usual d_{jk} and n_{jk}, or n_{jk}, $\bar{y}_{jk}$, and s_{jk}, and so it could be a lot of work to extract the additional statistics needed for a complicated model.

In summary, although these empirical priors using previous results sound like a good idea, mainly as a labour-saving device, they are not always easy to apply in a way that we can be comfortable will not inadvertently distort the analysis.

[†]...in theory at least; digital rounding error means that there may be *de facto* flat regions of parameter space when the proposed parameter values have either a very small prior density or very low likelihood. Sensible initial values will help us avoid them.

4.2.3   Deciding on a heterogeneity distribution

Software packages for non-Bayesian meta-analyses, such as RevMan or Stata, have to date only included normal distributions for the heterogeneity. This has some justification, because multiple competing (and unrelated) influences, some pushing a study's results up, and others down, will eventually combine to make a normal distribution, thanks to the central limit theorem.

However, there are many settings where we can imagine a definitively non-normal heterogeneity. It is well known that there are a number of genetic factors which influence endocrine and metabolic function and vary markedly in prevalence around the world. Suppose that one of these increased the effect seen from green tea extracts. A large number of studies, conducted in many parts of the world, would lead to a distinctly skewed or even bimodal (two peaks) distribution of study-specific population intervention effects.

In Bayesian meta-analysis, if we do not want to use a normal distribution for the heterogeneity, we can easily specify some other distribution. We can also try alternative heterogeneity distributions and compare them using information criteria, posterior predictive checks or leave-one-out cross-validation, to see which most closely describes the study statistics, as described in Chapter 2.

Any meta-analysis should justify the choice of heterogeneity distribution. This should be in terms of the observed distribution of study results (bearing in mind that many meta-analyses are based on relatively small numbers of studies, and so the distribution cannot be confidently known from them), and from the plausible explanations of factors influencing individual studies to be unlike the others. When the number of studies is very small, even just two or three, the heterogeneity distribution will act as an influential prior, whether it is intended to be "informative" or not [79]. Therefore, the choice is critical and must be approved by the wider project team. Sensitivity analysis, using alternative priors, is also important to give credence to the findings.

A close reading of the full-text papers sometimes provides clues about what factors might have contributed to inter-study variation, and therefore what distribution it might take . . . but then, sometimes it does not.

4.2.4   Elaborations

A final important consideration about this model is that it might serve as a starting point to set up a more realistic version, slightly more complex, that acknowledges all uncertainties (which, after all, is a major rationale for using Bayesian statistics). We noted above that it is close to the DerSimonian-Laird random effects meta-analysis, and in the original paper from 1986, its inventors wrote:

> In all our work we assume that the sampling variances are known, although in reality we estimate them from the data. Further research needs to be done in this area as there are alternative estimators that might be preferable to the ones we use.[53]

Their work was groundbreaking and far-reaching in its impact, but was always intended as a springboard to more subtle analyses. Some of the extensions in this chapter, such as accommodating outliers or considering a non-normal heterogeneity, should be considered in any random effects meta-analysis. Others, which we explore in Part 3 of this book, are tailored to particular problems.

4.3   Binary Outcomes and Counts

The thought process we went through above can be applied to any other statistics that you want to meta-analyse. First, how are the reported statistics going to be scattered around the study-specific effects (this gives a formula for the likelihood)? If we have odds ratios, for example, their logarithms will be approximately normally scattered around the study-specific log-odds-ratios: that is the sampling distribution and its standard deviation (standard error) can be calculated with Equation 1.18.

Next, the heterogeneity: perhaps the study-specific log-odds-ratios will be normally distributed around the underlying log-odds-ratio. It is a good idea to convert all reported statistics into a measure that will be most amenable to your meta-analysis, proceed as before, and then convert your findings back again when you are finished.

4.3.1 Binary outcomes

This DGP for log odds ratios ($\log \omega_{jk}$), with two levels of normal distributions, is comparable to DerSimonian-Laird:

$$
\begin{aligned}
&\text{Input parameters: } \mu_0, \theta, \tau \\
&\text{Input sample sizes: } n_{jk} \\
&\text{Data generation:} \\
&\qquad u_j \sim \mathrm{N}(0, \tau) \\
&\qquad \theta_j = \theta + u_j \\
&\qquad \therefore \theta_j \sim \mathrm{N}(\theta, \tau) \\
&\qquad \log \omega_{j\mathbf{Int}} = \mu_0 + \theta_j \\
&\qquad \log \omega_{j\mathbf{Ctl}} = \mu_0 \quad , \forall j \\
&\qquad \pi_{jk} = \mathrm{expit}(\log \omega_{jk}) \quad , \forall(j,k) \\
&\qquad d_{jk} \sim \mathrm{Binom}(\pi_{jk}, n_{jk}) \quad , \forall(j,k)
\end{aligned}
\tag{4.12}
$$

The final line produces the number of "events" that are observed in each arm of each study, d_{jk}. Although this has a binomial distribution, we do not have to work with the arm-based statistics, but rather with the intervention effect, $\log \omega_{jk}$.

The model can be succinctly stated in probability terms with priors and likelihoods, for example:

$$
\begin{aligned}
&\theta \sim \mathrm{N}(0, 2) \\
&\tau \sim \mathrm{N}^+(0, 2) \\
&u_j \sim \mathrm{N}(0, \tau) \\
&\hat{\theta}_j \sim \mathrm{N}(\theta_j, \widehat{\mathrm{SE}}(\hat{\theta}_j))
\end{aligned}
\tag{4.13}
$$

Once our random effects meta-analysis has inferred the rather obscure log odds ratio, we ought to convert it into statistics that can be more easily understood by our audience [214]. We exponentiate each posterior draw of $\log \omega_{jk}$ to get ω_{jk}, the odds ratio.

Another transformation that can be useful for communication purposes is to combine ω_{jk} with a selection of putative baseline risks in various patient groups, to derive a selection of risk ratios [93].

4.3.2 Counts of events

When studies report counts of events in a time period, or rates, then the intervention effect (contrast between arms) is usually in terms of a rate ratio. Like the odds ratio, this is a positive real number, and if we transform it by logarithms, we can use normal distributions to model it, just as above, replacing the log odds ratio with the log rate ratio.

The DGP is only different in some of the symbols that are traditionally used, and in the final line:

$$\text{Input parameters: } \mu_0, \theta, \tau$$
$$\text{Input participant time at risk: } T_{jk}$$
$$\text{Data generation:}$$
$$u_j \sim \mathrm{N}(0, \tau)$$
$$\theta_j = \theta + u_j \qquad\qquad (4.14)$$
$$\therefore \theta_j \sim \mathrm{N}(\theta, \tau)$$
$$\log \gamma_{j1} = \mu_0 + \theta_j$$
$$\log \gamma_{j2} = \mu_0 \quad , \forall (j, k)$$
$$d_{jk} \sim \mathrm{Poisson}(\gamma_{jk} T_{jk})$$

4.3.3   Survival or time-to-event data

Clinical trials very often report hazard ratios, arising from following participants until an event of interest happens, or the patient leaves the study, or is otherwise no longer eligible, or the study ends.

The log hazard ratio is, like the log odds ratio, approximately normal in its sampling distribution, and so can in the simplest case, be passed through the same DGP and model as log rate ratios, replacing one ratio for another.

Other approaches to time-to-event data, which are much more complicated, are discussed in Chapter 17.

4.4   Software Implementation

We will work with the green tea dataset in this section. To begin, we process the data file to obtain the derived variables that most of our software options will need:

```
greentea<-read.csv('data/cochrane_green_tea_weight_loss.csv')

greentea$md <- greentea$mean_tea-greentea$mean_control
greentea$pooled_var <- (((greentea$n_tea-1)*
                       (greentea$sd_tea^2))+
                       ((greentea$n_control-1)*
                       (greentea$sd_control^2))) /
                       (greentea$n_tea+greentea$n_control-2)
greentea$var_md <- (greentea$n_tea+greentea$n_control) *
                   greentea$pooled_var /
                   (greentea$n_tea*greentea$n_control)
greentea$se_md <- sqrt(greentea$var_md)
```

The various software implementations that follow have some differences in whether standard deviations, precisions or variances can be supplied. It is easier to assess (and elicit) priors on the standard deviation, and on this basis we select $\tau \sim \mathrm{t}^+(0, 1, 1)$ for the heterogeneity

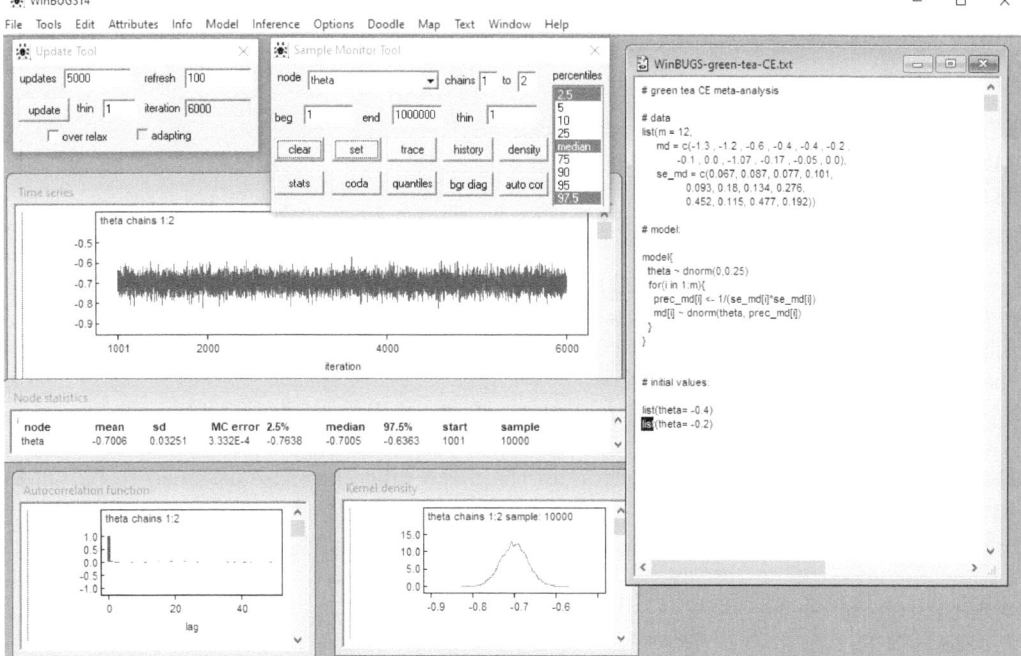

FIGURE 4.2
WinBUGS output for a (inappropriate) common-effect meta-analysis on the green tea data.

standard deviation. In terms of precision, this is quite close to $1/\tau^2 \sim \text{Gamma}(1, 0.8)$. However, we will vary, to show different priors, and sometimes because we are forced to do so by software constraints.

4.4.1 BUGS / JAGS

Figure 4.2 shows the result of applying a common effect meta-analysis to the green tea studies, which we calculated by hand in Section 3.2, but now using WinBUGS. The code is:

```
# data:
list(m = 12,
     md = c(-1.3 , -1.2 , -0.6 , -0.4 , -0.4 , -0.2 ,
            -0.1 , 0.0 , -1.07 , -0.17 , -0.05 , 0.0),
     se_md = c(0.067, 0.087, 0.077, 0.101,
               0.093, 0.18, 0.134, 0.276,
               0.452, 0.115, 0.477, 0.192))

# model:
model{
  mu ~ dnorm(0,0.5)
  for(j in 1:m){
    prec_md[j] <- 1/(se_md[j]*se_md[j])
```

```
    md[j] ~ dnorm(mu, prec_md[j])
  }
}

# initial values:
list(mu= -0.4)
list(mu= -0.2)
```

The posterior mean is -0.7006 kg.m^{-2}, with posterior standard deviation of 0.0325 kg.m^{-2}. This closely matches the previous hand calculations, because our priors are relatively uninformative. The result is an overestimate of the intervention effect, because the heterogeneity has been ignored.

The following code extends it to a random effects meta-analysis by adding a heterogeneity distribution with a standard deviation of τ, which is given a N$^+(0, 1)$ prior. Similarly to DerSimonian-Laird, the standard errors of the mean differences are assumed to be known without any uncertainty.

```
# data
list(m = 12,
     md = c(-1.3 , -1.2 , -0.6 , -0.4 , -0.4 , -0.2 ,
            -0.1 , 0.0 , -1.07 , -0.17 , -0.05 , 0.0),
     se_md = c(0.067, 0.087, 0.077, 0.101,
               0.093, 0.18, 0.134, 0.276,
               0.452, 0.115, 0.477, 0.192))

# model:
model{
  theta ~ dnorm(0,0.25)

  # heterogeneity SD:
  tau ~ dnorm(0,1)I(0,)
  # heterogeneity precision:
  tau_prec <- 1/(tau*tau)

  for(j in 1:m){

    # random effects:
    u[j] ~ dnorm(0, tau_prec)
    theta_u[j] <- theta+u[j]

    prec_md[j] <- 1/(se_md[j]*se_md[j])
    md[j] ~ dnorm(theta_u[j], prec_md[j])
  }
}


# initial values:
list(theta = -0.4, tau = 1)
list(theta = -0.2, tau = 1.2)
```

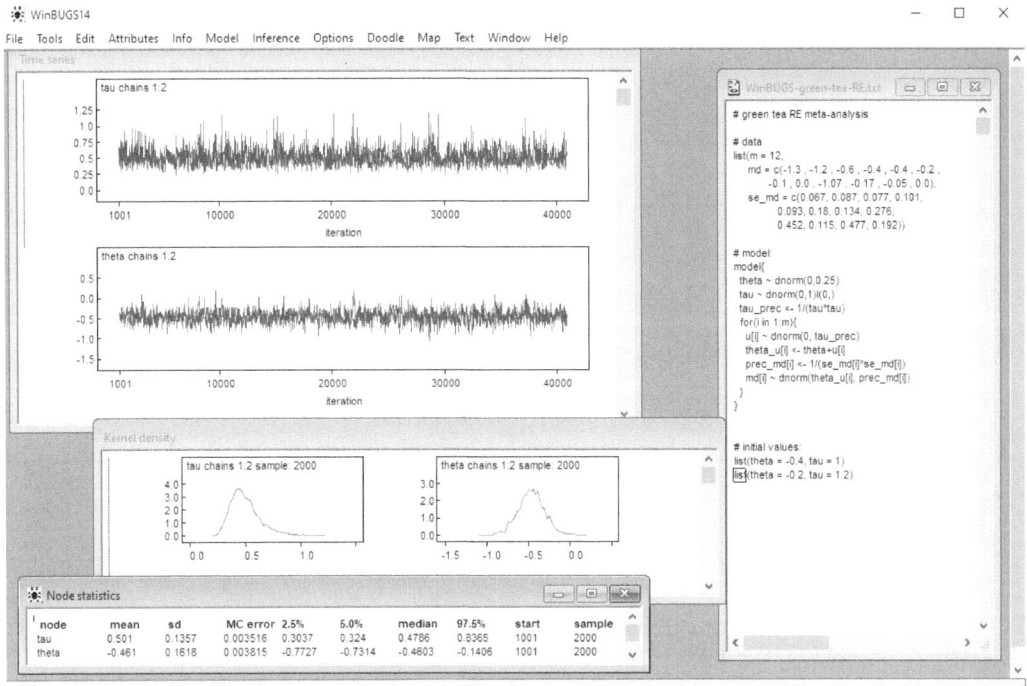

FIGURE 4.3
WinBUGS output for a random effects meta-analysis on the green tea data.

Once you are comfortable with this random effects code, try running it on the same data but with different heterogeneity distributions. Explore the impact it has on the results.

4.4.2 Stan code

Using the `cmdstanr` R package as interface, we program the Stan model as below. Note that each study has a study-specific population mean intervention effect (θ_j) given by `theta + u[j]`. The arguments for Stan's `student_t()` function are in the order: degrees of freedom, mean, scale, which is different to BUGS and JAGS.

```
stancode <- "
data {
  int m;
  array[m] real md;
  array[m] real se_md;
}
parameters {
  real<lower=0> tau;
  real theta;
  array[m] real u;
}
```

```
model {
  theta ~ normal(0,2);
  tau ~ student_t(1, 0, 1);
  u ~ normal(0,tau);
  for(j in 1:m) {
    md[j] ~ normal(theta+u[j], se_md[j]);
  }
}
generated quantities{
  array[m] real theta_u; // used for plotting
  for(j in 1:m) {
    theta_u[j] = theta + u[j];
  }
}"
```

We run this with the usual commands in `cmdstanr`:

```
stanmod <- cmdstan_model(write_stan_file(stancode),
                         compile = TRUE)

stanfit <- stanmod$sample(data=list(m    = NROW(greentea),
                                    md   = greentea$md,
                                    se_md = greentea$se_md),
                          iter_warmup=1000,
                          iter_sampling=5000,
                          chains = 2,
                          parallel_chains = 2)

stanfit$summary()

posterior_draws <- stanfit$draws()

mcmc_trace(posterior_draws, pars=c("theta",
                                   "tau",
                                   "u[1]",
                                   "u[2]""))
```

We could, in this small case, obtain traceplots, densities and so on, for all ten unknowns, but in general, if we have `theta`, `tau`, and two or three of the `u[j]`s, we will be able to spot any problems.

We can obtain a plot of posterior means and 95% credible intervals for any unknowns, that is similar to a forest plot in layout (Figure 4.4).

```
mcmc_intervals(posterior_draws,
               pars = vars(starts_with("theta_u"),
                           "theta"),
               point_est = "mean",
               prob = 0.5,
               prob_outer = 0.95)
```

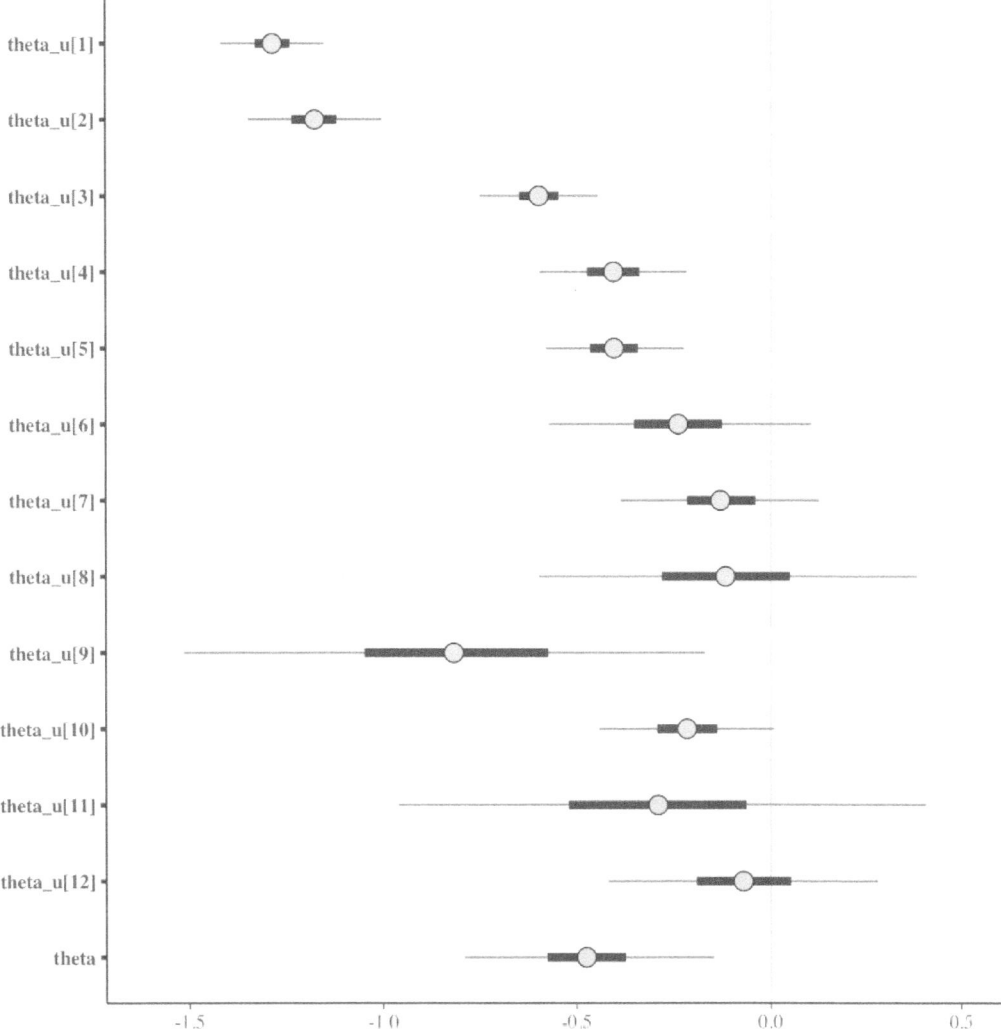

FIGURE 4.4

A forest plot-like visualisation of posterior means with 50% and 95% credible intervals from the green tea random effects meta-analysis. Studies appear in the order of the data.

The `pars` argument of the `bayesplot::mcmc_intervals()` function accepts partial matching code for unknowns' (parameters') names from `dplyr::vars()`, but you could also just supply a character vector, like `c("theta_u[1]", "theta_u[2]", ... "theta")`.

4.4.3 Stata code

To run a frequentist random effects meta-analysis in Stata, we need to change the `common()` option for `random()` instead. Suboptions that can be specified inside the brackets control the estimation process, including `mle` for maximum likelihood estimation, `reml` for the popular restricted MLE, `dlaird` for DerSimonian-Laird, and `sjonkman` for the Sidik-Jonkman (which we introduce below).

With the green tea data, the intervention effect is the variable `md` for mean difference, and its standard error is `se2`.

```
import delimited "cochrane_green_tea_weight_loss.csv", clear


meta esize n_tea mean_tea sd_tea ///
          n_control mean_control sd_control, ///
  esize(mdiff) random(dlaird) ///
  studylabel(study) eslabel("BMI change (kg/m^2)")

meta summarize

meta forestplot, nullrefline(lcolor(gray) ///
                             lpattern(dash) ///
                favorsleft("Favours ACEI") ///
                favorsright("Favours ARB"))

meta funnelplot, msymbol(Oh) mcol(black)

gen md = _meta_es
gen se2 = _meta_se^2
gen id = _n
```

In `bayesmh`, we keep the constant unknown `{md:_cons}`, which is θ, but add the random effects for each study, `U[id]`, which are θ_j. You must use a capitalised word for the name of the random effects vector, and the variable inside the square brackets is an integer that identifies group membership; in this setting, each study is its own group.

```
bayesmh md U[id], likelihood(normal(se2)) ///
                prior({md:_cons}, normal(0,25)) ///
                prior({U}, normal(0,{tau2})) ///
                prior({tau2}, t(0,2,1)) ///
                nchains(2) ///
                burnin(10000) ///
                mcmcsize(10000) ///
                thin(20) ///
                showreffects ///
                saving("stata_green_tea_chains.dta", replace) ///
                init1({md:_cons} -0.2 ///
                      {tau2}  0.5) ///
                init2({md:_cons} 0.2 ///
                      {tau2}  0.3)

bayesstats grubin
bayesgraph diagnostics {_cons}, title("Mean difference")
bayesgraph diagnostics {tau2}, title("Het. variance")
```

We have manually specified initial values for md:_cons and tau. Any unknowns that we do not initialise, Stata will do by default. Random effects parameters like U[id] are set to zero. Other parameters, if not specified, will be drawn from prior distributions if possible. More detail is given in the Stata [BAYES] manual.

To eliminate autocorrelation and slowly mixing chains, we thin the iterations to keep only every 20th. This takes a few minutes to run. We also save the retained iterations from the chains into a data file for later use (see Section 7.3.2). If we include the showreffects option as well, the iterations will include the "random effects" called U[id].

```
Gelman-Rubin convergence diagnostic

Number of chains       =              2
MCMC size, per chain =          10,000
Max Gelman-Rubin Rc  =         1.00129


     ------------------------
                 |         Rc
     ------------+-----------
md               |
        _cons |    1.00129
     ------------+-----------
         tau2 |   1.000664
     ------------------------
Convergence rule: Rc < 1.1
```

4.4.4   R bayesmeta and brms code

We now repeat the same procedure used for the common effect model in Section 3.6.4, but applying a random effects meta-analysis. We use a half-normal prior for the heterogeneity tau, with scale 0.5, which is equivalent to allowing tau to assume values less or equal to 0.98 with 95% probability. We report again the I^2, and the plots:

```
metaRE <- bayesmeta(y=dat[,"yi"], sigma=sqrt(dat[,"vi"]),
                    labels=dat[,"Study"],
                    mu.prior.mean=0, mu.prior.sd=4,
                    tau.prior=function(t){dhalfnormal(t, scale=0.5)})

metaRE$I2(tau=metaRE$summary["median","tau"])
[1] 0.2715443

forestplot(metaRE, exponentiate=TRUE, digits=3, zero=1, clip=c(0, 3))

plot(metaRE, prior=TRUE)
```

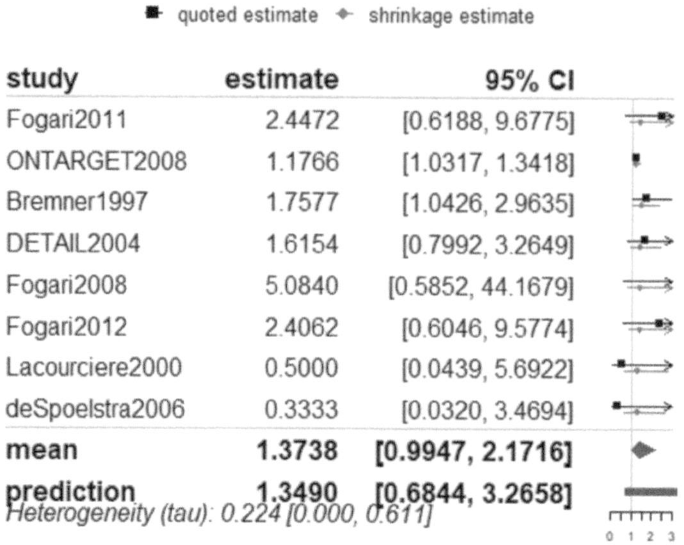

■ quoted estimate   ✦ shrinkage estimate

study	estimate	95% CI	
Fogari2011	2.4472	[0.6188, 9.6775]	
ONTARGET2008	1.1766	[1.0317, 1.3418]	
Bremner1997	1.7577	[1.0426, 2.9635]	
DETAIL2004	1.6154	[0.7992, 3.2649]	
Fogari2008	5.0840	[0.5852, 44.1679]	
Fogari2012	2.4062	[0.6046, 9.5774]	
Lacourciere2000	0.5000	[0.0439, 5.6922]	
deSpoelstra2006	0.3333	[0.0320, 3.4694]	
mean	**1.3738**	**[0.9947, 2.1716]**	
prediction	**1.3490**	**[0.6844, 3.2658]**	

Heterogeneity (tau): 0.224 [0.000, 0.611]

0 1 2 3

FIGURE 4.5
Forest plot of Bayesian random effects meta-analysis via `bayesmeta`.

The `pposterior()` function evaluates the area under the curve (posterior probability) equal to or less than the input provided to it. The probability of ACEI having a beneficial effect vs ARB is now slightly higher than the one we have estimated with the common effect model, but still rather small:

```
metaRE$pposterior(mu=0)
[1] 0.02231551
```

The bayesmeta package allowed us to fit a normal-normal hierarchical model, we now show how to fit a similar model using the `brms` package (Bayesian regression model using Stan) which is a powerful tool to fit many types of Bayesian regression models by running Stan in the background. Like Stata `bayesmh`, we have to present meta-analysis in a regression framework.

Before fitting the model, we specify the prior distributions of the overall effect size and the heterogeneity standard deviation. As we have done in `bayesmeta`, we assume a normal distribution with mean 0 and standard deviation 4 for the effect size. For `tau`, we use a half-normal centred at 0 with standard deviation 0.5. We use a function called `prior`, which takes two arguments, the distribution we want to assume and the class of priors.

For the effect size, we use an `Intercept` class as it is a fixed population-level effect. For the between-study heterogeneity we use class `sd`. We also need to manually calculate the standard error of the effect size which we need to fit the hierarchical model and use it as a weighting factor.

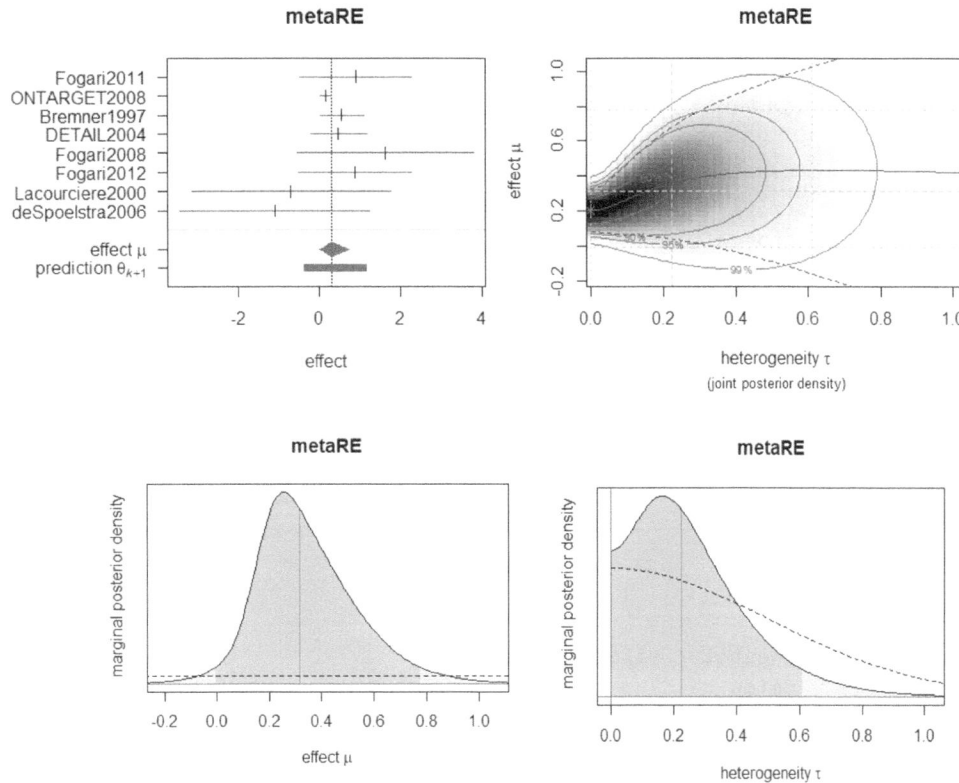

FIGURE 4.6
Exploratory plots of Bayesian random effects meta-analysis via `bayesmeta`.

```
library(brms)

priors <- c(prior(normal(0,4), class=Intercept),
            prior(normal(0,0.5), class=sd, lb=0))

# we calculate the standard error of the effect size:
dat$se_calc <- sqrt(dat$vi)
```

`brms` uses a regression formula notation in which an outcome (in our case, an observed effect size) is predicted by one or more predictors. A tilde ($\sim$) is used to specify that there is a predictive relationship.

Meta-analysis is a special case as we do not have any predictor variable so we type `1` in the place of predictor variable names. This is then an intercept-only model. In order to give studies with higher precision a greater weight we write `y | se(se_calc)`.

We fit a random effects model by adding the term (1|study) to the right side of the formula. If we were to use a common effect model, we can simply omit this term. The other arguments are the data to be used, the priors we have defined and the number of iterations of the MCMC algorithm:

```
meta_brms <- brm(yi | se(se_calc) ~ 1 + (1 | Study),
                 data=dat,
                 prior=priors,
                 iter=5000)
```

We can explore the results by simply using the function summary. Before examining those we need to be sure that the model has converged, firstly by checking the r-hat values of the parameter estimates, and secondly by a posterior predictive check.

```
> summary(meta_brms)

 Family: gaussian
   Links: mu = identity; sigma = identity
 Formula: yi | se(se_calc) ~ 1 + (1 | Study)
    Data: dat (Number of observations: 8)
    Draws: 4 chains, each with iter = 5000; warmup = 2500; thin = 1;
           total post-warmup draws = 10000

Multilevel Hyperparameters:~
Study (Number of levels: 8)
                Estimate Est.Error 1-95% CI u-95% CI Rhat Bulk_ESS Tail_ESS
sd(Intercept)       0.81      0.17     0.54     1.21 1.00      515     1290

Regression Coefficients:
                Estimate Est.Error 1-95% CI u-95% CI Rhat Bulk_ESS Tail_ESS
Intercept           0.34      0.29    -0.24     0.92 1.01      301      716

Further Distributional Parameters:
        Estimate Est.Error 1-95% CI u-95% CI Rhat Bulk_ESS Tail_ESS
sigma       0.00      0.00     0.00     0.00   NA       NA       NA

Draws were sampled using sampling(NUTS). For each parameter, Bulk_ESS
and Tail_ESS are effective sample size measures, and Rhat is the potential
scale reduction factor on split chains (at convergence, Rhat = 1).


> pp_check(meta_brms)
```

The posterior predictive plot is shown in Figure 4.7. Using the ranef() function, we can extract the estimated deviation of each study's effect size from the pooled effect:

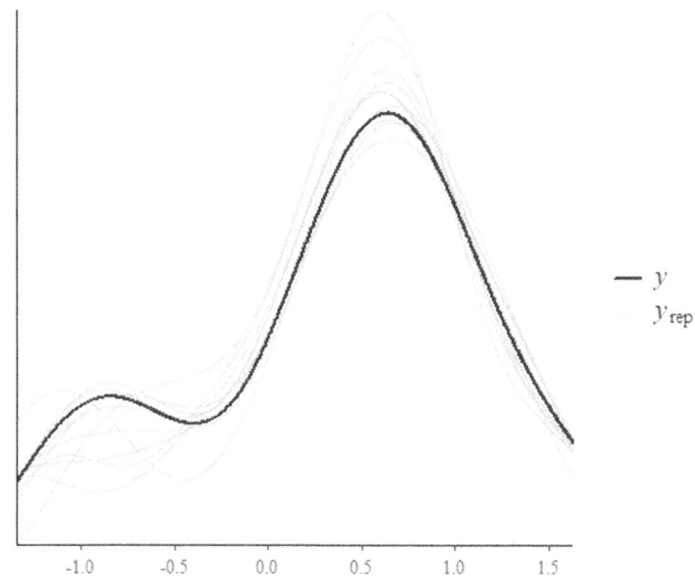

FIGURE 4.7
Posterior predictive plot of Bayesian random effects meta-analysis via `brms`.

```
> ranef(meta_brms)

$Study
, , Intercept

                 Estimate Est.Error        Q2.5       Q97.5
Bremner1997     0.2196776 0.2872923 -0.35467815   0.8054935
deSpoelstra2006 -1.3675028 0.3241007 -2.00496488 -0.7299749
DETAIL2004      0.1351304 0.2879105 -0.44042846   0.7200225
Fogari2008      1.2705810 0.2925913  0.69725509   1.8624526
Fogari2011      0.5494157 0.2898418 -0.02170003   1.1333982
Fogari2012      0.5329051 0.2897728 -0.04298676   1.1189481
Lacourciere2000 -1.0114403 0.3032202 -1.60928946 -0.4115518
ONTARGET2008    -0.1814135 0.2871107 -0.75447231   0.3998053
```

To fit a common effect model (see Section 3.6.4) we don't need any independent variables (predictors), unless we are fitting a meta-regression to the data. Therefore we have an intercept-only model which is:

```
priors <- c(prior(normal(0,4), class=Intercept))

meta_brms <- brm(yi | se(se_calc) ~ 1,
            data=dat,
            prior=priors,
            iter=5000)
```

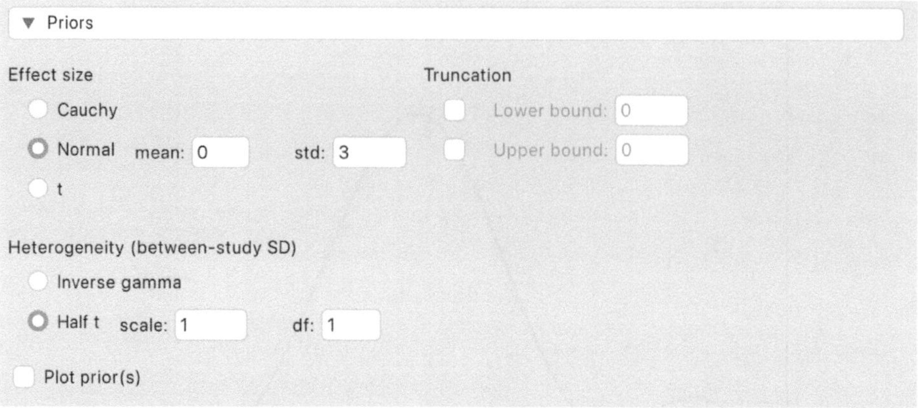

FIGURE 4.8
Prior input for JASP random effects meta-analysis.

Bayesian Meta-Analysis

Posterior Estimates per Model

		Mean	SD	95% Credible Interval		BF_{10}
				Lower	Upper	
Random effects	μ	−0.479	0.159	−0.802	−0.158	2.682
	τ	0.496	0.129	0.302	0.802	$5.883 \times 10^{+35}$[a]

Note. μ and τ are the group–level effect size and standard deviation, respectively.
[a] Bayes factor of the random effects H_1 over the fixed effects H_1.

FIGURE 4.9
Output for JASP random effects meta-analysis.

4.4.5 JASP

The input in the "Bayesian meta-analysis" dialog box is the same as we saw in Section 3.6.5 for common effect meta-analysis, except that we tick the "Random effects" option. In the priors, we can now choose a distribution for the heterogeneity standard deviation, either inverse gamma or half-t-distribution. In Figure 4.8, we choose $\tau \sim t^+(0, 1, 1)$.

Output is shown in Figure 4.9. The Bayes factor for the "effect size" is 2.682, which would be classified as "not worth more than a bare mention", according to Table 2.3. This has some correspondence with the larger credible interval, which extends close to the null value of zero. However, we would prefer to interpret in a holistic consideration of uncertainty, clinical importance, cost, risk of side effects, opportunity cost, and alternative treatments, before we choose what to give "more than a bare mention".

4.5   Case Study: The Green Tea Meta-Analysis

Let's explore the thought processes that should happen when you apply random effects meta-analysis to a real-life evidence base in the green tea meta-analysis. The Cochrane review is freely available in full online [136], but you do not need to read it to consider the questions below:

1. what would a clinical reader assume the global population of the green tea meta-analysis to be?

2. the Cochrane review listed the following inclusion criteria relating to study populations—what does this tell you about the global population in this evidence base:

"Participants were otherwise healthy male or female adults (18 years of age and older), who were classified by study investigators as overweight or obese (as defined by accepted standards such as BMI or percentage excess weight compared with ideal weight tables) at the beginning of the trial. Acceptable BMI values varied depending on the definition of overweight and obese in the country in which the study was conducted.

Studies were excluded if more than 25% of participants reported a co-morbidity requiring drug therapy, such as diabetes or CV disease, or were taking medications (other than those in the study) that might have affected weight gain or loss".

3. the Cochrane review describes the study populations that were obtained as follows—what, if anything, might be a factor behind heterogeneity, considering that the World Health Organisation defines overweight as BMI ≥ 25 and obesity as BMI ≥ 30:

"The 18 studies included in the review were all randomised controlled trials. Two thousand and seventy-six participants were randomised in total, with 1945 participants finishing their respective study. The trial duration ranged between 84 and 91 days and study size ranged between 19 and 270 participants. Nine of the 18 studies took place in Japan, and four were conducted in the Netherlands, while the rest took place in Australia, China, Taiwan, Thailand, and the US. Ten studies included both men and women, while five included only women and three included only men. Fifteen studies were weight loss studies, while the remaining three were weight maintenance studies. All studies used BMI as part of study inclusion criteria. In most cases, authors reported a BMI range that conformed with the WHO definition of overweight.

. . .

The range of BMI values for participant inclusion were noted for each study and are as follows:

- > 27
- > 25
- 25 to < 30
- 25 to 31
- 25 to 35
- 25 to 40
- 25 to 39.9
- 24 to 30
- 24 to 35
- 23 to < 30
- 22.5 to 30
- 22 to 30
- 21 to 39".

4. what can you learn about the study-specific ("local") population in Diepvens 2005, which you can read in full online at `https://doi.org/10.1079%2FBJN20051580` (you can also quickly assess some key points by just reading the abstract)?

5. to what extent will the differences among studies described so far influence the study-specific population mean differences, $\theta_j = \mu_{j\text{Int}} - \mu_{j\text{Ctl}}$? Bear in mind that increasing both arms' means does not change θ_j.

When you are ready, compare your ideas with ours, in the footnote below*. Remember that there is no right answer. What matters is that you are comfortable with justifying your conclusions.

We can see in the forest plot that there are some clear gaps between studies' confidence intervals; this is a clue that there is excess scatter coming from somewhere else: heterogeneity.

What would you expect to be different about the forest plot if there were negligible heterogeneity ($\tau \approx 0$)? (Our answer is in the footnote†.)

In the green tea meta-analysis (Figure 4.10), if we set aside the subgroups and analyse all studies together, using a DerSimonian-Laird random-effects meta-analysis, the heterogeneity variance estimate is $\tau^2 = 0.24$. The heterogeneity standard deviation is $\tau = \sqrt{0.24} = 0.49$.

Next to the τ^2 estimate at the bottom of the plot, there is also an I^2 statistic, which is the proportion of overall variance accounted for by heterogeneity. The value of 94.56% is very high.

Spending a little time exploring how the I^2 relates to the τ^2 estimate and the standard error around the overall estimate will help you to consolidate these ideas. First, take the estimated overall effect (-0.48) and its 95% confidence interval (-0.77 to -0.18). Considering that the 95% CI is the estimate ±1.96 standard errors, calculate the standard error. Next, square this to get an estimate of the *intra*-study variance (due to sampling error). Add this to τ^2 (*inter*-study variance) to get an estimate of the total variance. Finally, divide τ^2 by this total variance to find I^2.

Because the statistics we have are given to two decimal places, we must accept a degree of rounding error. We get a standard error of 0.15, intra-study variance of $0.15^2 = 0.023$, total variance of $0.24 + 0.023 = 0.263$ and I^2 of $0.24/0.263 = 0.91 = 91\%$.

4.5.1   Funnel plots for the green tea studies

We can use funnel plots to compare the observed study statistics with the theoretical sampling distribution in a common effect meta-analysis, and then a random effects meta-analysis with some estimate of τ^2.

In Figure 4.11, the central dashed vertical line is located at the common effect estimate of the mean difference, $\hat{\theta}$. The observed mean differences from the studies are shown as

---

*A clinical reader might think the conclusions reflect the outcome that can be expected for any overweight or obese person—which is implicitly their idea of the "global" population. However, the inclusion criteria clarify that the global population is adults who are overweight or obese, and who mostly do not have notable co-morbidities, so they are otherwise in good health. This is somewhat worrying for communication, as many patients seeking advice to lose weight in real life will have some co-morbidity. We suspect the authors were trying to avoid drug classes such as diuretics that might affect weight; whether they *interact* with green tea, and so change θ_j, is another question. The ranges of BMI in the studies are variable enough to be concerning, because we might imagine a larger effect is feasible in people who are more obese at baseline. It is also possible for there to be interactions between treatments and sex making the single-sex trials potentially different.

†The study estimates (the small squares) would only differ from each other (on the horizontal axis) by sampling error, so most of the confidence intervals would overlap, and they would be much more lined up above the diamond.

Study	Treatment N	Treatment Mean	Treatment SD	Control N	Control Mean	Control SD	BMI change (kg/m²) with 95% CI	Weight (%)
Kozuma 2005	107	-1	.6	119	.3	.4	-1.30 [-1.43, -1.17]	9.55
Takase 2008	44	-1.2	.5	45	0	.3	-1.20 [-1.37, -1.03]	9.43
Auvichayapat 2008	30	-3	1.7	30	-1.9	1.8	-1.10 [-1.99, -0.21]	5.22
Nagao 2007	123	-.6	.6	117	0	.6	-0.60 [-0.75, -0.45]	9.50
Takeshita 2008	40	-.5	.4	41	-.1	.5	-0.40 [-0.60, -0.20]	9.34
Kajimoto 2005	129	-.2	.5	66	.2	.8	-0.40 [-0.58, -0.22]	9.39
Suzuki 2009	18	-.2	.5	20	0	.6	-0.20 [-0.55, 0.15]	8.56
Hill 2007	19	0	.3	19	.2	.4	-0.20 [-0.42, 0.02]	9.22
Kataoka 2004	71	-.4	.8	71	-.3	.8	-0.10 [-0.36, 0.16]	9.05
Hsu 2008	41	-.1	2.8	37	0	.8	-0.10 [-1.04, 0.84]	4.96
Takashima 2004	10	-.5	.6	9	-.5	.6	0.00 [-0.54, 0.54]	7.37
Diepvens 2005	23	-1.5	.7	23	-1.5	.6	0.00 [-0.38, 0.38]	8.42
Overall							-0.48 [-0.77, -0.18]	

Heterogeneity: $\tau^2 = 0.24$, $I^2 = 94.56\%$, $H^2 = 18.37$

Test of $\theta_i = \theta_j$: Q(11) = 202.10, p = 0.00

Test of $\theta = 0$: z = -3.14, p = 0.00

Favours green tea | Favours control

Random-effects DerSimonian–Laird model
Sorted by: cochrane_mean_diff

FIGURE 4.10
The Cochrane green tea meta-analysis forest plot, without the subgroups of Japan and Outside Japan. The studies are ordered by the intervention effect estimates, $\hat{\theta}_j$.

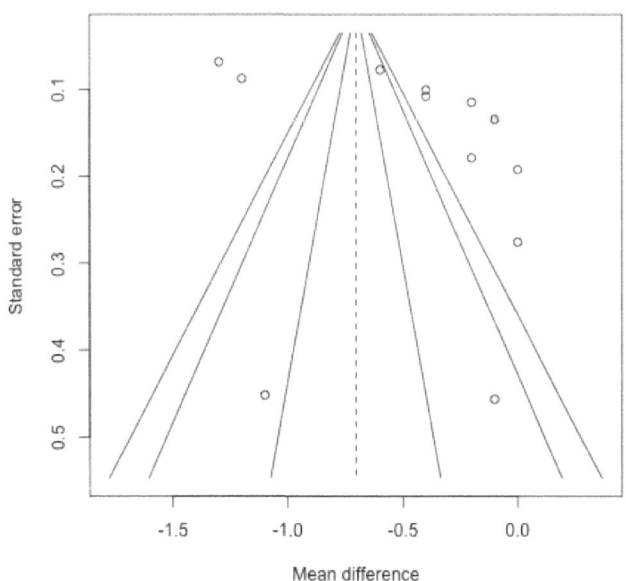

FIGURE 4.11
Study statistics (dots) compared to a common effect model (lines).

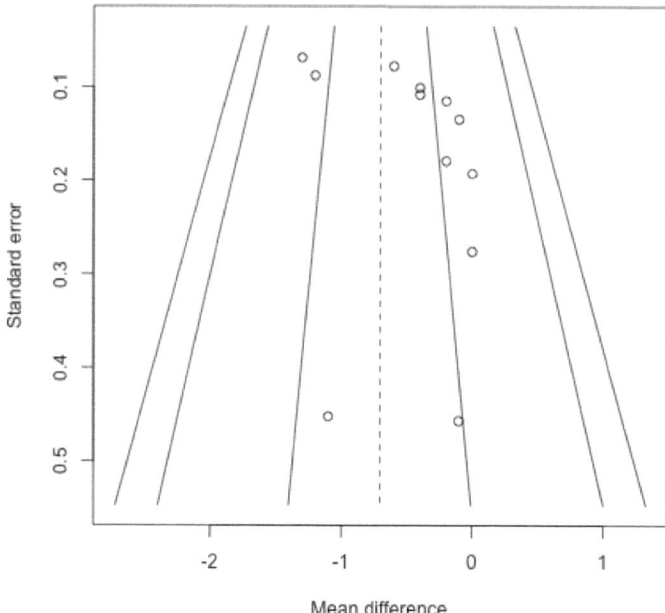

FIGURE 4.12
Study statistics compared to a DerSimonian-Laird random-effect model.

small circles. The curves and diagonal lines are, moving outward from the central estimate, the 50%, 90% and 95% central intervals of the sampling distribution.

We would expect to find about half of the studies/arms inside the 50% interval, but we do not, suggesting that there is wider scatter than sampling error can account for alone. This indicates heterogeneity.

We can compare this with a random effects model in Figure 4.12, here the DerSimonian-Laird. The intervals for the mean differences have been displaced outward from the central estimates by heterogeneity. Because τ^2 applies to all studies regardless of their size or standard error, the lines are not bent by it. This makes for a much more realistic model for the data, although there is some asymmetry in the mean differences, which might indicate publication bias, and we will return to that in Chapter 13.

It is worth noting that the model applies an expected distribution to the mean differences, but makes no demands on the study standard deviations. Heterogeneity acts on θ_j alone. However, there are some challenging problems in Part 3 of this book which may require more complicated models including the standard deviations.

4.5.2   Accommodating outliers

We saw in the previous section that there are one or two studies in the green tea meta-analysis (Auvichayapat 2008 and Hsu 2008) which have unusually high BMI standard deviations. These two are also the studies which did not have an upper limit to baseline BMI for recruitment. This kind of insight can guide us in shaping and, to some extent, explaining heterogeneity.

We can simply decide to accommodate them by a distribution that gives them more likelihood than the normal. The t-distribution (with low degrees of freedom) or Cauchy will provide this in a symmetric shape compared to the normal. The non-central chi-squared distribution does this for skewed and positive values, compared to the chi-squared. The negative binomial does this for positive natural numbers, compared to the Poisson.

This might be called a *robust* meta-analysis, and we will implement it in Section 4.6. When explaining a meta-analysis, we must help our audience to understand that robustness is always robustness *to* something—outliers, in this case—not a magic wand for all problems. The term is, in fact, used already for robustness to other problems. Because a more robust distribution allows for a certain number of outliers, it will not be pulled away from the main body of the evidence base in order to fit better to the outlier(s), so it is less affected by them.

4.6   A Model Analogous to (Hartung-Knapp-)Sidik-Jonkman

In Chapter 1, we introduced the t-distribution as the sampling distribution of a sample mean from normally distributed data, taking into account the fact that we must also estimate the sample standard deviation to calculate it. We can use the t-distribution in the same way in our random effects meta-analysis, because the studies' standard errors—$\widehat{SE}(\hat{\theta}_j)$—are themselves estimates, and so they add some additional uncertainty to the sampling distribution of $\hat{\theta}_j$ (or u_j, depending on your choice of parameterisation) and hence to the other parameters too.

The Sidik-Jonkman random effects meta-analysis is one of the best known of the frequentist formulas to estimate τ [229]. It is often paired with an adjustment of the standard error, to account for this additional uncertainty. This adjustment is sometimes called the Hartung-Knapp adjustment, or in combination with the Sidik-Jonkman estimator it is called the Hartung-Knapp-Sidik-Jonkman (HKSJ) random-effects meta-analysis [104, 105, 228].

HKSJ increases the variance of the pooled estimate to account for the uncertainty in the τ estimation [126]. It can be defined mathematically as an intercept-only weighted regression model, which makes a slightly weaker assumption than treating all variances as known [268].

Simulation studies have found that the HKSJ method performs better than conventional methods, especially when there are few studies or when study standard errors vary considerably [205]. However, in extreme cases, for example if there are only two studies, its confidence interval can become implausibly wide [276]. This can also be a concern in Bayesian meta-analysis, as it arises from a profound lack of information about τ, regardless of the statistical methods used.

To capture additional uncertainty, HKSJ-style, we can use a t-distribution, with $n_j - 2$ degrees of freedom. This approaches the problem in a simple way, tackling not the uncertainty in τ, but the uncertainty in $\widehat{SE}(\hat{\theta}_j)$, using the t-distribution as a long-established part of sampling distribution theory (see Chapter 1). In our BUGS model, it would simply be a case of changing the distribution from `dnorm` to `dt` in just one line of our code, and adding the degrees of freedom:

$$\theta \sim N(0, 2)$$
$$\tau \sim N^+(0, 1)$$
$$\theta_j \sim N(\theta, \tau) \tag{4.15}$$
$$\hat{\theta}_j \sim t(\theta_j, \widehat{SE}(\hat{\theta}_j), n_j - 2)$$

The BUGS data now includes n, the number of participants in each study (adding both arms together).

```
# data
list(m = 12,
     n = c(126, 89, 140, 81, 195, 38,
             142, 19, 60, 38, 78, 46),
     md = c(-1.3, -1.2, -0.6, -0.4, -0.4, -0.2,
             -0.1, 0.0, -1.07, -0.17, -0.05, 0.0),
     se_md = c(0.067, 0.087, 0.077, 0.101,
               0.093, 0.18, 0.134, 0.276,
               0.452, 0.115, 0.477, 0.192)))

# model:
model{
  theta ~ dnorm(0,0.25)

  # heterogeneity SD:
  tau ~ dnorm(0,1)I(0,)
  # heterogeneity precision:
  tau_prec <- 1/(tau*tau)

  for(j in 1:m){

    # degrees of freedom
    df[j] <- n[j]-2

    # random effects:
    u[j] ~ dnorm(0, tau_prec)
    theta_u[j] <- theta+u[j]

    prec_md[j] <- 1/(se_md[j]*se_md[j])
    md[j] ~ dt(theta_u[j], prec_md[j], df[j])
  }
}


# initial values:
list(theta = -0.4, tau = 1)
list(theta = -0.2, tau = 1.2)
```

The t-distribution requires three parameters: the mean, dispersion (not exactly the same as a standard deviation) and degrees of freedom. In this case, the degrees of freedom are fixed at $n_j - 2$, where n_j is the total of all participants in both arms of the jth study.

It is also important to choose the prior for τ carefully so that uncertainty in it is not overestimated. When there are few studies, a strongly informative prior, such as an expert opinion (see Chapter 6) or one based on related empirical heterogeneity [264, 263], may be essential.

4.6.1 "Fully Bayesian" models

It is also possible to carry out full inference for θ, τ, and σ, rather than taking σ as known from the standard error, or using the t-distribution. This has historically been called a "fully Bayesian" model [240], as every unknown gets a prior and a posterior. Rather than add more complication to this chapter, we hold it back until Chapter 11, where we have to use it to solve a particular problem.

4.7 Explaining Heterogeneity

Although intervention effects can be estimated with some precision because of the sample sizes in the individual studies, often on the order of 100s, or 1000s, we often have very few studies with which to estimate the heterogeneity. Prior distributions on the heterogeneity variance, standard deviation or precision therefore become very influential and should be chosen carefully, and with sensitivity analysis.

Turner and colleagues have analysed the heterogeneity reported by many clinical meta-analyses [264], which allows for an empirical prior. The logic is that, if we know nothing else about the heterogeneity that we might find in this evidence base, we should at least expect it to be like that which has been observed in other meta-analyses. A more general analysis by Roever and colleagues provided some R code and indicated a general utility of half-normal priors [206].

It is natural to question whether the heterogeneity distribution should always be normal [127]. In fact, a study of clinical meta-analyses suggests that between 15% and 26% were plausibly non-normal [153]. When we are using Bayesian sampling methods, such as MCMC, for our analysis, a change from normality is a trivial effort. More importantly, we should consider what the impact might be of getting it wrong [21]. Apart from the Central Limit Theorem (see Section 1.2), there is no theoretical reason why the normal distribution would be a safe default choice.

It is reasonable to assume that study-specific populations have their mean intervention effects (or other target parameters) pushed up or down by many competing and largely independent influences, and that in itself will make a normal distribution. However, it is also plausible that one factor would exert a very large influence compared to the others. For example, if disease severity varies between studies, there could be modest intervention effects in mildly affected people and the possibility of larger effects in those with more severe disease. That one strong influence might create a non-normal heterogeneity.

The heterogeneity in random-effects meta-analysis is in essence the same as a between-groups distribution in any multilevel model. However, there is an important difference, which limits how relaxed we can feel about the heterogeneity distribution. In most multilevel model applications, inference and prediction focus on the slopes that apply within-groups (or, confusingly for meta-analysts, "fixed effects"), and methodology has shown that the shape of the between-groups distribution does not impact strongly on the within-groups slopes [164]. Research into non-normal heterogeneity in meta-analysis shows that, although the overall effect size estimate is fairly robust to an incorrect assumption of normality [209], other inferences can be adversely affected [141], because heterogeneity is not just averaged over and ignored, but central to many inferences and predictions.

Most frequentist meta-analysis procedures quantify heterogeneity in a very simple way. We might obtain a point estimate of τ^2, without any information on uncertainty. This estimate of τ^2 might be used in a hypothesis test, such as Cochran's Q test, to make a binary decision as to whether there is or is no heterogeneity in the evidence base. In fact, it is hard to imagine different teams carrying out studies and *not* doing them in somewhat different ways that might impact on intervention effect [111].

In a Bayesian setting, the heterogeneity standard deviation (or variance, or precision) is an unknown like any other, and we obtain a posterior distribution, not just a point estimate. This gives us deeper insights, such as how clinically important the heterogeneity might be. Conversely, we could define *a priori* a minimal clinically important heterogeneity standard deviation, and then find the posterior probability that the true value exceeds this; Stangl and Berry describe this in their book at p.207 [243].

In the sections that follow, we consider how to go further than just quantifying heterogeneity, and actually try to explain it. Some reasons *why* we may find heterogeneity are held over to Part 3 of this book, as they involve more detailed methods and models: mixtures of study designs or risk of bias.

Unless disinterested clinical and statistical experts can be consulted to elicit causes of heterogeneity, then there will inevitably be an element of HARKing (Hypothesising After Results are Known), which greatly increases the risk of drawing incorrect conclusions from our heterogeneity analysis [179]. Any such findings should be treated as hypothesis generation, to be tested as future studies are added to the evidence base, rather than definitive insights.

4.7.1   Subgroups

We can model the heterogeneity but it is also important to try to understand how it arose. We might present meta-analyses with subgroups of similarly conducted studies, where there is an estimate of effect for each subgroup, and then an overall estimate too.

In the green tea studies (Table 3.1), the first eight rows were conducted in Japan, the last four elsewhere, and there does seem to be a difference between them, even though we do not know exactly why this is. In the original Cochrane review [136], they are presented in two subgroups for this reason. Figure 3.2 shows the original forest plot with two subgroups.

This is the simplest way to explain some of the heterogeneity, as shown in Figure 3.2. There is a meta-analytic estimate of θ^{JPN} and τ^{JPN} for the Japanese studies, and θ^{OJ} and τ^{OJ} for the studies from outside Japan. At the bottom of the forest plot, there is a combined θ and τ.

Frequentist random effects meta-analyses will estimate the two heterogeneity standard deviations by, in each subgroup, pooling the sampling distribution standard deviations (standard errors) from the studies according to some formula, then subtracting this from the total observed inter-study variation. The part left over is heterogeneity. This is then repeated for all studies together to give the "overall" estimates.

The problem with this is that the subgroup and overall calculations are not compatible; they represent different models. We are burdening the audience with the choice between subgroup results and overall results, when it is really our job to help them. Perhaps they will choose the one that matches their prejudices; these sorts of cognitive biases are part of human nature.

The Bayesian approach is to fit two normal distributions to the heterogeneity: one for each subgroup. This means that we can fine-tune the model further, and it forces us to think about what has led to the study statistics at hand (the data-generating process). If we wanted to show overall results too, that would require an entirely different model, and this prevents us from simultaneously presenting incompatible outputs.

The following subgroup model is comparable to DerSimonian-Laird so that you can focus on the subgroup logic:

$$\theta^{\text{JPN}} \sim \text{N}(0, 2)$$
$$\tau^{\text{JPN}} \sim \text{N}^+(0, 2)$$
$$\theta_j^{\text{JPN}} \sim \text{N}(\theta^{\text{JPN}}, \tau^{\text{JPN}})$$
$$\hat{\theta}_j^{\text{JPN}} \sim \text{N}(\theta_j^{\text{JPN}}, \widehat{\text{SE}}(\hat{\theta}_j^{\text{JPN}}))$$

$$\theta^{\text{OJ}} \sim \text{N}(0, 2)$$
$$\tau^{\text{OJ}} \sim \text{N}^+(0, 2)$$
$$\theta_j^{\text{OJ}} \sim \text{N}(\theta^{\text{OJ}}, \tau^{\text{OJ}})$$
$$\hat{\theta}_j^{\text{OJ}} \sim \text{N}(\theta_j^{\text{OJ}}, \widehat{\text{SE}}(\hat{\theta}_j^{\text{OJ}}))$$

(4.16)

The BUGS code is below. The data have been split into two parts for the two subgroups.

```
# data
list(m_JPN = 8, m_OJ = 4,
    md_JPN = c(-1.3, -1.2, -0.6, -0.4,
               -0.4, -0.2, -0.1, 0.0),
    se_md_JPN = c(0.067, 0.087, 0.077, 0.101,
                  0.093, 0.18, 0.134, 0.276),
    md_OJ = c(-1.07, -0.17, -0.05, 0.0),
    se_md_OJ = c(0.452, 0.115, 0.477, 0.192))

model {
  # Japanese studies:
  theta_JPN ~ dnorm(0, 0.25)
  tau_JPN ~ dnorm(0, 0.25)I(0,)
  tau_JPN_prec <- 1 / (tau_JPN * tau_JPN)

  for (j in 1:m_JPN) {
      theta_j_JPN[j] ~ dnorm(theta_JPN,
                          tau_JPN_prec)
      sampling_prec_JPN[j] <- 1 / (se_md_JPN[j] *
                              se_md_JPN[j])
      md_JPN[j] ~ dnorm(theta_j_JPN[j],
                      sampling_prec_JPN[j])
  }

  # studies from outside Japan:
  theta_OJ ~ dnorm(0, 0.25)
  tau_OJ ~ dnorm(0, 0.25)I(0,)
  tau_OJ_prec <- 1 / (tau_OJ * tau_OJ)

  for (j in 1:m_OJ) {
      theta_j_OJ[j] ~ dnorm(theta_OJ,
                          tau_OJ_prec)
      sampling_prec_OJ[j] <- 1 / (se_md_OJ[j] *
                              se_md_OJ[j])
```

```
        md_OJ[j] ~ dnorm(theta_j_OJ[j],
                        sampling_prec_OJ[j])
    }
}

# initial values:
list(theta_JPN = -0.3, theta_OJ = 0.3,
     tau_JPN = 0.2, tau_OJ = 0.4)
list(theta_JPN = 0.3, theta_JPN = -0.3,
     tau_JPN = 0.4, tau_OJ = 0.2)
```

This code assumes that you provide two vectors of mean difference estimates, md_JPN and md_OJ, and two of the standard errors, se_md_JPN and se_md_OJ. One vector contains the Japanese studies, the other those outside Japan.

This makes the two subgroups completely independent of each other, just like in the frequentist subgroup analysis (but with priors). Their heterogeneity distributions can have different means and standard deviations. That would indicate that local study populations come from a distribution in Japan that is entirely different to that elsewhere. Researchers might consider this and decide it is justified, because of some fundamental difference like the genetic hypothesis mentioned above. If this is the case, then this is the right model. However, it is really not one meta-analysis but two.

The posterior statistics output from WinBUGS is:

node	mean	sd	MC error	2.5%	median	97.5%
tau_JPN	0.573	0.203	0.002	0.311	0.530	1.088
tau_OJ	0.473	0.464	0.011	0.015	0.341	1.738
theta_JPN	-0.539	0.218	0.002	-0.967	-0.542	-0.093
theta_OJ	-0.230	0.343	0.004	-0.987	-0.206	0.429

If we are investigating two subgroups that are *not* expected to have different intervention effects, then we should do something different. Suppose that there is no known genetic factor affecting effectiveness of green tea extracts, but that we have found (from a close reading of the papers and interviewing researchers) that the Japanese studies prepare the product in a very consistent, traditional way, while those elsewhere are more inventive and vary considerably in the exact formulation. That might make us suspect that the subgroups share a single θ but have different τ parameters.

This is easily achieved:

$$\theta \sim \mathrm{N}(0,2)$$

$$\tau^{\mathrm{JPN}} \sim \mathrm{N}^+(0,2)$$
$$\theta_j^{\mathrm{JPN}} \sim \mathrm{N}(\theta, \tau^{\mathrm{JPN}})$$
$$\hat{\theta}_j^{\mathrm{JPN}} \sim \mathrm{N}(\theta_j^{\mathrm{JPN}}, \widehat{\mathrm{SE}}(\hat{\theta}_j^{\mathrm{JPN}})) \qquad (4.17)$$

$$\tau^{\mathrm{OJ}} \sim \mathrm{N}^+(0,2)$$
$$\theta_j^{\mathrm{OJ}} \sim \mathrm{N}(\theta, \tau^{\mathrm{OJ}})$$
$$\hat{\theta}_j^{\mathrm{OJ}} \sim \mathrm{N}(\theta_j^{\mathrm{OJ}}, \widehat{\mathrm{SE}}(\hat{\theta}_j^{\mathrm{OJ}}))$$

```
# common underlying effect:
theta ~ dnorm(0, 0.25)

# Japanese studies:
tau_JPN ~ dnorm(0, 0.25)I(0,)
tau_JPN_prec <- 1 / (tau_JPN * tau_JPN)

for (j in 1:m_JPN) {
    theta_j_JPN[j] ~ dnorm(theta,
                    tau_JPN_prec)
    sampling_prec_JPN[j] <- 1 / (se_md_JPN[j] *
                            se_md_JPN[j])
    md_JPN[j] ~ dnorm(theta_j_JPN[j],
                sampling_prec_JPN[j])
}

# studies from outside Japan:
tau_OJ ~ dnorm(0, 0.25)I(0,)
tau_OJ_prec <- 1 / (tau_OJ * tau_OJ)

for (j in 1:m_OJ) {
    theta_j_OJ[j] ~ dnorm(theta,
                    tau_OJ_prec)
    sampling_prec_OJ[j] <- 1 / (se_md_OJ[j] *
                            se_md_OJ[j])
    md_OJ[j] ~ dnorm(theta_j_OJ[j],
                sampling_prec_OJ[j])
}
```

Just as the model of Equation 4.20 and the accompanying code sets the mean of the heterogeneity within subgroups to be equal yet allows the standard deviations to differ, we can easily amend it to have shared standard deviations but different means.

The posterior statistics output from WinBUGS is:

node	mean	sd	MC error	2.5%	median	97.5%
tau_JPN	0.590	0.204	0.002	0.320	0.548	1.103
tau_OJ	0.492	0.407	0.008	0.023	0.402	1.567
theta	-0.407	0.187	0.003	-0.786	-0.401	-0.065

In this second subgroup model, we cannot obtain an overall τ or I^2, because we do not believe that the subgroups are related in that way. This is one example of how the Bayesian approach forces us to explicitly choose our models and justify them.

We should be extra cautious in interpreting subgroup results. Subgroups are often identified after seeing the study statistics, the allocation of individual studies to subgroups may be a little uncertain, and the number of studies in subgroups could be very small.

Together, these problems mean that there is considerable risk of higher than expected bias and uncertainty.

Spears and colleagues wrote an insightful letter on the subject, where they identify commentators on an RCT subgroup analysis picking one particular comparison for promotion and sharing, despite it not being the primary analysis, nor being designed to consider subgroups [237]. By comparing deliberately irrelevant subgroups, they show that the error rate is elevated in subgroups.

Another well-known example highlighted the risk of selecting interesting subgroup comparisons by analysing odds of death from cardiovascular disease by signs of the zodiac [118]. It is important to realise that the *selection* of interesting analyses, and the omission or low prominence of others, is the problem.

4.7.2   Fixed effects meta-analysis is an extreme case of subgroups

Taken to its extreme, subgrouping leads to every study having its own θ_j, without the effect of a shared heterogeneity distribution to act as a prior and "shrink" the studies with high standard errors towards the evidence base's centre of gravity. The prior on the θ_js could be diffuse or weakly informative, or could represent previous evidence or expert opinion. There is then no τ and θ arises as a weighted average of the θ_js, rather than as an unknown in the model. The generic inverse variance weighted formula could be used.

This is the fixed effects meta-analysis, which we listed as a less common option at the beginning of this chapter. To create it in a Bayesian context, we must consider the information available across the evidence base for each study's θ_j, and be prepared to justify the rather strong assumption that nothing about any one study's θ_j is informative about any other. This implies a tenuous standoff in our analysis plan: that the studies are all quite different, and yet that we want to pool their evidence into a single estimate.

If we construct such a model for the θ_js, there could yet be connections among other unknowns at study level. One example, not entirely incompatible with frequentist meta-analysis, would be a shared intra-arm standard deviation, σ (see Section 8.4). An epistemic unknown such as a bias common to some or all of the studies would be another, and this would be a good reason to choose a Bayesian model.

Bayesian output is a sample from a posterior distribution, and in this case there will be draws from each of the θ_js. To keep the analysis Bayesian, we must propagate uncertainty into the averaging of θ. The simplest way to do this is to calculate the point estimate $\hat{\theta}$ for each of the posterior draws, which will then provide a posterior distribution for θ. There will be no need to calculate a standard error of $\hat{\theta}$.

4.7.3   Subgroup differences are a special case of regression

As we start to investigate the nature of between-study differences, we are trying to use one variable, a characteristic of the trials, to predict the locations of the trial statistics. We will use x_j for a variable that is defined for each trial. This variable might be a detail of how the trials were conducted, or the baseline participant statistics. In this simple case above, it is a binary variable telling us whether trial j took place in Japan or not. We could write it as 1 for Japan and 0 for Outside Japan.

This variable, x_j, predicts the intervention effect within each subgroup; to be precise, it predicts the mean of the within-subgroup heterogeneity distribution that applies to study j:

$$\theta|x_j = \beta_0 + \beta_1 x_j \tag{4.18}$$

In this equation, studies do not all have the same underlying θ. Note that the left-hand side is $\theta|x_j$ (we would say "theta given x j"), a true underlying intervention effect that is predicted by variable x in study j, not θ_j, a study-specific population intervention effect. Because x_j is either 0 or 1, this formula leads to two values of θ_j, using the notation from Equation 4.20:

$$\theta^{OJ} = \beta_0$$
$$\theta^{JPN} = \beta_0 + \beta_1 \tag{4.19}$$

This is simply equivalent to the mathematical notation and BUGS code above, but it allows us to extend our model of the heterogeneity further.

If we have more than two subgroups, we could write a subgroup meta-analysis model in this same regression style, by having binary indicator variables, one fewer than the number of subgroups, and assigning one of the subgroups to be a baseline where all the indicator variables are 0.

It also accommodates a continuous value of x_j, which could be a predictive value drawn from baseline participant statistics or study characteristics. This is called *meta-regression*.

4.7.4 Meta-regression

The purpose of this form of regression is causal understanding, not prediction at any cost. For this reason, meta-regressions should be confined to examination of *a priori* hypothesised causal relationships, rather than trying many potential predictor variables and choosing the most predictive one.

Finding associations with dose, or duration of treatment, or achieved reduction in an objective mediator [110], can provide insights that nuance the interpretation of the intervention effect itself. For example, trials of cholesterol reduction achieve a variety of measured reductions in serum cholesterol (the objective mediator) after some period of time, and this is correlated with the log odds ratio of ischaemic heart disease events (the outcome under consideration) [255].

It is important to realise that all we are doing in meta-regression is allowing the mean of the heterogeneity distribution to move up and down a sliding scale (the straight line in Figure 4.13). In the beginning of this chapter, we had one mean of the heterogeneity distribution, θ, which was common to all studies. The variance in the study statistics could be said to be divided into a part explained by sampling distribution and another unexplained part called heterogeneity.

Then, we split the evidence base into two subgroups. Each had their own θ^{JPN} or θ^{OJ}. Variance was now split three ways: sampling error, between subgroups and within subgroups.

The meta-regression model is just like this, but with the mean sliding up and down the prediction line. The three parts are the explained sampling error, the explained meta-regression line, and the unexplained heterogeneity. You can also think of it as the residual variance above and below the meta-regression line, which is split into sampling error and unexplained heterogeneity.

If study characteristics, such as attrition ("loss to follow-up"), explain some of the heterogeneity, this will allow us to estimate the size of the bias created in the affected studies, and also to provide an estimate of the unbiased intervention effect.

On the other hand, if participant characteristics, such as baseline BMI in the green tea studies, explain some of the heterogeneity, it would suggest that variable is an effect modifier. This would mean that there is evidence that green tea is consistently more effective in high baseline BMI people.

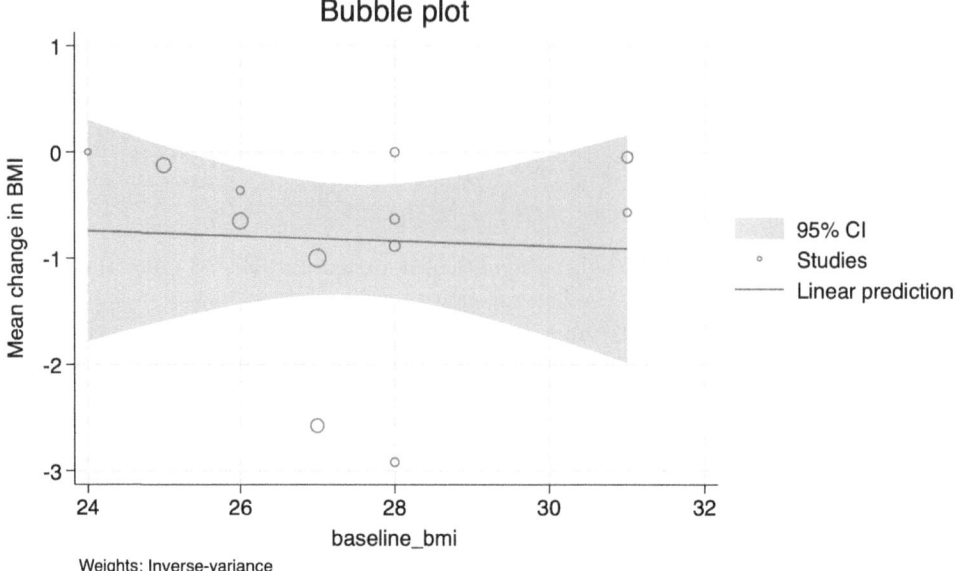

FIGURE 4.13
Bubble plot of green tea studies with the (frequentist) meta-regression line superimposed. The size of the bubble is proportional to the sample size.

Centring the predictor variable, x_j, so that a 0 value is in the middle of the observed values in the evidence base, helps interpretation. Our meta-regression line will have an intercept of β_0 and a slope of β_1, and the interpretation of β_0 is as the predicted intervention effect $(\theta|x_j)$ when $x_j = 0$. This helps us to set meaningful priors for it.

$$\beta_0 \sim N(0,2)$$
$$\beta_1 \sim N(0,1)$$
$$\tau \sim N^+(0,2)$$

$$\theta|x_j = \beta_0 + \beta_1 x_j$$
$$\theta_j \sim N(\theta|x_j, \tau)$$
$$\hat{\theta}_j \sim N(\theta_j, \widehat{SE}(\hat{\theta}_j))$$

(4.20)

In the BUGS code below, we use meta-regression to investigate the relationship between the mean baseline BMI in each study (see discussion in Section 4.5), and the intervention effect. Figure 4.13 gives an indication, from Stata, of what a frequentist meta-regression would show: there is no evidence of a relationship.

```
# data
list(m = 12,
     baseline_bmi = c(27, 28, 27, 28,
                      26, 26, 25, 24,
                      28, 31, 31, 28),
```

```
      md = c(-1.3, -1.2, -0.6, -0.4,
             -0.4, -0.2, -0.1, 0.0,
             -1.07, -0.17, -0.05, 0.0),
   se_md = c(0.067, 0.087, 0.077, 0.101,
             0.093, 0.18, 0.134, 0.276,
             0.452, 0.115, 0.477, 0.192))

# model:
model{
beta0 ~ dnorm(0, 0.25)
beta1 ~ dnorm(0, 1)

tau ~ dnorm(0, 0.25)I(0,)
het_prec <- 1 / (tau * tau)

for (j in 1:m) {
    theta_given_base[j] <- beta0 + beta1 * baseline_bmi[j]
    theta_j[j] ~ dnorm(theta_given_base[j], het_prec)
    sampling_prec[j] <- 1 / (se_md[j] *
                                se_md[j])
    md[j] ~ dnorm(theta_j[j],
                  sampling_prec[j])
}
}

# initial values:
list(beta0 = 0.2, beta1 = -0.2, tau = 0.4)
list(beta0 = -0.2, beta1 = 0.2, tau = 0.3)
```

Pause to think about how this code could also be used for two subgroups with a binary x_j in the place of `baseline_bmi[j]`. Also, consider how we could have a formula with coefficients that predicts the heterogeneity standard deviation (or variance, or precision).

The posterior statistics output from WinBUGS is:

node	mean	sd	MC error	2.5%	median	97.5%
beta0	-0.024	1.469	0.012	-2.889	-0.022	2.854
beta1	-0.016	0.054	4.324E-4	-0.122	-0.016	0.089
tau	0.519	0.142	0.001	0.313	0.494	0.869

Remember that more than one characteristic may vary between studies, making it hard, if not impossible, to attribute study differences to a cause. Nevertheless, we can usefully serve our audience by demonstrating the competing evidence for different causes of between-study variation, as a resource for hypothesis generation for future studies. Furthermore, the inclusion criteria for studies should not be the only consideration. Stephen Senn explains this well [225]:

"The inclusion criteria for a randomised clinical; trial cannot be used as a means of generalising the results because the patients recruited are rarely a representative sample of patients who could be recruited. Using the results from clinical trials requires recognising that they are experiments. Judgements as to how the results should be used rely on theory and the use of appropriate scales and are inevitably potentially fallible".

4.8   Interpreting Heterogeneity

Now that we have added heterogeneity to the common effect models of Chapter 3, we should revisit the interpretation ideas of Section 3.7, and consider what else we can say about heterogeneity.

4.8.1   Centre of the posterior distribution

Like any variance (or standard deviation, or precision), we should expect the posterior distribution of heterogeneity to be skewed. The mean will be higher than the median, and more easily influenced by unusual posterior draws.

The mode will probably be lower than the mean and median; because of the connection between the posterior mode and the maximum likelihood estimate*, this is related to the fact that maximum likelihood non-Bayesian meta-analysis under-estimates heterogeneity [125].

It is also possible for the mode to be zero, which is sometimes reported in maximum-likelihood meta-analyses. A Bayesian random effects meta-analysis of the ACEI versus ARB evidence base shows this pattern (code for this is available online). As Bayesians, we should be cautious about reporting one point estimate, as our goal is understanding of uncertainty.

It is very common to see a point estimate provided for heterogeneity variance or standard deviation, with no acknowledgement of uncertainty. In part, this is a legacy of the early random effects models, where uncertainty in heterogeneity was not fully explored, if at all. However, with Bayesian methods, we have the opportunity to comment in detail on the uncertainty in our understanding of heterogeneity, and we should do so.

Therefore, showing a graph of the posterior density and indicating the central estimate is likely to be more informative than simply giving one value.

We should also compare the heterogeneity *variance* to the study standard errors, to understand in context how large the between-study variation is. Note that the variance has a special property in that it can be decomposed into sources of variation (between- and within-study, in this case), with individual variations that add to the total variance.

4.8.2   Interval containing a certain probability

Because of the skewness of the posterior, if we provide an interval such as the 95% credible interval, we must make sure that we give the central estimate too. The difference between the central estimate and the upper limit of the credible interval will, most of the time, be larger than the difference between the central estimate and the lower limit, making asymmetry evident. A graph is likely to bring this to audience attention more clearly than three numbers.

When we are decomposing a total variance into parts, like heterogeneity, or any multi-level model, some formulas for the frequentist confidence interval can result in a lower limit

---

*As the prior approaches flatness, the posterior approaches the likelihood (normalised to integrate to one and thus behave like a probability distribution)—see Section 2.2.

of zero[†]. This has led to a habit in some meta-analysis audiences of looking at heterogeneity confidence intervals to see if they touch zero[‡]. This is related to the fallacy that common effect or random effects meta-analyses can be chosen empirically [23]. A Bayesian credible interval might get close to zero but should not exactly be equal to it, which echoes Higgins' assertion—which we agree with—that heterogeneity should be expected and quantified [111].

4.8.3 Probability of being above or below a certain threshold

It is more productive to consider, and to engage the audience in considering, whether the size of the heterogeneity exceeds some threshold of clinical importance. To help them define that threshold *a priori*, you can provide simulated forest plots, using the data-generating process code, for various values of τ.

4.8.4 Predictive inference for a future trial

The steps described in Section 3.7.5 for predicting a future trial in a common effect meta-analysis are similar for random effects. The only additional step is to simulate the study-specific population mean intervention effect, θ_j from the heterogeneity distribution, and then simulate the observed study statistic, $\hat{\theta}_j$, around θ_j, using the sampling distribution.

4.8.5 Sensitivity analysis with priors

Bear in mind that the heterogeneity distribution that we choose for our model is in fact a prior for θ_j. We might try out some different heterogeneity shapes, if there is reason to do so (see Section 4.7), and if we do, then we should show the prior densities side by side or superimposed in a graph. We should also show the posteriors that result in the same way. If we find little impact on $P(\theta|\boldsymbol{Y})$ and little impact on $P(\tau|\boldsymbol{Y})$, then we can clearly demonstrate that it is safe to proceed with one of the models only (the easiest to interpret and communicate, we would suggest in general).

[†]Some, in fact, result in negative lower limits, which might then be brushed under the carpet by being replaced with a zero. Crude asymptotic approximations like this were a necessary evil in the days of pencils and desk calculators.

[‡]The warped logic goes like this. Confidence intervals are related to p-values. If the confidence interval touches zero, then we can't reject the null hypothesis that there is no heterogeneity, right? So, by Occam's Razor, we should use a common effect meta-analysis. (Wrong. Hypothesis testing, especially *post hoc* like this, does not inform us of the existence of a cause in reality.)

Part II

Getting Inputs and Crafting Outputs

5

How to Extract Statistics from Published Papers

Learning objectives

After reading this chapter, you will be able to:

1. transcribe statistics from publications accurately and fully, recording any concerns and calculations

2. identify which statistics to extract for your meta-analysis

3. recognise when reported study statistics are not totally trustworthy

4. deduce the required statistic via a formula if other inputs are available

5. use a prior distribution to incorporate any remaining uncertainty

6. use your project team and expert advisors to agree and approve a course of action

The success of a meta-analysis depends on the quality of the study statistics that are its inputs. As Bayesian meta-analysts, you may find that you have to extract additional information from studies, even if someone else has done standard outcome extraction as part of the systematic review.

Some of the specialised models that follow in Part 3 of this book will require additional specific information, but in this chapter, we consider how to convert one statistic into another, and how to read between the lines when not enough information is given. We also share some practical tips that we have acquired over the years.

The first course of action when not enough information seems available is to contact authors and request what you need. However, it is quite common not to get results this way. People have moved, data is no longer in their possession, and so on*.

Your goal is to get the statistics you need to relate all the studies to one another. Don't drop studies just because they don't provide exactly the statistic that you wanted: meta-analysis is part of systematic review, not the other way round, so we meta-analysts must do our best to use all the studies that were included in the review. This chapter gives a collection of techniques to help with this.

If you believe that one or more studies must be dropped, this should be proposed to the rest of the project team and agreed in the larger context of the systematic review. The rationale for the decision must be fully documented.

---

*Some study authors may offer data in exchange for authorship. Be careful about this: you and your collaborators need the freedom to critique the studies in the evidence base impartially and without anyone exercising a veto.

DOI: 10.1201/9781003375821-5

Sometimes, a Bayesian meta-analysis requires more than the usual statistics at the end of the intervention or follow-up. Extracting statistics at all time points in each study can provide helpful information if the statistic you really hope to have is missing or ambiguous (see Chapter 11). Also, it is sometimes useful to model the statistics in individual arms of a study, rather than the contrasts (see Chapter 8). The most obvious example of this is network meta-analysis (see Chapter 9).

If you have individual patient data (IPD) from one or more studies, then you should be able to calculate exactly the statistic that you need (see Chapter 10). The ideas in this chapter apply when you have to work with the published statistics only ("aggregate data meta-analysis").

5.1   Practicalities

Transparency and an audit trail are key parts of meta-analysis workflow. Keep a log where you note down considerations and concerns about all the studies, plus any calculations and assumptions. Capture any thoughts or concerns about study conduct, unit of randomisation, population, baseline characteristics, or risk of bias.

Be careful to capture the units in which studies measured their data, the direction of comparisons (differences or ratios), and the definitions of denominators in percentages. These can all vary between, or even within, studies, while not obviously changing the numbers.

Efforts to improve the reproducibility of systematic reviews have produced two useful areas of work which you should be aware of. Firstly, Ivimey-Cook and colleagues have published advice on data extraction workflow and R packages to assist [124]. Secondly, Jadad and colleagues published a simple flowchart for decision-makers to compare systematic reviews and select one to guide them [128]. This is popular but has been criticised recently for lacking detailed guidance for its implementation [157].

Sometimes, one study will produce multiple papers. You should consider whether the papers analyse truly different data, or just look at the same data in different ways, for example subgroups of the participants or interim time points. Only the former really warrants inclusion of more than one paper, and we must be very careful to avoid duplication. If the same data are included in two different forms, it will bias the meta-analysis.

Studies with more than two arms—perhaps one control arm and two different intervention arms—would traditionally be included in meta-analysis by either combining the two intervention arms into one, or splitting the control and treating it as two studies [112]. You can take a more authentic approach than this by analysing the study at arm level, rather than its contrasts between arms; we discuss this in detail in Chapter 8.

You may find that some of the scales employed are interpreted in the opposite direction to others. Perhaps high values mean a good outcome in some scales and a bad outcome in others. It is up to you to reverse the sign of the mean differences so that they are consistent. In continuous outcomes, the variances and standard errors will be unchanged, so the rest of the task of standardisation still remains to be done at this point.

It takes time and effort to become familiar with a paper, to understand exactly what was done in the study. We suggest allowing plenty of time to read and extract statistics, and to add any observations that might be useful to your data extraction log. It is better to take longer than expected on one study before moving on to the next, than to rush and then have to return to it later. Once you have moved on, you will probably find (if you are like Robert and Gian Luca) that you forget the details quickly and have to repeat the effort of reading and understanding, which will be wasted time and energy[†].

5.1.1 Avoiding transcription errors

When extracting statistics, you will almost certainly make notes on paper and then type some of those numbers into your software. It is crucial to minimise human error at that stage. Here are some of the practical ideas that we use:

1. write differences (from baseline, or between arms, or both) with a + sign or a − sign; the same can apply to logarithms of ratios or any other value that might be positive or negative

2. write a confidence interval with the word "to" in the middle, not a dash, which could be mistaken for a minus sign

3. when you are writing in a table, draw a horizontal line after every third line; this helps you not to slide between lines by mistake as you look left and right

You may also choose ways to modify your handwriting when transcribing, to avoid confusion, for example between 5 and S, 1 and l, 0 (zero) and O (upper-case o), 7 and 1, and so on.

How many decimal places are relevant? Sometimes, a paper may report a statistic to many more decimal places than the original data could ever have. For example, systolic blood pressure is only ever recorded in integers, usually units of millimeters of mercury (mmHg). Summary statistics such as the mean could have many decimal places, though more than one or two is *spurious precision*, and there is nothing gained from feeding it into your meta-analysis. When you are rounding off decimal places, remember to round up for 5 or greater, and down otherwise: for example, 114.33591 mmHg becomes 114.3359 or 114.336 or 114.34 or 114.3 or just 114 mmHg.

5.1.2 Checking

"One thing we regretfully learn about work with numbers is the need for checking. Late-caught errors make for painful repetition of steps we thought finished".—John Tukey, "Exploratory Data Analysis", p.10 (1977) [261]

Ideally, you should use *double-extraction*, where two people independently extract statistics and then check and correct any disagreements. This reduces errors substantially [36]. In one study, single-extraction and double-extraction differed in some way in 28% of papers, with the differences in statistics of particular variables varying between 17% and 78% of papers [31].

This perhaps reflects both the ease with which subtle details can be missed or misunderstood, and also the surprising extent to which somewhat subjective judgements are required in systematic reviews. The fact that some variables appear to be inherently harder to interpret at the point of extraction is also both a useful warning to systematic reviewers and meta-analysts and a reassurance that we are all working in a difficult setting, and we will sometimes make mistakes, regardless of experience. Reproducibility and transparency are especially important in these situations.

[†]Robert's former colleagues, carrying out systematic reviews for UK health service guidelines in the 2000s, would plan to complete two papers per day: one in the morning and one in the afternoon. Robert was the project manager as well as statistician and so would often urge them to go faster, which they wisely resisted. Taking your time and getting a deep understanding of the evidence base is very valuable.

After standardisation

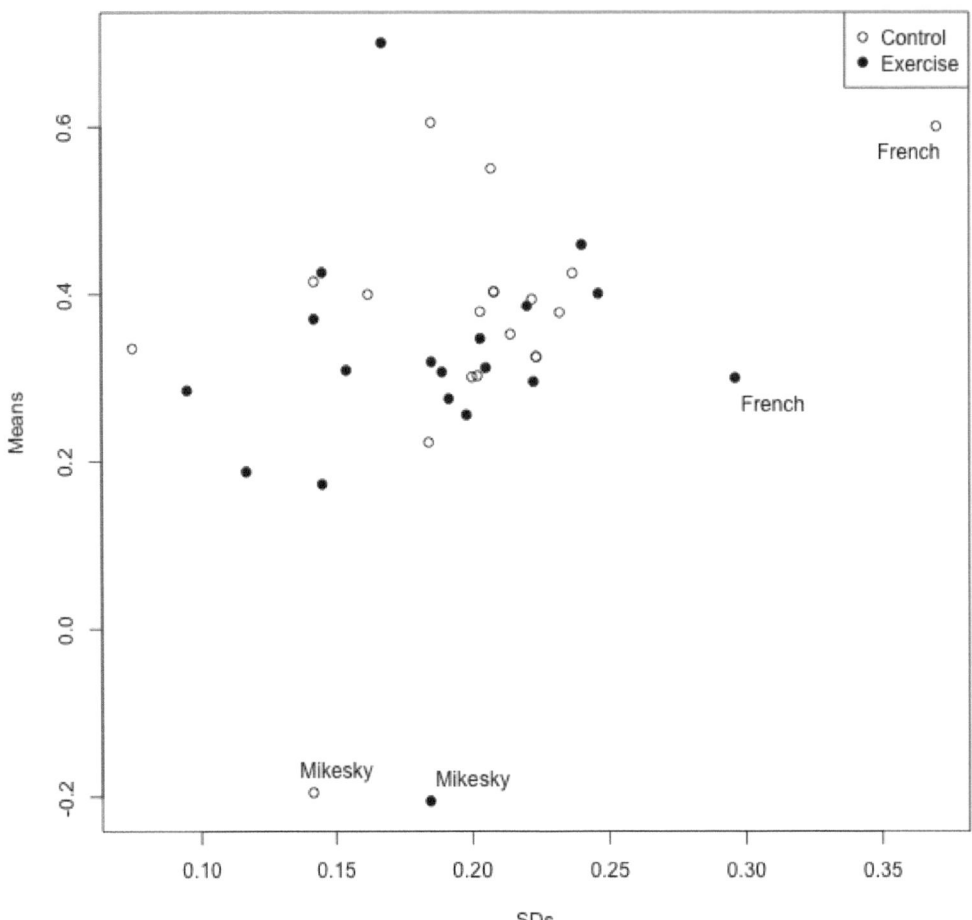

FIGURE 5.1

Arm means and standard deviations for the meta-analysis of exercise and osteoarthritis pain; this is a transformed preliminary extraction of data, not the version of the data used in the final review.

We would like to emphasise this message: if you are not sure how to interpret a particular published statistic, it is not your fault. Publications should be unambiguous and give enough detail to be reproducible. Note the problem, discuss it with the project team and advisors, and ask the authors if possible.

It is also important to pause to think about what the numbers really mean: what they stand for. When extracting statistics at scale, it is easy to fall into a kind of autopilot mindset, where any number is copied down without curiosity about how trustworthy it might be.

It can be helpful to plot the statistics from all studies, all arms or all timepoints, to look for any unexpected discrepancies, where one study does not match the pattern of the others. In Figure 5.1, we show all the means and standard deviations of standardised pain scales (from 0 to 1, with a higher meaning worse pain), from each arm of each study in the osteoarthritis meta-analysis [119].

This shows two unusual points (arising from the same study by Mikesky and colleagues [170]) at the bottom, with impossible negative means. There are also two unusual points on the right with outlier standard deviations (arising from the same study by French and colleagues [78]). This helps us to identify papers that require deeper investigation. The values may be correct, but even so, we might decide that the papers are not comparable with the others, and either exclude or subgroup them.

In this case, the Mikesky *et al* statistics [170] turned out to be an extraction error: we had recorded changes from baseline rather than the pain score at the end of the intervention. This was easily corrected. The French *et al* study [78] required closer consideration and team discussion; the most likely reason was that the outcome scale was pain on exertion, rather than overall assessment of pain in daily life. It seems reasonable that there will be greater intra-arm variability in this. It is then a judgement call to say whether this makes the results comparable enough for inclusion; we felt it did, and retained the statistics as they stand.

Sometimes, the fault for the wrong number belongs with the authors of the papers, not us meta-analysts. Identifying that there is a problem is technically challenging, and the decision on how to act requires the input of the whole study team and advisors. An example will clarify some of the issues.

Among the osteoarthritis papers, in an open-access account of a randomised controlled trial of tai chi, by Wang and colleagues [273], there is a likely typographic error, though it is not obvious at first. In their Table 1, the means and standard deviations of the WOMAC* pain scale are shown along with other outcomes and demographics at baseline. Note that baseline statistics are not those shown in Figure 5.1. The version of WOMAC used in this study produced values from 0 (no pain) to 500 (maximum pain).

At baseline, the tai chi arm had a mean of 209.3, and a standard deviation of 58.5, while the control arm had a mean of 220.4 and a standard deviation of 101.0. The difference between the standard deviations is considerable, but each arm had only 20 participants. Other outcomes did not have such large differences in standard deviations. Graphs of the means with error bars ($\pm$ standard deviation) did not show any noticeable difference between arms' standard deviations at baseline (see Figure 3 in the paper, which we reproduce here as Figure 5.2 [273]). Is the table or the graph correct? We investigate those graphs further in Section 5.5.1, where we find that there are still more surprises about this paper.

It seems plausible that the figure in the table is a typo. Instead of 58.5, perhaps it should be 85.5? There is no way of knowing for sure. In Section 5.5.1, we consider replacing it with a prior distribution based on the graphs in the paper. Another approach would be to do a sensitivity analysis with some alternative values. Yet another is to discuss it in the project team or with subject expert advisors, choose one value, and document the reason carefully. However you approach such problems, the decision and other relevant information must be written down in your data extraction log. Remember also to contact authors if you can.

Another reason to be cautious is that studies do not always report methods perfectly. In an RCT of stem cell transfer after heart attack [132], published in a prominent medical journal, the authors calculate means (of left ventricular ejection fraction, a measure of heart function) in the two arms, divide one by another, and then describe it as an *odds ratio*. All twenty-one authors seem to have been quite certain about this, as it is repeated in the methods, results, tables and even the abstract. These results were appropriately re-calculated as a mean difference in left ventricular ejection fraction by two meta-analyses [44, 284].

---

*Western Ontario and McMaster knee and hip osteoarthritis index: `https://www.womac.com/womac/`

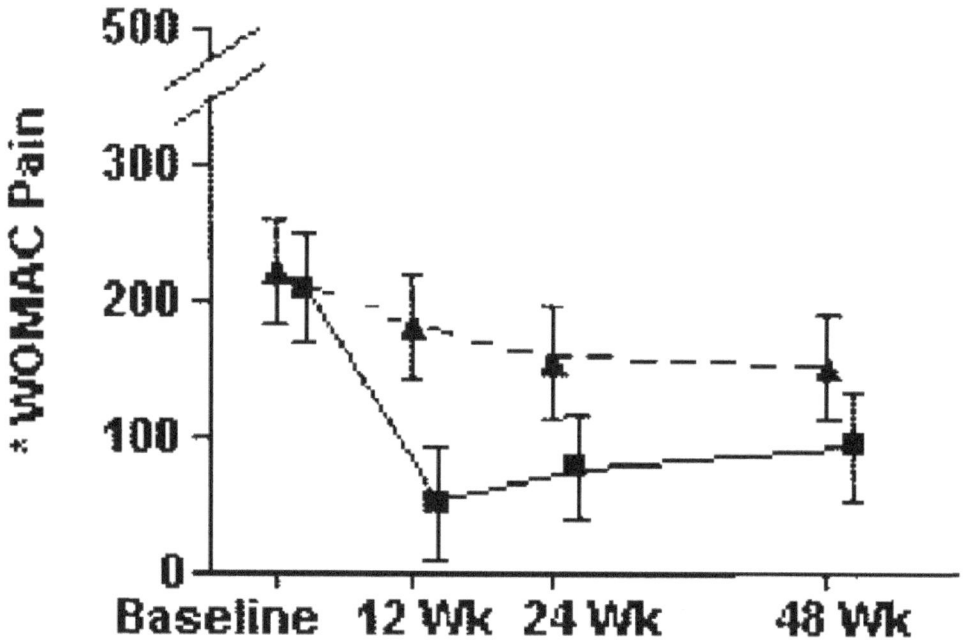

FIGURE 5.2
Enlarged detail of Figure 3 from Wang *et al* [273]. Square markers indicate the tai chi group
and triangles indicate the control group. The pixelation seen here is from the original image
even in the digital paper. (Reproduced with permission of John Wiley and Sons, Inc.)

If a study has produced multiple publications, even if you have not included all the papers, it is often fruitful to examine them all for any helpful insights. However, contradictions
can also come to light in this way [76], creating even more questions.

5.2   Selecting Study Statistics

It is not always obvious which statistics to extract for the purpose of meta-analysis. A study
may have used multiple outcome measures for the same underlying concept, for example.

A very important consideration is to make the study statistics as comparable as possible
in terms of PICO (see Section 3.1).

Studies should either all assess efficacy via a per protocol analysis, or effectiveness via
an intention to treat analysis. If there has been some covariate adjustment, by regression,
weighting or stratification, then this should be as comparable as possible between the studies.

A useful way of thinking about the compatibility of these studies is in terms of their
estimands. These are the quantities which they were attempting to estimate. Per protocol

and intention to treat analyses are discussed, along with other estimand differences, in Chapter 16.

Consider the time scale over which you want to assess the intervention or risk factor. Extract the statistics closest to that time scale, bearing in mind that "end of intervention" or "final follow-up" can mean very different things in different studies. You may choose to set aside some studies from meta-analysis (though not narrative review) if they cannot provide comparable time points. As stated above, any such decision to exclude a reviewed paper from the meta-analysis needs to be discussed and agreed by the whole review team. However, the possibility remains of conducting multiple meta-analyses for multiple time points, or of estimating a time-response curve (see Chapter 17).

Studies may report change from baseline or statistics at a particular time point. If there is enough information, you may be able to convert one into the other (see Section 5.3), to keep study statistics comparable. However, it is also possible to use the mixture of these statistics after standardisation. It can also be argued that the contrast between arms of the studies is comparable in either method, assuming that there has been no gross covariate imbalances, or failure of allocation concealment in RCTs, so if you are comfortable with this, document the decision and treat the statistics together.

We have mostly discussed randomised controlled trials up to this point. These have the benefit to the trialist of an easily obtained causal estimate. They also have the benefit to the meta-analyst of a simple model, because the arm statistics are independent of each other, and the observations are independent of each other too.

Not every study design has these advantages [274]. Cluster randomised trials have independence (in theory, at least) between clusters and arms, but not necessarily between participants. Crossover trials use the same participant in both arms. Stepped wedge trials and related designs do this too at the level of clusters. Quantitative study design is a complex and evolving field, which we can only begin to consider in the scope of this book.

5.3 Converting One Statistic into Another

When the statistic that a study reported is not exactly what you want, you can use formulas to convert it. For example, we know that the 95% confidence interval of a sample mean $\bar{y}$ with standard error $\widehat{SE}(\bar{y})$ has lower and upper limits given by:

$$
\begin{aligned}
LCI(\bar{y}) &= \bar{y} - 1.96\widehat{SE}(\bar{y}) \\
UCI(\bar{y}) &= \bar{y} + 1.96\widehat{SE}(\bar{y})
\end{aligned}
\tag{5.1}
$$

(see Section 1.2.1).

If a study reports the estimate and the confidence interval, but we need the standard error for our meta-analysis, then we should reverse the formula:

$$
\widehat{SE}(\bar{y}) = \frac{UCI(\bar{y}) - LCI(\bar{y})}{3.92}
\tag{5.2}
$$

Every formula comes with some assumptions, and some of them are quite rough approximations. In general, let sensitivity analysis guide your decisions on when to trust an approximate formula.

A general procedure could follow these steps:

1. identify what statistic you can obtain

2. find the formula for calculating it

3. if you have all the inputs, except the statistic you need, rearrange it algebraically

4. if not, can you justifiably assume a value? or do a simple sensitivity analysis?

5. some statistics are loosely related to others, though not through a formula that pins it down precisely (in mathematics, these are called one-to-one mappings)— we consider such a case next, relating the standard deviation to the inter-quartile range

6. alternatively, consider imputing the required statistic from an opinion prior; sometimes, we can specify a conditional distribution given other unknowns, and we follow this approach in Chapter 11.

The Cochrane handbook has advice on converting statistics in a wide range of situations, though they do not encompass Bayesian methods; we explain the important techniques here. Some conversion functionality is available in the R function `meta::metagen`.

A different situation arises when all studies summarise the data adequately, but not using the same statistics, for example if some studies report mean change in a depression scale, and others define some participants as "responders" to treatment. This situation is dealt with in Chapter 14.

5.3.1 One-to-one mappings

We saw above how the standard error and the confidence interval are related directly, given the observed mean, through a formula for a one-to-one mapping. As long as you have some understanding of rearranging algebra, you can manipulate such formulas into the direction that you need for your meta-analysis. We list some more one-to-one mappings in this section.

5.3.1.1 Arm-based statistics and contrasts

Arm-specific statistics are sometimes desired, either for a specific model, or because it is what the software requires. At other times, the contrast between arms is needed. When the contrast is given, and only one of the individual arm statistics, you can subtract (in the case of a difference), or divide (in the case of a ratio), to obtain the missing arm statistic. To illustrate this, suppose we are given an odds ratio ($\hat{\theta}_j$) and a proportion in the intervention arm ($\hat{p}_{j\mathbf{Int}}$), but need the proportion in the control arm:

$$\hat{\omega}_{j\mathbf{Int}} = \frac{\hat{p}_{j\mathbf{Int}}}{1 - \hat{p}_{j\mathbf{Int}}}$$

$$\hat{\theta}_j = \frac{\hat{\omega}_{j\mathbf{Int}}}{\hat{\omega}_{j\mathbf{Ctl}}}$$

$$\therefore \hat{\omega}_{j\mathbf{Ctl}} = \frac{\hat{\omega}_{j\mathbf{Int}}}{\hat{\theta}_j} \tag{5.3}$$

$$\therefore \hat{p}_{j\mathbf{Ctl}} = \frac{\hat{\omega}_{j\mathbf{Ctl}}}{1 + \hat{\omega}_{j\mathbf{Ctl}}}$$

Remember that, if you are given a *log* odds ratio, logarithms are traditionally to base $e \approx 2.718$, which is the `ln` function in pocket scientific calculators. If you are unsure what base a `log` function uses in your software, you can try `log(2.718)`. If it is to base e, you will get a number very close to 1.

5.3.1.2 Arm-based and contrast standard deviations and standard errors

When arms are independent of one another, for example in a randomised controlled trial, we can apply Equation 1.12 to add or subtract variances.

When there is some correlation, for example in paired arms[†], then we must use Equation 1.15 instead.

It requires knowledge of the correlation between the arms, r_j, and sadly, this is rare in study reports and papers. Sometimes, other information allows us to reverse-engineer it somehow. We consider some of these techniques, but if we cannot calculate it, Bayesian analysis allows us to plug in a probability distribution for the missing correlation instead, and thereby acknowledge the uncertainty.

The prior may be based on expert opinion, the distribution of correlations in the known studies, or a conditional distribution given other statistics, such as we consider in Section 5.3.2. As correlations can take a value between -1 and $+1$, but we usually have reason to strongly expect it to be positive or negative, you could use a truncated distribution such as the normal (in BUGS):

```
corr ~ dnorm(0.5,1)I(-1,1)
for(j in 1:m) {
  mean_diff[j] <- mean_int[j] - mean_ctl[j]
  sd_diff[j] <- sqrt(sd_int[j]*sd_int[j] +
                sd_ctl[j]*sd_ctl[j] -
                2*sd_int[j]*sd_ctl[j]*corr)
}
```

Alternatively, you could fix it as positive or negative and use a beta distribution, or instead compute a transformed version of it (Equation 5.4) and apply the prior to that. This function is the inverse hyperbolic tangent, also known as Fisher's z-transformation.

$$\frac{1}{2} \log \left(\frac{1 + r_j}{1 - r_j} \right) \tag{5.4}$$

5.3.1.3 Pooled standard deviation

In a meta-analysis of a continuous outcome, the pooled standard deviation, $s_{j\bullet}$ (Equation 3.1), will be required. Calculating it requires the arm-specific standard deviations, and the arm-specific sample sizes. Priors could be used to replace any one of these if they are unavailable (see Chapter 11).

Conversely, if arm-specific standard deviations are required, but the pooled standard deviation is available, the challenge is to know how to split it into arms. You could assume equality, or use a prior for one arm and then determine the other from that.

If the pooled standard deviation is required, but no arm-specific standard deviations are given, you might calculate it from a t-test statistic, if that is given. One formula for the

---

[†]An example of paired data in RCTs occurs when participants have one of a pair of organs, or one side of the body, receive the treatment first. Identical twins are also sought-after in epidemiological risk factor studies for this reason.

t-statistic to compare two arm means is:

$$t_j = \frac{\bar{y}_{j\text{Int}} - \bar{y}_{j\text{Ctl}}}{s_{j\bullet}\sqrt{\frac{1}{n_{j\text{Int}}} + \frac{1}{n_{j\text{Ctl}}}}}$$

(5.5)

$$\therefore s_{j\bullet} = \frac{\bar{y}_{j\text{Int}} - \bar{y}_{j\text{Ctl}}}{t_j\sqrt{\frac{1}{n_{j\text{Int}}} + \frac{1}{n_{j\text{Ctl}}}}}$$

This formula does not make the assumption of "equal variances" and can be used regardless of arm-specific standard deviations or sample sizes. It may not be the formula used by the trialists, but reversing it will produce a figure of $s_{j\bullet}$ that can be used for meta-analysis of contrasts.

In the absence of information on sample sizes for each arm, it is often a justifiable approximation to assume equal sizes.

5.3.1.4 Change from baseline

Change from baseline is related to the statistics at baseline and end of intervention or follow up, along with the correlation between time points, using Equation 1.15. See Section 11.5.1 if conversion is not possible.

5.3.1.5 Standardised mean differences and effect sizes

The standardised mean difference (SMD) is typically a mean difference between arms, divided by the pooled (intra-arm) standard deviation. This expresses the difference in units of standard deviations.

The motivation for using SMDs is that different outcome scales, measuring the same underlying construct, will all be brought onto one shared scale, enabling quantitative comparisons. However, it can be difficult to justify the assumption that the various scales used in the evidence base, after simple arithmetic manipulation, will be comparable.

SMDs are one particular case of an *effect size*. Effect size statistics are popular in some disciplines (such as psychology) more than others, and have perhaps increased in popularity in recent years, as part of a wide movement against statistical significance or p-values [275, 192].

If a study with continuous outcomes only reports an effect size, you may still be able to use it as a measure of standardised mean difference. There are many effect size statistics that have been proposed, including among the most popular for continuous outcomes: Cohen's d, Hedges' g, and Glass' Δ. For binary outcomes, there are also measures based on the chi-squared statistic, such as Cramér's V [24]. The popularity of these effect sizes varies greatly between fields, and they are particularly common in psychology research [145].

If you do not want to use standardised mean differences, you can rearrange the equation if the other inputs are known. Formulas for these effect size statistics are easily found online.

5.3.1.6 Dichotomised continuous outcomes

Some studies, especially in medicine, make the mistake of splitting continuous-valued outcomes into "responders" and "non-responders", then proceeding to odds ratios or risk ratios in terms of this dichotomised binary variable [102]. Where you clearly have some studies reporting the continuous variable, and others reporting the same variable dichotomised, you should preferably extract the continuous value statistics such as the mean and standard deviation.

When this is not possible, extract all the available statistics, and relate the two likelihoods to each other (see Chapter 14). To do this, it is important to extract from any dichotomising studies what thresholds they set, and how they were calculated. They can be classified into three types [95]:

1. absolute threshold: above or below a value of the outcome after intervention

2. relative-difference threshold: above or below a difference from baseline to after intervention

3. relative-ratio threshold: above or below a ratio between baseline and after intervention

A case study showed a number of complex and ambiguous threshold definitions in published RCTs [95], so you should read papers carefully and identify the thresholds. This is discussed in full in Chapter 14.

There are several approximations to convert an odds ratio to a standardised mean difference, and *vice versa*. These have largely been evaluated in terms of the bias and variance of their point estimates, and found to be acceptably accurate [50]. However, the standard errors can easily be shown by simulation to be quite inadequate. Example R code is given on the website. Therefore, we cannot recommend using any of these simple conversions for Bayesian meta-analysis.

5.3.1.7 Other epidemiologic statistics

In the context of a two-arm study reporting a binary outcome, all data can be drawn in a two-by-two table, and this table can be summarised into a single statistic in many different ways. Some that are popular in epidemiology for communication will not be useful for meta-analysis, and should be converted to a log odds ratio instead. We must assume here that the entire two-by-two table, comprising:

1. $p_{j\mathbf{Ctl}}$ and $p_{j\mathbf{Int}}$, the *risks* or proportions in the control and intervention arms respectively

2. $n_{j\mathbf{Ctl}}$ and $n_{j\mathbf{Int}}$, the sample sizes

is not provided, otherwise you can simply calculate the log odds ratio and its standard error directly instead (see Equations 1.17 and 1.18).

In the statistics that follow, both ns and one of the ps would be required to derive the log odds ratio and its standard error. As described above, we might also use a prior on one of the ps and then derive the other.

The *absolute risk reduction* is:

$$p_{j\mathbf{Ctl}} - p_{j\mathbf{Int}} \tag{5.6}$$

The *number needed to treat* (or *number needed to harm*, depending on the context) is:

$$\frac{1}{p_{j\mathbf{Ctl}} - p_{j\mathbf{Int}}} \tag{5.7}$$

The *risk ratio*, or relative risk,, which we introduced in Chapter 1, is:

$$\frac{p_{j\mathbf{Int}}}{p_{j\mathbf{Ctl}}} \tag{5.8}$$

The *relative risk reduction* (sometimes this is called the *preventable risk fraction*) is:

$$\frac{p_j\text{Ctl} - p_j\text{Int}}{p_j\text{Ctl}} = 1 - \frac{p_j\text{Int}}{p_j\text{Ctl}} \tag{5.9}$$

This can also be evaluated as a relative risk increase, when it is sometimes called the *attributable risk fraction*:

$$\frac{p_j\text{Int} - p_j\text{Ctl}}{p_j\text{Int}} = 1 - \frac{p_j\text{Ctl}}{p_j\text{Int}} \tag{5.10}$$

It is worth bearing in mind that the names of some of these epidemiologic statistics imply causal interpretation, which may not be justified, unless the studies were designed to support it (see Chapter 16). More recent developments may give similar-sounding measures of attributable or preventable risk, yet not arise from these formulas [110].

5.3.2   Medians and quartiles: an example of loosely associated statistics

Studies reporting a median and quartiles, or inter-quartile range (IQR: the difference between the 75th centile and the 25th centile), can be converted to mean and standard deviation with some assumed distribution shape for the participant level data. However, we should be cautious here: one of the reasons why scientists use medians and quartiles is precisely because their data were not normally distributed.

Sometimes, we can be quite confident about the distribution of the participant data. Blood pressure, for example, is well-known to have a normal distribution. You should look for external data and references that support such an assumption, and ask expert advisors in the field.

In a normal distribution, the bottom 25% of the data should lie below $\mu - 0.6745\sigma$, and the top 25% above $\mu + 0.6745\sigma$. This means that the IQR should be 1.349σ. You can find these with quantile functions, such as `qnorm` in R, `invnormal` in Stata, or indeed a book of statistical tables [176].

Remember, however, that studies are often not performed in the general population. A study reporting a blood pressure measurement might recruit participants who have been recommended some intervention to lower their blood pressure. It might also have a hard lower limit to blood pressure for recruitment. The resulting distribution at the end of the intervention, or at follow-up, is hard to predict, but it is unlikely to be normal, and more likely to be positively skewed.

A further caveat comes from small sample sizes. The conversion above will be approximate for small n_{jk}. A small simulation experiment can provide us with the sampling distribution of the conversion factor (IQR/SD) between the observed IQR and the observed standard deviation. This shows that, even in normally distributed data, the conversion factor is biased downward in small sample sizes. The variance of the sampling distribution grows with smaller sample sizes, as we would expect, but there is also slight negative skewness too, notable for $n < 20$.

Here is some R code to simulate normal data and compute their IQRs, repeatedly. We can then estimate the bias, variance and skewness of the sampling distribution of the conversion factor $\frac{IQR(x)}{SD(x)}$. this then gives us an idea of the uncertainty inherent in the conversion, which we might try to capture in our Bayesian model.

TABLE 5.1

An example of statistics of a sampling distribution of a conversion factor, in this case IQR/SD, from 1,000,000 simulations with each sample size and data from $N(0, 1)$.

n_{jk}	Mean	SD	Skewness
10	1.2048	0.3173	-0.2367
20	1.2746	0.2486	-0.0836
30	1.2986	0.2120	-0.0967
40	1.3107	0.1868	-0.0632
50	1.3185	0.1694	-0.0699
60	1.3235	0.1554	-0.0482
70	1.3272	0.1447	-0.0554
80	1.3300	0.1358	-0.0368

```
iter <- 1000000
ns <- seq(from=10, to=80, by=10) # sample sizes
nns <- length(ns)
conversions <- matrix(NA,nrow=nns,ncol=iter)

for(i in 1:nns) {
        for(j in 1:iter) {
                x <- rnorm(ns[i], 0, 1)
                conversions[i,j] <- IQR(x)/sd(x)
        }
}

bias_conversion <- apply(conversions, 1,
                    function(z) {mean(z)-1.349})
sd_conversion <- apply(conversions, 1, sd)
skew_conversion <- apply(conversions, 1,
        function(z){ mean(((z-mean(z))/sd(z))^3) })
```

Table 5.1 shows the means and standard deviations obtained from the simulation study. Given the fairly small skewnesses, we could use a normal distribution to represent the uncertainty around a study arm's standard deviation, given the IQR. If we have a study reporting IQRs with $n_{jk} = 20$, we should use a prior distribution for the standard deviation of:

$$s_{jk} \sim N\left(\frac{IQR_{jk}}{1.2746}, 0.2486\frac{IQR_{jk}}{1.2746}\right) \tag{5.11}$$

Note how the sampling standard deviation of 0.2486 is for a data standard deviation of 1, so in practice we must inflate it proportionally to the estimated data standard deviation.

This approach can be used with a wide range of data distributions and conversions between observed statistics, even when no statistical theory has been published on the particular subject. Remember that your goal is to estimate the observed (but unreported) standard deviation, not the population standard deviation.

You should also consider how many simulations are needed for precision [173]. With 1,000,000 data from $N(0, 1)$, we can expect a Monte Carlo error (see Section 2.5.2) for the means of $\frac{1}{\sqrt{1,000,000}} = 0.001$, which seems acceptable in this context. However, it will be larger for the standard deviations and larger still for the skewnesses, which are based on the sums of data squared and cubed, respectively, thus inflating any error. The skewness figures in Table 5.1 do not increase monotonically, probably as result of this error, though they give a rough impression of the scale of the problem.

The same logic we used with quartiles can be applied to any quantile of an assumed distributional shape. However, you should be cautious about using the range, or minimum and maximum, which are frequently reported. These extreme values may have been changed a great deal within the study by excluding outliers, and you might not necessarily agree with those cleaning decisions, though papers and reports might not provide any evidence that it happened. Also, the theory relating them to the population is not as simple as we have seen above for IQRs.

5.4   Using Priors in Lieu of Statistics

We discuss the question of unreported statistics in depth in Chapter 11, but in this chapter, there is a specific need for priors as part of the extraction process. These might form part of the calculation for the statistic that we really need, or its standard error.

We will present an example with statistics for a continuous-valued variable. The problem is expanded further in Chapter 11, including when the statistic is discrete valued, probably a count.

As an example, consider the conversion from change from baseline ($\bar{y}_{jk1} - \bar{y}_{jk0}$) to mean at end of intervention ($\bar{y}_{jk1}$), in Section 5.3.1.4. If you have every part of the calculation except the correlation between baseline and end of intervention outcomes (including `sd_change_int[j]`, `sd_baseline_int[j]`), then the correlation will be drawn from a prior, and used to calculate the end of intervention outcomes. BUGS code will look something like this:

```
corr ~ dbeta(4,2)
var_change_int[j] <- sd_change_int[j] * sd_change_int[j]
var_baseline_int[j] <- sd_baseline_int[j] * sd_baseline_int[j]
var_end_int[j] <- var_change_int[j] -
                  var_baseline_int[j] +
                  2 * sd_change_int[j] *
                      sd_baseline_int[j] *
                      corr
sd_end_int[j] <- sqrt(var_end_int[j])
```

This applies a rearranged version of Equation 1.15. You may gain more understanding from comparing it with the code in Section 5.3.1.2. The intervention arm is shown, and the control arm would be a copy of all but the first two lines. The beta distribution enforces a positive correlation and has a slight preference for strong correlations*. We are also applying

---

*This prior is used here to illustrate the process and code; it is *not* recommended in general, and you should consider each prior you use in context. For most evidence bases, this prior will inject too much uncertainty, because other studies will provide information about the correlation that you should expect.

the same correlation to all arms and studies, though we have little choice in that. If some studies provide information about the correlation, see Chapter 11.

5.5 Reconstructing a Statistic

5.5.1 Getting numbers from graphs

Graphs in publications often give away a surprising amount of information. You may be able to use them to obtain the required statistic, or to clarify a point of ambiguity. Dotplots with error bars, scatterplots, Kaplan-Meier charts and line charts are all potentially useful in this technique.

Some generic software exists to extract data values from graphics, including graphreader (`http://www.graphreader.com`), PlotDigitizer (`https://plotdigitizer.com`) and Web-PlotDigitizer (`https://automeris.io/WebPlotDigitizer.html`). However, we recommend doing it manually, for safety. It is important to be able to observe and check every step of the process.

We recommend that you take a screenshot of the graph and open it in any raster graphics editor software, such as Microsoft Paint (which is part of all Windows installations), GIMP (which is free) or Photoshop. The task will be to identify the pixel numbers where points of interest lie. Be aware that some software counts vertical pixels from 0 at the top, downwards.

A worked example will help to clarify the process, using graphics from the osteoarthritis study mentioned above, by Wang *et al* [273], which is open-access. We want to compare the standard deviation of WOMAC pain scores at baseline between their Table 1 and their Figure 3. We saved the screenshot of the top left panel of their Figure 3, which shows mean ± standard deviation as markers and error bars, for the tai chi and control groups, at baseline, 12, 24 and 48 weeks. This was a PNG file of 864 by 634 pixels, but the original image in the paper was low-resolution and added additional pixelation (see Figure 5.2).

The horizontal axis was well-aligned with the horizontal in the file and no rotation was needed. We used GIMP (GNU Image Manipulation Program, `https://www.gimp.org/`, a freeware image editor) to obtain vertical pixel numbers (counting downward from the top) for the vertical axis ticks at WOMAC 0 and 300. These were 560 and 224 pixels respectively. Any vertical pixel number, x, in that range can be converted to a WOMAC pain score by:

$$300\frac{560 - x}{560 - 224} \tag{5.12}$$

```
pixel2womac <- function(x) { 300*(560-x)/(560-224) }
```

Note that the numerator is $560 - x$ and not $x - 560$ because the pixel numbers count downward from the top. The edges of the tai chi baseline marker were at pixels 316 and 334, meaning that the WOMAC score is somewhere between 202 and 218, plausibly at the midpoint of 210 [†].

[†]This measures the top and bottom of the square or triangle in the graph, but close examination of the lines, which presumably join the exact locations of the true point estimates, suggests that they do not pass through the centre of those markers. Neither the paper nor the protocol name the software used for statistical analysis (though sometimes graphs are made in other packages anyway). At this level of convolution, even we lose interest in this detective work.

The error bars extended to T-shaped terminals, each about 4 pixels high. The top covered pixels 278 to 282, and the bottom 367 to 371. Taking the midpoint for each, we find the mean plus standard deviation was 250, suggesting a standard deviation of 40. The mean minus standard deviation was 171, suggesting a standard deviation of 39.

Their Table 1 cited a standard deviation of 58.5 for the tai chi group, which seemed small in comparison to others, but now, having examined the graph in detail, we find it is not implausible any more. Instead, the control group standard deviation, reported as 101.0 in their Table 1, looks implausible, considering how similar the two groups' error bars look in their Figure 3. There are many twists and turns as we scrutinise published papers closely.

5.5.2   Deducing integers

If a study reports counts but leaves one out that you need, you may be able to deduce it, or at least pin it down to within a narrow range. This builds on the idea that a proportion, or percentage, is a numerator over a denominator. If we need the numerator (for example), and we are often given the denominator (the sample size) and a percentage, then we can work out the numerator.

For small denominators, the percentage identifies the numerator exactly: only one natural number is compatible. But as the denominator grows, and the percentage is rounded off, there may be more than one candidate.

Suppose the denominator is $n_{jk} = 205$, and we are given a percentage of 11%. We can see that all the percentages in the paper are rounded off to integers, so we can be confident that the numerator we seek produced a percentage between 10.5% and 11.4999...%.

There are two candidates, 22 (leading to 10.73%) and 23 (11.22%). You must then decide whether this could really influence the results enough to warrant inclusion with a prior. When findings of the meta-analysis are close to some decision-making threshold, any small difference is worth incorporating. This and other issues of unreported counts are explored in Section 11.4.

6

Eliciting Priors

Learning objectives

After reading this chapter, you will be able to:

1. understand the process of eliciting priors and its use

2. decide whether eliciting expert priors would be useful for your work

3. choose and justify a method for elicitation and conversion

4. explain to experts what information they need to provide

5. convert the information provided into a prior distribution

6. recognise when to call on a statistician for more advice in fitting a distribution to the expert opinions

---

Expert opinion can be usefully employed in Bayesian analysis, and meta-analysis is no different. Sometimes, the goal of the analysis is to estimate expert opinion in the light of new data, and updating an expert opinion prior into an expert opinion posterior provides this. It is also possible to work with a prior that represents a panel of experts, either by averaging, consensus, or some other more esoteric methods. This chapter addresses the task of obtaining expert opinion prior distributions and preparing them for use in your Bayesian meta-analyses.

6.1 When to Use Expert Opinion Priors

The posterior will be influenced by both the likelihood and the prior. If the likelihood is more concentrated in a narrow range of values, perhaps because there are many observations in the data, then the prior will have comparatively little influence.

In a meta-analysis, if there are many studies, each quite large in sample size, then the prior for treatment effect or heterogeneity variance will not matter much. However, some unknowns might still have limited information, such as treatment effect differences between subgroups, and they will benefit the most from informative priors.

When information is limited, an expert opinion is worth considering. This chapter describes the methods needed to elicit those opinions and convert them into a useful probability density which can be used in a Bayesian model.

We must acknowledge that you will sometimes encounter people who are highly sceptical about prior distributions, and fearful that results might be manipulated by them. Setting

---

out on a career in Bayesian statistics can seem so dominated by this antagonism that it is surprising we got to page 147 before mentioning it.

The attitudes towards opinion priors differ greatly between professions, specialisms and fields of study. This does not seem related to attitudes to Bayes in general. In machine learning, for example, Bayesian thinking is common, but opinion priors are unfashionable.

The decision to use these priors is one that you should take with all the collaborators on a project, and you should document the rationale for it carefully. You will almost certainly be challenged about it at some point. This does not mean you should avoid expert opinion priors, but it does mean that you are responsible for justifying your decisions. It is the Bayesian analyst's duty to be transparent and clearly describe the use of priors and sensitivity analysis.

We will discuss mostly probability *density* functions (PDFs) in this chapter—that is to say, continuous-valued unknowns—as that is the most common target for eliciting opinions. Discrete and categorical unknowns have probability *mass* functions (PMFs) instead, but once you understand the principle for PDFs, it can be applied simply to PMFs; in fact, eliciting priors for discrete-valued unknowns is even easier.

6.2   Eliciting One Person's Opinion

We will consider working with one expert first. The analyst's goal is to obtain a prior probability density function. Whatever is fed into your software as a prior must match the definition of a probability density function, notably that the area under the curve should be 1. The simplest way to achieve this is to use one of the standard families of probability densities, such as the normal distribution, the gamma, beta, log-normal and so on.

Suppose we want to ask our expert advisor for their opinion about the treatment effect for a new drug. Treatment effects, as a mean, should in theory have a normal prior, and that will be completely specified by the mean and standard deviation. The expert will probably not be able to give us a mean and standard deviation straight away. Instead, they might be able to answer some questions about how they feel about the probability of various treatment effect values. Our task will then be to convert those answers into a mean and standard deviation.

There are some different ways that we can ask the expert for these probabilities. We will look at one as an example, but the general principle should be to use a consistent and systematic method for all the unknowns and all the experts. There are some established and peer-reviewed frameworks for this, which we can confidently regard as validated.

There are problems in human judgement that will induce bias and introduce noise to any elicitation of expert opinions. A book by O'Hagan and colleagues details many of these issues and the elicitation methods that try to minimise them [180]. A central consideration is that the order in which the questions are asked can influence (subconsciously) the expert's response, and this has been shown in psychological research.

A simple order of questions could be determined by starting with the domain of the unknown: the interval in which we assume it must lie. Some unknowns, like proportions, have *hard constraints* to the domain, and we should choose a distribution accordingly. For example, a proportion can never, ever go outside [0, 1], and it would not make sense to elicit a distribution such as a normal without truncating it.

Others may have *soft constraints* that we can apply in order to fit a more plausible probability distribution. For example, we can confidently state that the effect of a vaccine is either zero or to decrease the incidence of the disease*, but we cannot be so certain as to forbid the computer from trying out a proposed value that increases the incidence. We should choose a prior distribution that allows negative values, even if we then make them improbable.

Having defined the domain, we can ask questions that recursively bisect it. An example shows this most clearly:

1. Give a value that splits the probability into a 50% chance of the true value being above it, and 50% below it

2. If the true value must be *below* this, give a value that splits the probability again (this is the 25th centile)

3. If the true value must be *above* this, give a value that splits the probability again (this is the 75th centile)

4. ...and so on, if you feel confident in the reliability of the judgements, to obtain 12.5, 37.5, 62.5 and 87.5 centiles

5. after this, further bisection is likely to become unreliable

O'Hagan and colleagues point out the difficulty that experts have in judging the tails of distributions [180]. This means that it would be unreliable to ask for extreme centiles like the 1st and 99th, even though they would, in theory, be useful.

Clearly, the person who asks the questions ought to be skilled in doing so, in order to minimise bias and noise. You, the meta-analyst, might not be the best person for the job, so consider who in your team would be well placed to do this task.

Another important consideration is how the expert is briefed beforehand [180]. They need to know exactly what the PICO definition of the meta-analysis is, and their answers should focus on that. They should be familiar with the evidence base in general, but not to the extent of simply citing all the studies that will be in the meta-analysis. They should probably not be someone already closely involved with the project.

This is a particular concern in Bayesian meta-analysis: many experts in the subject area will know about research that has been done, and are likely to already know the studies, and to have a good idea of how the meta-analysis might come out. They would not provide a prior, but an informed guess at the likelihood or the posterior! For this reason, it can be a good idea to recruit someone who is either not very research-active, or who works in a closely related topic. In this hypothetical scenario about osteoarthritis, a consultant rheumatologist who mostly sees patients with other conditions, and is not involved in pharmaceutical trials, might be a good choice. We will see below that there are advantages to consulting a panel of experts rather than pinning your hopes on one.

It is also helpful to hear some insight into the expert's thought process and how they arrive at the decisions. Certainly, you should introduce any elicitation process as a conversation where you need to understand *why* a certain value is chosen.

6.2.1 Turning elicited quantiles into a distribution: the SHELF method

In the previous section, we obtained centiles, which is a common way of describing *quantiles*. This just means that we provided a probability, and the expert gave us in exchange a value for the unknown true treatment effect. There are other methods for elicitation, and we

---

*This implies that the log rate ratio lies in $(-\infty, 0]$. The round bracket shows that it is greater than $-\infty$, and the square bracket shows that it is less than *or equal to* 0. You might see this sort of constraint written (but not in this book) in set theory style: $\in \mathbb{R}^-$, which just means that it is an element of the set of negative real numbers. It is helpful to be aware of these notation options in case you encounter them.

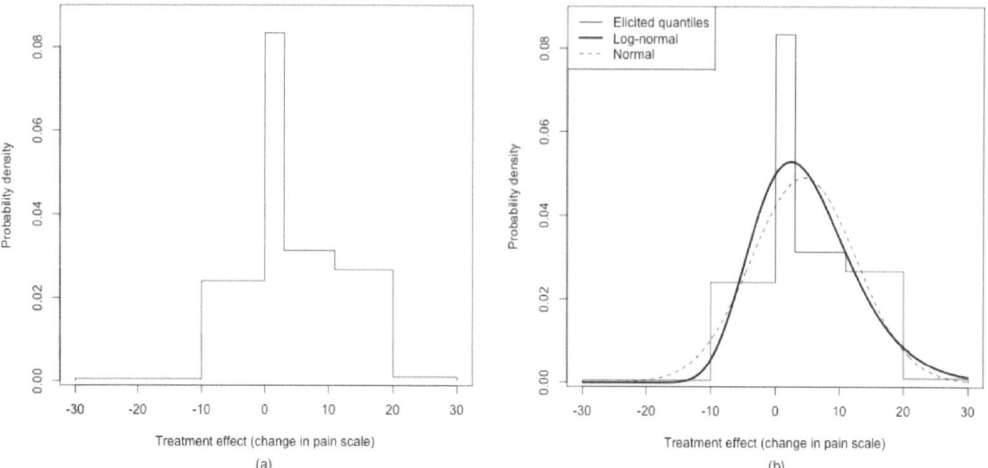

FIGURE 6.1
Histogram of (a) elicited quantiles, and (b) superimposed normal and log-normal distributions that best fit it.

will list some below, but for now let's continue with our example and try to turn it into a distribution.

We can put the elicited centiles onto a scale where positive-valued changes are desirable and negative ones are not. Suppose that we elicited the 25th, 50th and 75th, and we also define soft constraints and set them as the 1st and 99th:

- the 1st centile is -10

- the 25th centile is 0

- the 50th centile is +3

- the 75th centile is +11

- the 99th centile is +20

We can see at a glance that there will be a lot of probability density between the 25th and 50th centiles, because they are close together (0 and +3). The distribution will not be symmetric, so we should consider some skewed distributions. A histogram, with only these five cutpoints, will not be very informative (Figure 6.1, left).

When we elicit quantiles, we can use the SHeffield ELicitation Framework (SHELF) method [182]. This includes an R package, SHELF, which finds the best parameters to fit your quantiles for a selection of common distributions. There is a lot of documentation and advice at https://shelf.sites.sheffield.ac.uk/

The R package loads an interactive page in the browser, into which you can enter your probabilities and quantiles, and receive the details of the best-fitting of several candidate probability density functions (Figure 6.2). There is one additional requirement, which is not unique to SHELF. We must supply a lower and upper limit to the possible values[†]. This allows us to use distributions with a lower or upper limit, like the log-normal or beta.

[†]Mathematically, this is the *domain* of the PDF. Some software will return a probability density of zero if it is asked for a value outside the domain, while others may issue an error, or return some non-numeric code.

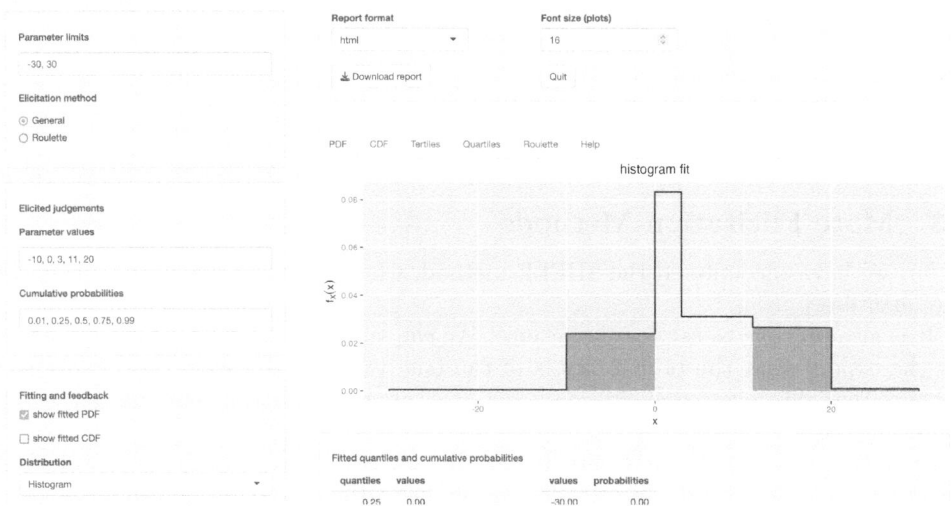

FIGURE 6.2
Part of the SHELF interactive interface in the browser (running the R package in the background); the probabilities and quantiles are entered at left, and various distributions can be fitted to them by selecting from the drop down menu at bottom left.

For the quantiles above, the best normal distribution has mean 4.43 and standard deviation 8.13. The log-normal distribution is the closest fit of all the candidate distributions, however, and that has two parameters: location 3.53 and spread 0.227. You can compare these to the elicited quantiles in Figure 6.1 on the right. You will probably agree that, while they are not terrible, they are not very faithful representations of the histogram either. We will list some more flexible options below.

The choice of these "limits" requires a little judgement about hard constraints. For our 0-100 pain scale, obviously the only hard limit is a treatment effect of -100 or +100, but that would be extreme. In practice, we must simply fit a distribution to the quantiles, and so we just have to allow distributions to fit the data without missing anything more than negligible probability off either end.

The log-normal, for example, needs a lower limit; it is only defined for non-negative values. We can shift this to start instead at -30, for example. SHELF does this automatically. To do it manually for a distribution with a lower limit θ_{min}, we must replace the value of the unknown θ with $\theta - \theta_{min}$.

Consider the log-normal distribution we obtained from SHELF. This is defined with a lower limit of -30, and that anchors the distribution so that it is defined for any values ≥ -30. We can express the density as:

$$(\theta - (-30)) \sim \text{LogN}(3.53, 0.227)$$

The beta distribution has both a lower and an upper limit, and we can shift it to a desired lower limit and then stretch it or squash it to reach the upper limit. To make a beta distribution fit to lower and upper limits, θ_{min} and θ_{max}, we transform θ into $(\theta - \theta_{min})/(\theta_{max} - \theta_{min})$. This is always between 0 and 1.

Suppose the unknown value can be between -30 and 30. The beta density for a value θ will be:

$$\frac{\theta - (-30)}{30 - (-30)} \sim \text{Beta}(\alpha, \beta)$$

6.3   More Elicitation Methods

So far, we have encountered the SHELF method, which asks experts to turn probabilities into quantiles.

It is also possible to ask for the reverse. We can supply some value of the unknown ans ask the expert what the probability is of the true value being below this. There is some evidence that this reversed elicitation is not as easily understood by experts as the SHELF approach [180].

In theory, we can ask the expert directly for statistics, such as the mean and standard deviation. This would directly provide a normal distribution. It could also be turned into the required parameters for any two-parameter distribution, like the beta, though to do so may require a little algebra, and you might prefer to seek out someone trained in statistics to do that.

If you are eliciting distributions from only a few statistics, it might be a good idea to then generate random pseudo-data, draw a histogram (of the usual type, with 20-30 bins) and feed that back to the expert so that they can confirm or edit it accordingly. Few people can produce reliable statistics to order from their imaginations!

Another quite flexible method that experts can understand involves providing a selection of pre-determined bins, and asking them to allocate votes to the bins. In the example of the pain scale, we might allow 5-point wide bins:

- $-30 \leq \theta \leq -25$

- $-25 < \theta \leq -20$

- $-20 < \theta \leq -15$

- ... and so on through to ...

- $+25 < \theta \leq +30$

We could give the expert 100 "votes" to be distributed as they see fit. Sometimes this is called a stones-in-bins approach.

In general, if you have some elicited information, and you want to fit a particular distribution to it, then it can probably be done. You may need to find a statistician and ask them to run a maximum likelihood estimate on it*.

6.4   Not Assuming Any Distribution

We can also take a non-parametric approach, and not shoehorn our elicited values into any off-the-shelf distribution. Whatever we do in this case, our task is fundamentally one of smoothing the elicited histogram.

---

*Good tools for this are `bbmle` in R, `mlexp` in Stata, or `scipy.optimize` in Python. The topic of maximum likelihood estimation is beyond the scope of this book.

One approach is to use kernel density, which is readily available in all statistical software. The R function `density()` provides this, and in Stata, you can use `kdensity`.

If you are using the stones-in-bins approach, kernel density will replaces each of the n stones, at values $\theta_i, 1 \leq i \leq n$, with a smooth shape like a probability density function, called a kernel, then adds the heights of those kernels together. For simplicity here, we will describe using the normal probability density function, $N(\theta_i, \sigma_k)$ as the kernel function.

The kernel density will simply be the average of the individual kernels:

$$\frac{\sum_{i=1}^{n} N(\theta_i, \sigma_k)}{n} \tag{6.1}$$

This produces a valid probability density function because each of the kernels is itself a probability density function, which is to say that the area under the curve is one. If you use other kernels, you may need to multiply the end result by some *normalising constant* to get a valid probability density function. However, in MCMC algorithms, we need only produce the posterior density times some constant, so for any of the software that we consider in this book, the normalising constant can be omitted. In fact, you can even forget about dividing by n in Equation 6.1, although it does help to remind us humans of what we are doing.

When you elicit a histogram using SHELF, you do not start with stones (votes) but just bins of higher or lower density. The kernels can be centred on the midpoints of histogram bins, or can be evenly spaced or randomly scattered throughout the bins. This is because we do not have an exact location, θ_i, for each kernel, only that it belongs to a certain bin. Figure 6.3 (left) uses uniformly randomly distributed values within each histogram bin to calculate a kernel density, and the number of values inside each bin is proportionate to the area under the bin (density times width: you know this already if you started with quantiles).

To implement kernel density priors, you need to add to your model code a sum of kernels. Each kernel will be centred on a value that you supply as extra "data". While kernel density

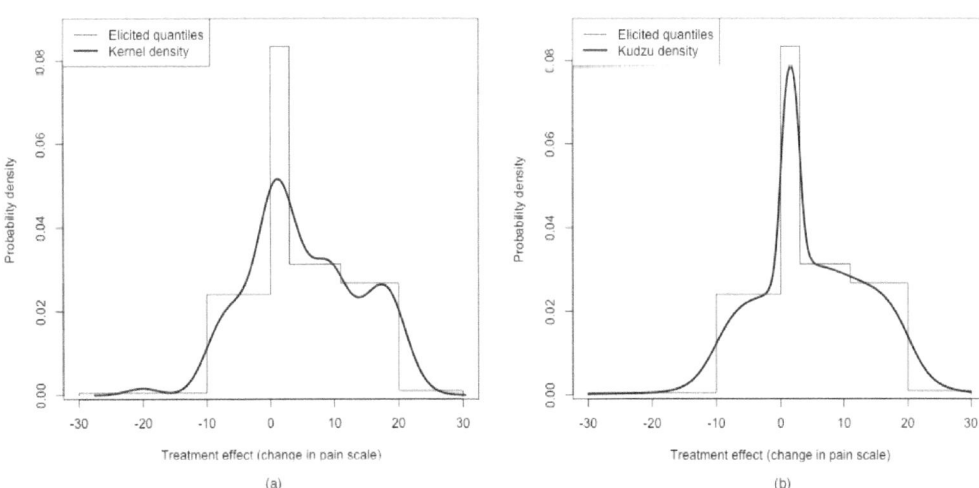

FIGURE 6.3
Histogram of (a) elicited quantiles with superimposed kernel density and (b) kudzu density. In both methods, the extent of smoothing can be increased or decreased.

is a good option to keep close to the original shape of the elicited histogram, it is a more challenging coding task than supplying a single parametric prior. Examples are given online.

Another option is to replace the sharp edges of the histogram bins with smooth ramp shapes, such as the expit or inverse logistic function:

$$\frac{1}{1 + e^{-\theta}} = \frac{e^\theta}{1 + e^\theta} \qquad (6.2)$$

This is implemented in the kudzu density function [96] (Figure 6.3, right).

When you adopt one of these flexible approaches, it is very important to generate a graph of the density, compared to the elicited histogram, to double-check that it does not accidentally misrepresent the prior opinions. These methods might sometimes create distributions with local peaks and troughs, which might cause trouble for any sampling algorithm.

6.5   Panels of Experts

We have discussed eliciting opinions from one expert. In practice, most projects prefer to use a panel, to reflect a range of opinions and to avoid any individual's bias.

The work involved in finding several experts, getting their commitment to the project, organising interviews or meetings as required, and combining their views into a prior, is not trivial, and should be built into project planning, and therefore any business case or funding application. It might be a good idea to involve a researcher with experience of either consensus processes or qualitative research in focus groups.

The output from the panel can be multiple priors—one per expert—which are then mixed together like kernels were in Section 6.4, or it could be one distribution which is the best fit to the multiple expert histograms, or it could be one prior which the experts have all agreed on. This determines the method used for the panel process.

For multiple priors or one best fit, each expert can be dealt with in isolation from the others, requiring only a repetition of the process we outlined above for one expert.

For a consensus, we should provide some feedback to the panel, and hence there must be at least two rounds of the elicitation and discussion. There are two consensus processes which the Bayesian analyst can adapt for this.

In the Delphi process [20], the panel members are first consulted independently of one another. This is when elicitation takes place. Then, all their priors are compiled into a report, which compares them to one another and notes any differences of opinion among the panel members. This report is circulated for everyone to read, and then a second round of elicitation takes place. The experts are able to take other panel members' views into consideration and might amend their priors if they think others have important insights.

The Nominal Group Technique is similar, but after being initially consulted independently, and having a report circulated, the panel members meet and discuss the reasons for their differences of opinion [20]. A face-to-face meeting may be more productive for this, compared to video conferencing, because of the way that people are more open to new ideas in person. They might propose any amendments to their priors at the meeting, so it is helpful if there is a system allowing rapid distribution-fitting and feedback[†], so more rounds of discussion can take place if needed, without convening a third meeting.

[†]Robert's experience of developing clinical guidelines (2000–2006) included Nominal Group Technique consensus sessions to amend recommendations. A voting hardware (clicker) system allowed us to set a consistent threshold for approval, with frantic calculations taking place during lunch and coffee breaks, but

In the SHELF system [182], which is similar to Delphi, experts see each other's priors and are asked to then consider what prior would be suggested by a rational impartial observer (RIO), who might enter the room at that point and sum up the opinions.

6.5.1 Managing the panel

Selecting the panel and managing their interactions is critical. It is important to bring together different schools of thought, as well as different professions, generations and levels of experience. Of course, it is not feasible to represent every possible combination, but it is vital that everyone who is consulted can see that their views are being taken seriously.

Much has been written about group dynamics for decision-making [139], and also about the important task of including the experiences of patients and carers [215]. Importantly, an impartial chair or facilitator is valuable if there is any chance of conflict. We should expect a degree of robust disagreement, but at the same time, we must not tolerate attempts to derail the process or bias the results. Choosing a facilitator who is perceived to be independent from the researchers can be helpful.

Some attempts have been made to develop methods to measure or adjust for different human habits in answering questions, including innate tendencies to optimism or pessimism, or to the strength with which views are expressed. None of these is a magic wand that can eliminate the tricky and multi-faceted task of understanding human rationales and trying to bring a group to consensus. If you are interested, then some of the methods you might want to look into are:

- self-assessment of confidence, then weighting accordingly [154]

- calibration of how strong (far from neutrality) opinions are by asking "seed questions" first, which all experts are expected to agree on [154]

- hierarchical models that "shrink" unusual opinions towards the group average [154]

- summary by an independent "supra-Bayesian" assessor [22, 154]

- dividing responses into "feeling" and "uncertainty" using combined uniform-binomial (CUB) models [196]

6.5.2 Don't forget ...

Finally, whatever method is used to elicit and process expert opinions, Bayesian analysts must remember to do sensitivity analysis with somewhat different priors.

---

now a faster and easier turnaround could be achieved in the context of prior elicitation with smartphones, an online survey, and a distribution-fitting and plotting script.

7

Writing up your Meta-Analysis

Learning objectives

After reading this chapter, you will be able to:

1. identify appropriate guidelines and checklists to help you write

2. plan how to share sufficient code and data to make your Bayesian meta-analysis reproducible

3. critique and review other people's published Bayesian meta-analyses

4. produce forest plots of posterior distributions from Bayesian meta-analysis

---

It is the duty of every practitioner of statistics both to calculate accurately and to communicate effectively. We have already seen, particularly in Chapter 5, the great scope for confusion and ambiguity in published research. Your meta-analyses must rise above this poor standard, and this chapter will cite various sources of relevant guidance and exemplars of good practice to help you.

Any research publication should justify all decisions taken in a transparent way, and give enough information that an interested party could reproduce the study. A Bayesian meta-analysis should meet these requirements in terms of both the Bayesian analysis and the meta-analysis. A scoping review of Bayesian meta-analysis between 2005 and 2016* found generally poor standards of reporting [94]. Recent reviews continue to confirm this [61].

7.1 Guidelines

The EQUATOR network is a collaboration to provide one port of call for reporting guidelines [68]. These tend to have a health focus, but can be readily applied to other fields too. The PRISMA checklist is applicable to meta-analyses; there are also guidelines proposed for meta-analysis in the economic setting [107]. The relevant EQUATOR guidelines for Bayesian analyses in general are the Bayesian Analysis Reporting Guidelines (BARG) [142], created in 2021. There are also four relevant older checklists: ROBUST (Reporting Of Bayes Used in clinical STudies) [246], BaSiS (Bayesian Standards in Science) [14], WAMBS (When to

---

*An update is underway at the time of writing [218].

worry and how to Avoid the Misuse of Bayesian Statistics) [52], and BayesWatch, from the influential Health Technology Assessment report by Spiegelhalter *et al* [240].

Because Bayesian methods have advanced rapidly in recent years, older checklists should be considered carefully before being used as assurance of contemporary good standards. Table 2 in the ROBUST paper provides a helpful side-by-side comparison of three of the older checklists [246].

We can identify some recurring features from guidelines and checklists:

1. description of the available data, including any shortcomings and challenges

2. rationale for using a Bayesian approach

3. interpretation of the prior

4. source(s) of the prior; justification for assumptions; prior predictive checks (if relevant)

5. prior formulas

6. sensitivity analyses

7. likelihood formulas; justification for assumptions

8. a priori definition of thresholds for evaluating probabilities (see Section 2.3.3)

9. details of software used

10. details of sampling algorithm and settings such as the number of chains, discarded warmup iterations, random number generator seeds, initial values—the simplest way to achieve this is to share the code

11. convergence statistics, Monte Carlo error, posterior predictive checks, and other diagnostics (see Section 2.5)

12. details of how the posterior sample has been summarised (see Section 2.3)

13. summary statistics of the posterior

To this list, we should add the challenge of data extraction, which is peculiar to evidence synthesis (see Chapter 5): explain and justify all choices in data extraction [36]. There should also be documentation of checks done to ensure that Bayesian sampling algorithms have executed as expected, including r-hat statistics, traceplots, and prior/posterior predictive checking (see Section 2.5).

A recent review and report has also urged the transparent reporting of processes for elicitation of expert priors [234]. The more recent BARG guidelines add to this the need for sharing of code and study statistics so that analyses can be run by readers. An example of how this can be delivered online is explored below.

A good way to provide this information, when the main publication does not allow space for it, is as an analysis plan, preferably pre-specified before data collection. Academic studies may publish this as part of a protocol.

It is unfortunately common for applied peer reviewed journals to limit the space available for papers, and statistical methods sections are often cut to make way for substantive background and interpretation. In this age of online-first publication, there is no reason not to place an appendix of complete information online, including the code for your Bayesian software. For future-proofing, it may be wise to place this both on the publisher's website and your own personal or institutional website. Below, we describe an exemplary publication of a Bayesian meta-analysis.

The scoping review highlights one recently emerged problem that is cause for concern [94]: that network meta-analyses (and occasionally others too) often report a mixture of non-Bayesian meta-analyses of pairs of interventions, and then a Bayesian network meta-analysis. This is inadvisable as there is the potential to confuse readers and leave them the task of choosing from competing syntheses of the evidence base. If there is a defensible rationale for a mixture of Bayesian and non-Bayesian methods, state it clearly.

For general guidance on publishing systematic reviews and meta-analyses, the PRISMA guidelines are the international standard. Along with various relevant extensions, including individual patient data, network meta-analyses, and protocols, the latest versions of these guidelines are best accessed directly from EQUATOR [67].

Another, older, checklist for reviewers provides a number of useful insights for writing up [1].

To make a Bayesian meta-analysis truly reproducible, you should make the code and the study statistics available. Because study statistics (aggregate meta-analysis inputs) are not at individual human level, and are typically already in the public domain, there should be few barriers to this. If the meta-analysis contains some individual participant data, then sharing may not be possible for ethical and data governance reasons.

The additional items for a *Bayesian* meta-analysis should include:

- clarify which decisions were made *a priori*

- share study statistics

- justify model specification, for example heterogeneity distribution

- investigation of heterogeneity (see Section 4.7)

- present secondary (*a posteriori*) meta-analyses as hypothesis-generating

  Additional considerations for network meta-analyses are discussed in Chapter 9.

7.2   Online Supporting Information

Of the 312 Bayesian meta-analysis papers examined in the 2005-2016 scoping review, a report on management of uterine fibroids stood out as clearly the best publication in terms of clarity, completeness of information, and reproducibility [103]. Although the report is 409 pages in length, this is in large part because there are several different systematic reviews and very extensive appendices. The highlight for meta-analysis reproducibility lies in the sharing of all code and study stats, along with detailed rationale and exposition of the models, in an online repository [74]. This includes Jupyter Notebooks, an interactive format for combining code, data, output, graphics, and commentary [135].

Although the way that this study gathered all information together was by Jupyter Notebooks hosted on GitHub, the excellence of this publication is in the careful curation and explanation of the analyses. You can share your detailed information in any file format and on any server[†]. We do not recommend making them "available on request", and we do recommend making an effort to make them as comprehensible as possible to your fellow humans (as the BARG suggests, through annotation, meaningful variable names, and file names).

The HEDCO Institute at the University of Oregon, USA, maintain another form of exemplary online information in their Evidence Hub at `https://hedcoinstitute.uoregon.`

[†]There are alternatives to GitHub that are not owned by a large tech company, and other ways that you can self-host repositories, not least of all by simply making compressed `.zip` files.

`edu/evidence-hub`. Although their work has not included Bayesian meta-analysis to date, they show how it is possible to improve impact and outreach by providing complex information in a layered, easily accessible, and continuously updated format.

For example, their review of studies on a four-day school week across the USA is summarised in an interactive webpage for exploring the database of studies [109]. This allows users to select settings most relevant to them and to scroll through study PICO characteristics and findings.

The Metapsy website provides trial filtering and meta-analysis (not Bayesian) in one interface, with modern interactive controls [251].

7.3 Data Visualisation

Data visualisation in meta-analysis is an aid to communication. No plot is essential, but usually they help readers and reviewers a great deal.

The forest plot is the classic meta-analytic format (see Section 3.3). From a random effects (or fixed effects) Bayesian model, the study-specific unknowns and the overall intervention effect can be shown in a similar way (see Figure 4.4 and accompanying code for the R package `bayesplot`). Common effect meta-analyses could show the observed study statistics and their reported confidence intervals along with the combined intervention effect. Generating a diamond shape is possible but there is no special need for it; a dot and horizontal error bars will be as clear if not clearer.

Other plots are not universally used or understood; you should decide on a case by case basis. The funnel plot is quite common in considering publication bias and we will revisit it in Chapter 13.

For the Bayesian aspects of meta-analysis, prior and predictive checks, such as we showed in Section 2.5.4, may be useful, as well as density plots of the posterior, perhaps highlighting regions [148]. If meaningful values of the intervention effect, heterogeneity standard deviation, or other unknowns have been defined a priori, it will be useful to annotate the density plots of the posteriors at these values. One example might be a minimum clinically important difference, another the estimated effectiveness of an established intervention.

DuMouchel and Normand set out several innovative and potentially useful graphs in a book chapter from 2000 [62].

We will now consider how the outputs from Bayesian meta-analysis, mainly posterior summary statistics, can be fed into standard meta-analysis functions in R and Stata. Although this produces familiar formats without requiring any manual creation of shapes and layouts, it may be preferable to take a different approach so that the Bayesian outputs are visually distinct to remind viewers that the meta-analysis was not a standard non-Bayesian one.

We will skip the step of loading posterior means and credible intervals into R / Stata, as this is relatively simple and will depend on your preferred Bayesian software. We assume that the study-specific effect estimates, whether as reported by the studies (common effect model), or shrunken by the heterogeneity (random effects), is in a variable called `post_effect`, and the lower and upper limits of the 95% confidence or credible intervals are in `post_lci` and `post_uci`.

7.3.1   Standard graphics in R

We start from the point in Section 4.4.2 where the green tea random effect meta-analysis has been run in `cmdstanr`. We can extract the posterior statistics and feed them into the functions of the `forestplot` package*

```
# obtain posterior draws from the chains:

standraws <- stanfit$draws(variables=c("theta", "theta_u"))
poststats <- posterior::summarise_draws(standraws,
                        mean,
                        ~quantile(.x,
                                probs=c(0.025,
                                        0.975)))


# put the overall estimate to one side:

theta_stats <- unlist(poststats[1,-1])


# get the theta_u statistics into a format that forestplot will recognise:

theta_u_stats <- data.frame(mean = poststats[-1, 2],
                        lower = poststats[-1, 3],
                        upper = poststats[-1, 4],
                        study = greentea$Study)
colnames(theta_u_stats)[c(2,3)] <- c("lower", "upper")
theta_u_stats$poststats <- paste0(round(theta_u_stats$mean, 2),
                        " (",
                        round(theta_u_stats$lower, 2),
                        ", ",
                        round(theta_u_stats$lower, 2),
                        ")")


# call the forestplot functions:

theta_u_stats |>
    forestplot(labeltext = c(study, poststats),
            clip = c(-3, 1),
            xlog = FALSE) |>
    fp_add_lines() |>
    fp_add_header(study = c("", "Study"),
            poststats = c("Posterior mean", "(95% CrI)") |>
                fp_align_center()) |>
    fp_append_row(mean  = theta_stats[1],
            lower = theta_stats[2],
            upper = theta_stats[3],
```

---

*In a departure from R code elsewhere in this book, the `forestplot` package only really makes sense if we use the piping syntax convention of passing objects from left to right. Here, we use the native R pipe operator, `|>`, but you can also use the `%>%` operator from the `magrittr` package, which appears in much writing and tutorial material for Tidyverse R packages.

```
                study = "Overall effect",
                poststats = paste0(round(theta_stats[1], 2),
                                   " (",
                                   round(theta_stats[2], 2),
                                   ", ",
                                   round(theta_stats[3], 2),
                                   ")"),
             is.summary = TRUE)
```

Graphs should be saved immediately into a raster format such as .png, and a vector format, particularly .svg. SVG files can be edited in a vector graphics editor package such as Inkscape (which is freeware) or Adobe Illustrator, and can then be exported to raster formats in any desired resolution. To save in the PNG format, we can wrap the forestplot code in a call to a png device, like this:

```
png("modified_forestplot.png", width=1200, height=600)
theta_u_stats |>
  forestplot(labeltext = c(study, poststats),
             clip = c(-3, 1),
             xlog = FALSE) |>
  fp_add_lines() |>
  fp_add_header(study = c("", "Study"),
                poststats = c("Posterior mean", "(95% CrI)") |>
                  fp_align_center()) |>
  fp_append_row(mean  = theta_stats[1],
                lower = theta_stats[2],
                upper = theta_stats[3],
                study = "Overall effect",
                poststats = paste0(round(theta_stats[1], 2),
                                   " (",
                                   round(theta_stats[2], 2),
                                   ", ",
                                   round(theta_stats[3], 2),
                                   ")"),
                is.summary = TRUE)
dev.off()
```

The final line, dev.off(), closes the connection to the .png file. We can do the same with SVG, for which we recommend using the svglite package, as the result is simpler and more easily edited afterwards. The result is shown in Figure 7.1.

7.3.2   Standard graphics in Stata

We can construct a bespoke forest plot in Stata by manipulating the data stored in special variables created by the meta set command. Be careful with these actions as they overwrite the effect size and confidence interval limits.

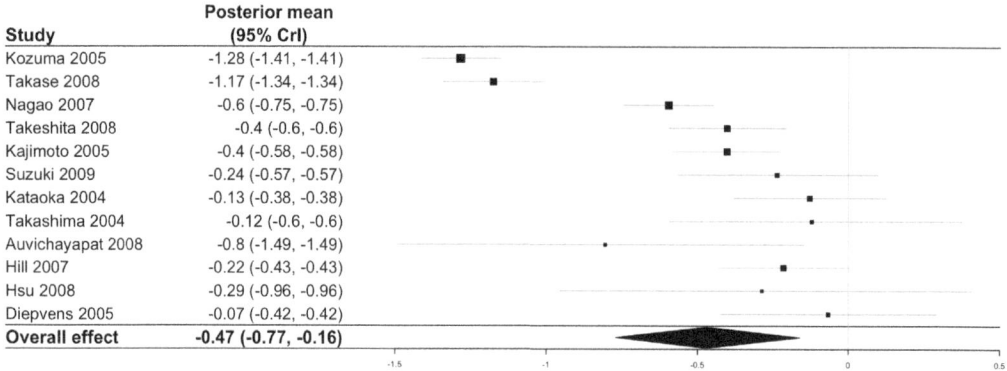

FIGURE 7.1
Modified Bayesian random effects forest plot from R `forestplot` package.

Starting from where the code in Section 4.4.3 left off, we can store the means and 95% credible interval for the overall effect size directly from `e(mean)` and `e(cri)` (see "Stored results" under `help bayesmh` for details).

```
global postmean_theta = e(mean)[1,1]
global postlci_theta = e(cri)[1,1]
global postuci_theta = e(cri)[2,1]
```

Next, we create a 12-by-6 empty matrix called `posterior`, and fill each row with the summary statistics for each element of `{md:_cons}+{U[id]}`, in other words, each study's shrunken effect. The six columns are the mean, standard deviation, Monte Carlo standard error, median, lower 95% credible interval, and upper 95% credible interval. Then, we can add the columns of this matrix to the current dataset by `svmat`; they will be called `posterior1` to `posterior6`.

```
matrix posterior = J(12,6,.)

forvalues i=1/12 {
  bayesstats summary ({md:_cons}+{U['i'.id]})
  matrix posterior['i',1] = r(summary)
}

svmat posterior
```

We can then overwrite the `meta set` special variables, which begin with underscores. Finally, we specify many modifications of the forest plot, including disposing of the standard overall effect and all the tests and statistics of heterogeneity, imposing a custom overall effect diamond for our posterior statistics (using the global macros we stored earlier), and labelling everything sensibly. The final result is in Figure 7.2.

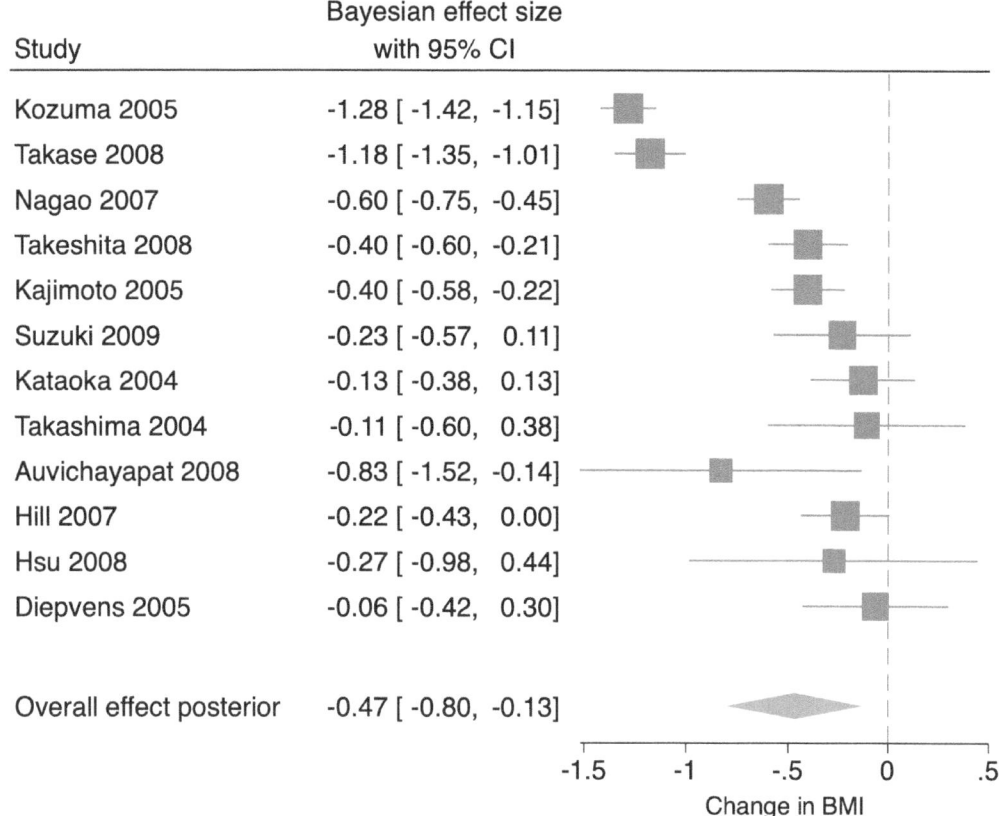

FIGURE 7.2
Modified Bayesian random effects forest plot from Stata.

```
replace _meta_es = posterior1
replace _meta_cil = posterior5
replace _meta_ciu = posterior6

meta forestplot _id _esci _plot, ///
  columnopts(_esci, supertitle("Bayesian effect size")) ///
  nullrefline(lcolor(gray) ///
              lpattern(dash)) ///
  xtitle("Change in BMI") ///
  customoverall($postmean_theta $postlci_theta $postuci_theta, ///
                label("Overall effect posterior")) ///
  nooverall noohetstats noohomtest noosigtest nonotes

graph save "modified-forestplot.gph", replace
graph export "modified-forestplot.png", replace
graph export "modified-forestplot.svg", replace
```

It is worth pointing out that it is helpful to save graphs immediately in the native Stata `.gph` format (which can be manually edited in Stata, if later required), a raster format such as `.png`, and a vector format, particularly `.svg`. SVG files can be edited in a vector graphics editor package such as Inkscape (which is freeware) or Adobe Illustrator, and can then be exported to raster formats in any desired resolution.

Part III

Specific Problems

8

Using Arm- and Time-Based Statistics

Learning objectives

After reading this chapter, you will be able to:

1. compute an arm-based meta-analysis for statistics from randomised controlled trials, so as to respect randomisation

2. consider relevant models for non-randomised studies

3. compute an arm-based meta-analysis for single arm statistics, such as prevalence or incidence rates

4. represent multiple study statistics, such as from different arms or time points, as a multivariate distribution with a mean vector and covariance matrix

---

More sophisticated models of the evidence base often require the statistics from studies to be broken down into more detail. Instead of just having a mean difference, and its standard error, from each study, we might benefit from extracting the mean and standard deviation in the control group, and the same in the intervention group. Likewise for binary outcomes, we can model the sample size and the count of events in each group.

The same applies to different study designs, and for more than two-group comparisons. We will refer to such models as *arm-based*. So far in this book, we have emphasised contrast-based models, which use a point estimate comparing two arms, and its standard error, from each study. Most meta-analyses are analysed on this basis, and we will take care in our arm-based models not to break the familiar assumptions of the contrast-based approach.

In the case of randomised controlled trials, the contrast can be interpreted as an estimate of intervention effect. We used that term throughout Parts 1 and 2 of this book, referring to simple study designs. If you are meta-analysing non-randomised studies, then any causal interpretation has to be done with caution and is likely to involve some untestable assumptions. To be as general as possible from now on, we will refer to *contrasts*.

Just as we might extract statistics at multiple arms, we can also extract for multiple arms and time points. If we extract the statistics not just at the endpoint but at baseline and any interim time points, we will have a lot more information on each study, which could be useful to inform more complicated models. Meta-analysis at multiple time points is an emerging topic and we return to it in Chapter 17.

8.1   Motivation

Some of the more complicated models that may need arm-based meta-analysis include network meta-analysis, where multiple intervention options are compared, though not every option appears in every study (Chapter 9). Some problems of unreported statistics (Chapter 11) might also need information from other studies' arms for the same intervention to impute the missing statistic.

Studies with binary outcomes and rare events can also run into trouble, even with simple meta-analysis models. With one or more zeros in the two-by-two table that determines odds ratios and risk ratios, the calculations either fail completely (consider how Equations 1.17 or 3.6 would have to divide by zero) or have to make some heuristic adjustment such as adding 0.5 to each cell's count [47]. Sometimes, we have seen studies report such an adjusted point estimate, but omit the standard error.

Arm-based Bayesian models are regarded as a useful approach to this problem [131]. In an arm-based model, we develop the data-generating process, just as we did in Sections 3.5, 4.1.1, and 4.3.1, but instead of computing a likelihood for the true contrast given the observed contrasts, we do so for the true contrast given the individual arm statistics.

Sometimes we have heard the objection that any evidence synthesis at the level of the individual arms is wrong because it "breaks randomisation" [55]. Randomisation between the arms is certainly central to clinical trials' claim to be the most reliable form of evidence. It is worthwhile considering exactly what "breaking randomisation" means in simple terms.

Suppose that we are combining statistics from two studies. Study 1 recruited people with mild disease and relatively good outcomes, and for some practical reason had a small control group and a large intervention group. Study 2 is the opposite, with severe disease, relatively poor outcomes, a large control group and a small intervention group. If we break the studies into arm statistics and combine the arms, Study 1's intervention group dominates, and Study 2's control group. This leads to relatively good outcomes in the pooled intervention estimate and relatively poor outcomes in the pooled control estimate. This will over-estimate the intervention effect. Unfortunately, although in this thought experiment we are able to spot the imbalances between studies which lead to bias, there could be others that are not so easy to spot.

The reason why this goes wrong is that arms of different studies, even if they have the same intervention, are not *exchangeable*. Exchangeability is a concept that underpins a lot of statistics, but learners often find it difficult to grasp. Simply put, with some simplification, if we can shuffle the individual numbers in some part of our analysis, with no impact on the result, then they are exchangeable. Within one arm of one RCT, we can shuffle the participants: the order in which they appear in our spreadsheet makes no difference. In a paired analysis such as a crossover trial, that would not be the case. Each participant's data need to stay paired. The same is true of time series or geo-spatial data. When our data are not exchangeable, we always need to use a model that takes that into account.

In meta-analysis of RCTs, the study contrasts are exchangeable but the individual arms are not. Non-randomised studies are also not exchangeable at the level of the arms, to the extent that they sample somewhat different populations and use somewhat different interventions and controls over, somewhat different periods of time, and so on. Although in theory, you could argue that your non-randomised evidence base is made of entirely comparable studies, this is hard to verify in full.

The important distinction is between a likelihood evaluated for each arm, but built from contrast estimates, and a model with separate unknowns for each arm, which would break from the contrast-based methods we have seen so far [55, 281].

The evidence base might also contain some single-arm studies. To combine these with multi-arm studies that each have a comparable arm*, we will have to break studies into arms and work at that level [231]. Recently, there has been much interest around including single-arm data from routinely collected sources such as electronic patient records (in the health care setting). These data sources have been called *real-world evidence*.

We recommend careful consideration of the external validity of such data sources. This is related to the idea of *historic controls*, and more broadly, *borrowing external information*. They require an arm-based approach because an intervention arm and a "real-world" control arm will not have drawn participants from the same population.

In this chapter, we will show how arms can be combined, but when some studies, or arms, are randomised and others are not, there could be bias in the arm and contrast statistic, arising from how the intervention is prioritised in the "real-world". This combination of different study designs is addressed in Chapter 15.

As we progress through the models, we will show code for means (continuous outcome variable), and for counts (binary or count outcome variable). We will also reflect on the model choices for non-randomised studies, such as cohort, case-control and case series. Finally, in Section 8.6, we consider how these models can be used on statistics from single arms, for example to estimate an incidence rate of some event in the untreated population by looking at a collection of control arms.

8.2 Common Effect Models

The fundamental idea in any arm-based model is that we are going to assume an underlying data-generating process just as we did for contrast-based meta-analysis in Chapters 3 and 4, but evaluate the likelihood in each arm.

8.2.1 Common effect models: continuous outcomes

We will start with a common effect model for a continuous-valued outcome in randomised controlled trials with two arms each, building from Equation 3.7:

$$\text{Data-generating process}:$$
$$y_{ij\textbf{Ctl}} \sim \text{N}(\mu_j, \sigma_{j\textbf{Ctl}})$$
$$y_{ij\textbf{Int}} \sim \text{N}(\mu_j + \theta, \sigma_{j\textbf{Int}})$$
$$\text{Likelihood}:$$
$$\therefore \bar{y}_{j\textbf{Ctl}} \sim \text{N}\left(\mu_j, \frac{\sigma_{j\textbf{Ctl}}}{\sqrt{n_{j\textbf{Ctl}}}}\right) \tag{8.1}$$
$$\therefore \bar{y}_{j\textbf{Int}} \sim \text{N}\left(\mu_j + \theta, \frac{\sigma_{j\textbf{Int}}}{\sqrt{n_{j\textbf{Int}}}}\right)$$
$$\text{Prior required for}:$$
$$(\mu_1, \mu_2 \ldots \mu_m) \in \mathbb{R}$$
$$\theta \in \mathbb{R}$$

---

*In this chapter, we explain arm-based models for an evidence base with two types of arm: intervention and control. Later, in Chapter 9, we will consider network meta-analysis, where a more relevant description might be "multi-arm studies where each a comparable arm with at least one other study".

This assumes one shared σ, which is the intra-arm standard deviation. As in previous chapters, we might use the reported standard errors or standard deviations for this, taking them at face value as perfectly known, or we might apply a Sidik-Jonkman style adjustment for the uncertainty in σ. In Section 8.4, we will estimate σ as another unknown. We are also assuming the normal distribution of the data, as before, and the uncorrelated nature of randomised arms.

It is important to notice how the intervention arm data and their mean, $\bar{y}_{ij\mathbf{Int}}$, have a sampling distribution with mean determined by two inputs: θ, which is common to all studies, and by the *study-specific* control group population mean, μ_j. These μ_js are fixed effects: they do not share a heterogeneity distribution. They are more likely to have diffuse or weakly informative priors, unless you have opinion priors for them.

If we instead used a single shared μ, we would be pulling all study control arms towards the overall mean of control arms, which could introduce bias if there are imbalances between arms. A random effects model with heterogeneity on the control arm means would potentially make this worse by actively shrinking small studies' posterior samples towards the centre of the heterogeneity distribution [281].

This is an example of BUGS code for the above model, with diffuse priors (which you should adapt to your own data):

```
# Priors:
theta ~ dnorm(0, 0.0001)
for(j in 1:m){
        mu[j] ~ dnorm(0, 0.0001)
}


# Derived variables:
for(j in 1:m) {
        mu_int[j] <- mu[j] + theta
        prec_mean_ctl[j] <- 1 / pow(se_mean_ctl[j], 2)
        prec_mean_int[j] <- 1 / pow(se_mean_int[j], 2)
}


# Likelihood:
mean_ctl[j] ~ dnorm(mu[j], prec_mean_ctl[j])
mean_int[j] ~ dnorm(mu_int[j], prec_mean_int[j])
```

Compare this with another approach, where the two arms' unknown population means are completely unconnected, and a contrast is evaluated afterwards, which will lead to the bias previously discussed, if there are arm imbalances:

$$\text{Data (unobserved)}:$$
$$y_{ij\mathbf{Ctl}} \sim \mathrm{N}(\mu_{\mathbf{Ctl}}, \sigma)$$
$$y_{ij\mathbf{Int}} \sim \mathrm{N}(\mu_{\mathbf{Int}}, \sigma)$$
$$\text{Statistics (observed)}:$$
$$\therefore \bar{y}_{ij\mathbf{Ctl}} \sim \mathrm{N}(\mu_{\mathbf{Ctl}}, \frac{\sigma}{\sqrt{n_{j\mathbf{Ctl}}}}) \tag{8.2}$$
$$\therefore \bar{y}_{ij\mathbf{Int}} \sim \mathrm{N}(\mu_{\mathbf{Int}}, \frac{\sigma}{\sqrt{n_{j\mathbf{Int}}}})$$
$$\text{Derived posterior}:$$
$$\theta = \mu_{\mathbf{Int}} - \mu_{\mathbf{Ctl}}$$

The sampling distribution (likelihood) used above includes known study statistics in the calculation of the unknown mean of the sampling distribution for the intervention arm. This blending of knowns and unknowns—or data and parameters, if you prefer those terms—can baffle some software that prefers to keep them separate. In Stata, for example, you would need to use the more complicated `llevaluator` syntax to implement this model.

8.2.2 Common effect models: binary and count outcomes

If we construct the same model for binary outcomes, we must use a binomial likelihood in each arm. The probability of an event in the intervention arm is the study-specific log odds in the control arm (μ_j), plus the shared log odds ratio of the intervention effect (θ).

$$\text{Data-generating process}:$$
$$y_{ij\textbf{Ctl}} \sim \text{Binom}(\text{expit}(\mu_j), 1)$$
$$y_{ij\textbf{Int}} \sim \text{Binom}(\text{expit}(\mu_j + \theta), 1)$$
$$\text{Likelihood}:$$
$$\therefore d_{j\textbf{Ctl}} \sim \text{Binom}\left(\text{expit}(\mu_j), n_{j\textbf{Ctl}}\right) \tag{8.3}$$
$$\therefore d_{j\textbf{Int}} \sim \text{Binom}\left(\text{expit}(\mu_j + \theta), n_{j\textbf{Int}}\right)$$
$$\text{Prior required for}:$$
$$(\mu_1, \mu_2 \ldots \mu_m) \in \mathbb{R}$$
$$\theta \in \mathbb{R}$$

In BUGS, we can set priors that are not as enormously spread out, because a log odds of 20 is extremely close to a probability of 100%.

```
# Priors:
theta ~ dnorm(0, 0.01)
for(j in 1:m){
        mu[j] ~ dnorm(0, 0.01)
}

# Derived variables:
for(j in 1:m) {
        mu_int[j] <- mu[j] + theta
        pi_ctl[j] <- 1/(1+exp(-1*mu[j]))
        pi_int[j] <- 1/(1+exp(-1*mu_int[j]))
}

# Likelihood:
d_ctl[j] ~ dbin(pi_ctl[j], n_ctl[j])
d_int[j] ~ dbin(pi_int[j], n_int[j])
```

It may be possible to work directly with a study-specific probability π_j for the control arm, times a shared risk ratio (θ, relative risk):

Data-generating process :
$$y_{ij\mathbf{Ctl}} \sim \mathrm{Binom}(\pi_j, 1)$$
$$y_{ij\mathbf{Int}} \sim \mathrm{Binom}(\pi_j \theta), 1$$
Likelihood :
$$\therefore d_{j\mathbf{Ctl}} \sim \mathrm{Binom}\,(\pi_j, n_{j\mathbf{Ctl}}) \tag{8.4}$$
$$\therefore d_{j\mathbf{Int}} \sim \mathrm{Binom}\,(\pi_j \theta, n_{j\mathbf{Int}})$$
Prior required for:
$$(\pi_1, \pi_2 \ldots \pi_m) \in [0, 1]$$
$$\theta \in \mathbb{R}^+$$

or even a study-specific probability for the control arm, plus a shared risk difference:

Data-generating process :
$$y_{ij\mathbf{Ctl}} \sim \mathrm{Binom}(\pi_j, 1)$$
$$y_{ij\mathbf{Int}} \sim \mathrm{Binom}(\pi_j + \theta), 1$$
Likelihood :
$$\therefore d_{j\mathbf{Ctl}} \sim \mathrm{Binom}\,(\pi_j, n_{j\mathbf{Ctl}}) \tag{8.5}$$
$$\therefore d_{j\mathbf{Int}} \sim \mathrm{Binom}\,(\pi_j + \theta, n_{j\mathbf{Int}})$$
Prior required for:
$$(\pi_1, \pi_2 \ldots \pi_m) \in [0, 1]$$
$$\theta \in [-1, 1]$$

but in both these models, it is possible to arrive at a probability for the intervention group which is outside the possible range $[0, 1]$, which will cause your Bayesian sampling software to stop and issue an error. We may use priors or (in Stan) variable definitions to keep π_j and θ in the range, but we cannot easily constrain $\pi_j \theta$ or $\pi_j + \theta$. It is preferable to obtain the log odds ratio and convert it afterwards for a range of baseline risks [93].

If the outcome is a count of events per unit of time, geographical area or person-years at risk, then a Poisson likelihood is called for, with μ_j a control arm log rate for study j, and θ acting as a log rate ratio. t_{ijk} the time (or area) at risk[†] for observation / participant i, in study j and arm k, which we add together into a total for each arm as $t_{jk} = \sum_{i=1}^{n_{jk}} t_{ijk}$. We also need to add together the count of events for all the participants in each arm: $d_{jk} = \sum_{i=1}^{n_{jk}} d_{ijk}$.

The Poisson distribution has only one parameter, the expected number of events, which will be the rate, multiplied by the time (or area). Further, the expected number of events for all the participants in an arm is simply the sum of the expected numbers of each participant. This kind of model is ideally suited to events that you can reasonably treat as independent of each other. Dealing with zero counts is a common reason for the adoption of Poisson likelihoods in non-Bayesian meta-analysis [241], although being able to link multiple statistics arising from underlying counts—such as risk ratio, risk difference, and incidence risk ratio—is also desirable [9].

[†]This is also called an exposure variable. If you are using regression-focused software such as Stata `bayesmh` or `brms`, take care over whether you should supply t_{ijk} or $\log t_{ijk}$

Data-generating process :
$$d_{ij\mathbf{Ctl}} \sim \text{Poisson}(e^{\mu_j} t_{ij\mathbf{Ctl}})$$
$$d_{ij\mathbf{Int}} \sim \text{Poisson}(e^{\mu_j + \theta} t_{ij\mathbf{Int}},)$$

Likelihood :
$$\therefore d_{j\mathbf{Ctl}} \sim \text{Poisson}\left(e^{\mu_j} t_{j\mathbf{Ctl}}\right) \tag{8.6}$$
$$\therefore d_{j\mathbf{Int}} \sim \text{Poisson}\left(e^{\mu_j + \theta} t_{j\mathbf{Int}}\right)$$

Prior required for:
$$(\mu_1, \mu_2 \ldots \mu_m) \in \mathbb{R}$$
$$\theta \in \mathbb{R}$$

8.3   Random Effects Models

We suspect that, most of the time, an evidence base for meta-analysis will have some evidence of heterogeneity or reason to suspect it exists. The heterogeneity we saw in previous chapters was a distribution of study-specific contrasts such as $\theta_j \sim \text{N}(0, \tau)$. We can easily apply this to the models we set out above, for example in the binary outcome case, with a half-t prior on τ:

Data-generating process :
$$\theta_j \sim \text{N}(\theta, \tau)$$
$$y_{ij\mathbf{Ctl}} \sim \text{Binom}(\text{expit}(\mu_j), 1)$$
$$y_{ij\mathbf{Int}} \sim \text{Binom}(\text{expit}(\mu_j + \theta_j), 1$$

Likelihood :
$$\therefore d_{j\mathbf{Ctl}} \sim \text{Binom}\left(\text{expit}(\mu_j), n_{j\mathbf{Ctl}}\right) \tag{8.7}$$
$$\therefore d_{j\mathbf{Int}} \sim \text{Binom}\left(\text{expit}(\mu_j + \theta_j), n_{j\mathbf{Int}}\right)$$

Prior required for:
$$(\mu_1, \mu_2 \ldots \mu_m) \in \mathbb{R}$$
$$\theta \in \mathbb{R}$$
$$\tau \in \mathbb{R}^+$$

```
# Priors:
theta ~ dnorm(0, 0.01)
tau ~ dt(0,0.1,1)I(0,)
prec_tau <- 1 / pow(tau,2)
for(j in 1:m){
        mu[j] ~ dnorm(0, 0.0001)
        theta_j[j] ~ dnorm(theta, prec_tau)
}

# Derived variables:
for(j in 1:m) {
        mu_int[j] <- mu[j] + theta_j[j]
```

```
        pi_ctl[j] <- 1/(1+exp(-1*mu[j]))
        pi_int[j] <- 1/(1+exp(-1*mu_int[j]))
}

# Likelihood:
d_ctl[j] ~ dbin(pi_ctl[j], n_ctl[j])
d_int[j] ~ dbin(pi_int[j], n_int[j])
```

Crucially, there is no heterogeneity on μ_j (`mu[j]`), for the reasons described above [281]. A beta-distributed heterogeneity on arm probabilities has also been suggested for binary data, but we believe that would likely exhibit some of the same problems [131].

This is the Poisson model with heterogeneity:

$$\text{Data-generating process}:$$
$$\theta_j \sim \mathrm{N}(\theta, \tau)$$
$$d_{ij\mathbf{Ctl}} \sim \mathrm{Poisson}(e^{\mu_j} t_{ij\mathbf{Ctl}})$$
$$d_{ij\mathbf{Int}} \sim \mathrm{Poisson}(e^{\mu_j + \theta_j} t_{ij\mathbf{Int}})$$
$$\text{Likelihood}:$$
$$\therefore d_{j\mathbf{Ctl}} \sim \mathrm{Poisson}\left(e^{\mu_j} t_{j\mathbf{Ctl}}\right) \qquad (8.8)$$
$$\therefore d_{j\mathbf{Int}} \sim \mathrm{Poisson}\left(e^{\mu_j + \theta_j} t_{j\mathbf{Int}}\right)$$
$$\text{Prior required for}:$$
$$(\mu_1, \mu_2 \ldots \mu_m) \in \mathbb{R}$$
$$\theta \in \mathbb{R}$$
$$\tau \in \mathbb{R}^+$$

```
# Priors:
theta ~ dnorm(0, 0.01)
tau ~ dt(0,0.1,1)I(0,)
prec_tau <- 1 / pow(tau,2)
for(j in 1:m){
        mu[j] ~ dnorm(0, 0.0001)
        theta_j[j] ~ dnorm(theta, prec_tau)
}

# Derived variables:
for(j in 1:m) {
        mu_int[j] <- mu[j] + theta_j[j]
        rate_ctl[j] <- exp(mu[j]) * t_ctl[j]
        rate_int[j] <- exp(mu_int[j]) * t_int[j]
}

# Likelihood:
d_ctl[j] ~ dpois(rate_ctl[j])
d_int[j] ~ dpois(rate_int[j])
```

8.4 "Fully Bayesian" Models

The models we set out above for continuous outcomes did not have any new sophistication in terms of the observed standard deviations and standard errors of the mean. As before, those are either taken at face value (the DerSimonian-Laird approach), or the uncertainty in them can be included in a t-distribution for the means (the Sidik-Jonkman approach). However, the reason you might adopt an arm-based model could be that you need to guess at some unreported statistics by drawing on information in other studies, and the missing statistic is very often the standard deviation or standard error.

The sampling distribution of a standard deviation, assuming normally distributed data, requires a couple of stepping stones before we can relate it to an off-the-shelf probability density. An observed sample standard deviation of s must be squared to become the variance, s^2. Then, the ratio between the sample variance and the population variance, multiplied by $n-1$ (where n is the number of observations), has a chi-squared sampling distribution (Equation 8.9).

$$\frac{s^2(n-1)}{\sigma^2} \sim \chi^2(n-1) \tag{8.9}$$

In the chunk of BUGS code below, this chi-squared distributed variable is called `variance_x2`:

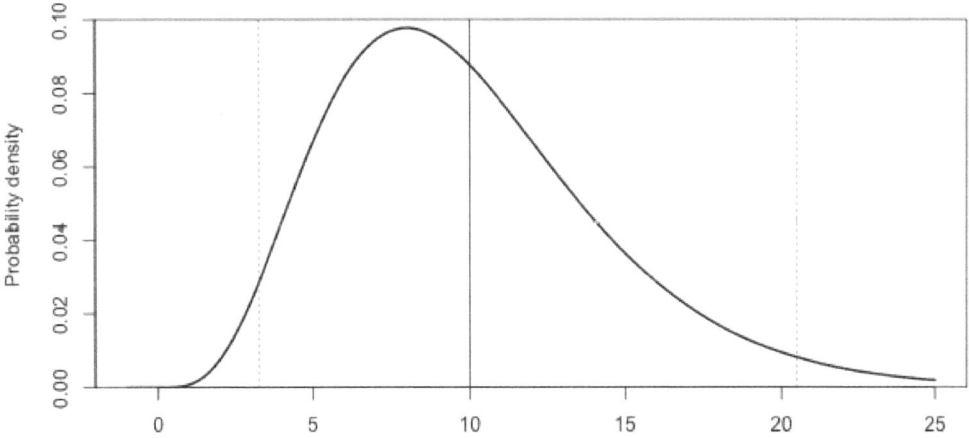

FIGURE 8.1
The chi-squared distribution with $n = 11$, therefore 10 degrees of freedom; the solid vertical line is at the mean and the dotted lines at the edges of the central 95% of the distribution.

```
# Prior:
sigma ~ dt(0,0.01,1)I(0,)

# Likelihood:
for(j in 1:m) {
  variance_x2[j] <- s[j]^2 * (n[j]-1) / sigma^2
  df[j] <- n[j]-1
  variance_x2[j] ~ dchisqr(df[j])
}
```

By including inference for the unknown population standard deviation, we are treating all sources of uncertainty in the same way, by applying priors to them and hence obtaining posterior distributions. This is what makes such a model "fully Bayesian" [240].

We can add this inference to one of our existing models for a continuous outcome. First, let's assume that all studies, and all arms, drew from (sub-)populations with the same standard deviation (σ), even if their means differed:

$$\text{Data-generating process}:$$
$$y_{ij\text{Ctl}} \sim \mathrm{N}(\mu_j, \sigma)$$
$$y_{ij\text{Int}} \sim \mathrm{N}(\mu_j + \theta, \sigma)$$
$$\text{Likelihood}:$$
$$\therefore \bar{y}_{j\text{Ctl}} \sim \mathrm{N}\left(\mu_j, \frac{\sigma}{\sqrt{n_{j\text{Ctl}}}}\right)$$
$$\therefore \bar{y}_{j\text{Int}} \sim \mathrm{N}\left(\mu_j + \theta, \frac{\sigma}{\sqrt{n_{j\text{Int}}}}\right) \tag{8.10}$$
$$\therefore \frac{s_{jk}^2(n_{jk}-1)}{\sigma^2} \sim \chi^2(n_{jk}-1)$$
$$\text{Prior required for:}$$
$$(\mu_1, \mu_2 \ldots \mu_m) \in \mathbb{R}$$
$$\theta \in \mathbb{R}$$
$$\sigma \in \mathbb{R}^+$$

Of course, it is hard to believe that means differ but standard deviations never do. A more relaxed model would have two unknown population standard deviations, one for all intervention arms and one for all control arms. Meta-analyses with subgroups could justifiably divide it further.

It is also tempting, having learnt how to make random effects models with heterogeneity, to apply it to other aspects of our models too. Imagine a model with study-specific σ_js drawn from a heterogeneity distribution. Two important considerations should temper our enthusiasm. Firstly, what distribution would be justified? Secondly, will it make enough of a difference to be worth the effort? By "effort", we mean not only coding and checking it, but convincing colleagues, reviewers, and your audience of the merits of the rather unusual, and possibly unique, model you settle on.

8.5 Correlation Structure and Multiple Time Points

An alternative way of conceiving of the multiple arms is to view the patient data, and hence the study statistics, as drawn from a *multivariate distribution*. This is a little harder than the material we have covered before, conceptually and mathematically, so if you find it tough, we suggest you put a bookmark on this page and come back to it when you need it. It may make more sense later, after you have more hands-on experience of Bayesian meta-analysis.

We will begin with the subject matter of the chapter so far, two arms in a randomised study, and expand from there. The multivariate distribution idea can be very helpful and a compact way of capturing our likelihood model. The range of off-the-shelf multivariate distributions is not as great as the univariate (one variable) distributions, and if you find you need a bespoke one, it is certainly time to call for expert statistical help, as the mathematics becomes convoluted quickly.

We are just considering the sampling distribution part of the model. For two arms with a continuous-valued outcome variable, the control arm will (as the sample size grows large) have a normal sampling distribution. The intervention arm is similar but for the addition of θ, the contrast unknown:

$$\bar{y}_{j\mathbf{Ctl}} \sim \mathrm{N}\left(\mu + u_j, \widehat{SE}(\bar{y}_{j\mathbf{Ctl}})\right)$$
$$\bar{y}_{j\mathbf{Int}} \sim \mathrm{N}\left(\mu + u_j + \theta, \widehat{SE}(\bar{y}_{j\mathbf{Int}})\right) \tag{8.11}$$

If we wanted to use a common effect model, we could simply remove the random effects u_j. We will see in Chapter 9 that there are models that require a *fixed effects* approach, where we directly estimate a $\mu_j = \mu + u_j$ for each study, and in those cases, we can just make that substitution.

Each study is reporting two means: the control and the intervention arm. We can consider those two means as arising from a *multivariate normal* (MVN) distribution. This has a vector of two means, one for each arm, and a matrix of variances and *covariances*. In general, for z variables, there will be a vector of z means and a $z \times z$ covariance matrix.

To avoid confusion, we will write σ_X^2 for the population variance of a variable X (or whatever symbol the variable has). The population correlation of any two variables, X and Y, is ρ_{XY}. Their covariance is $\rho_{XY}\sigma_X\sigma_Y$. That is the population correlation of the two variables, times the population standard deviation of each. For our two arm study, because it is randomised, the data in the two arms will be uncorrelated.

If the participant-level data are bivariate normal (two arms), there is only one kind of correlation, so we can just write it as ρ. We call this distribution bivariate (two variables), and we can write it like this:

$$\begin{bmatrix} \bar{y}_{j\mathbf{Ctl}} \\ \bar{y}_{j\mathbf{Int}} \end{bmatrix} \sim \mathrm{MVN}\left(\begin{bmatrix} \mu + u_j \\ \mu + u_j + \theta \end{bmatrix}, \begin{bmatrix} \sigma_{j\mathbf{Ctl}}^2 & \rho\sigma_{j\mathbf{Ctl}}\sigma_{j\mathbf{Int}} \\ \rho\sigma_{j\mathbf{Ctl}}\sigma_{j\mathbf{Int}} & \sigma_{j\mathbf{Int}}^2 \end{bmatrix}\right) \tag{8.12}$$

Take a close look at the correlation matrix. The variances (standard deviations squared) are down a diagonal line from top left to bottom right. In matrix algebra, this is simply called *the diagonal*. The covariances are *off-diagonal*.

So, for randomised studies, we know that $\rho = 0$, and the covariance matrix simplifies to:

$$\begin{bmatrix} \sigma_{j\mathbf{Ctl}}^2 & 0 \\ 0 & \sigma_{j\mathbf{Int}}^2 \end{bmatrix} \tag{8.13}$$

In this case, we call the individual variables (sampling distributions, in this case) *independent*, and we could simply evaluate the likelihood of one ($\bar{y}_{j\mathbf{Int}} \sim \mathrm{N}(\mu + u_j + \theta, \sigma_{j\mathbf{Int}})$), then the likelihood of the other ($\bar{y}_{j\mathbf{Ctl}} \sim \mathrm{N}(\mu + u_j, \sigma_{j\mathbf{Ctl}})$), as shown in Equation 8.11, and add the two log likelihoods together. More complex multivariate structures will not be so simple, though.

8.5.1 Non-zero correlations

Studies that have some pairing of data between arms, such as pre-post designs, crossover trials, or within-human comparisons of healthy and affected organs, will have non-zero correlations between arms.

Using these in multivariate meta-analysis requires the covariance matrix to either be specified, based on the intra-study covariances [277], or to be estimated in a fully Bayesian way from the study data. One's preference for these options probably mirrors the alternative methods for network meta-analysis, which we touch on in Section 9.1.1.

However, unless we have individual participant data (IPD), we are unlikely to have much success in estimating all the correlations. If you want to try exploring the feasibility of this kind of meta-analysis, it will be vital to collaborate with an experienced statistician. Not every symmetric matrix is a valid covariance matrix *, so guessing covariance matrices, or initial values for them as unknowns, can lead to impossible values that will produce an error from your software.

8.5.2 Time points

If you are interested in using information from multiple time points in studies, then this too can be represented by a multivariate distribution. Even in randomised studies, we expect there to be quite strong correlation among time points. This additional information can be useful to impute unreported statistics (Chapter 11), deal with dichotomising studies (Chapter 14), or consider a time-response curve for interventions (Section 17).

We could drop or simplify the cumbersome subscripts to ρ if there is no scope for ambiguity. Here is the multivariate normal for three time points in an independent arms design:

$$
\begin{pmatrix} y_{ijk1} \\ y_{ijk2} \\ y_{ijk3} \end{pmatrix} \sim \mathrm{MVN} \left(\begin{pmatrix} \mu_{jk1} \\ \mu_{jk2} \\ \mu_{jk3} \end{pmatrix}, \right.
$$

$$
\left. \begin{pmatrix} \sigma_{jk1}^2 & \rho_{1,2}\sigma_{jk1}\sigma_{jk2} & \rho_{1,3}\sigma_{jk1}\sigma_{jk3} \\ \rho_{2,1}\sigma_{jk2}\sigma_{jk1} & \sigma_{jk2}^2 & \rho_{2,3}\sigma_{jk2}\sigma_{jk3} \\ \rho_{3,1}\sigma_{jk3}\sigma_{jk1} & \rho_{3,2}\sigma_{jk3}\sigma_{jk2} & \sigma_{jk3}^2 \end{pmatrix} \right) \right) \tag{8.14}
$$

This assumes that all studies and arms have the same set of correlations (ρ) relating two time points. That assumption could be relaxed, at the cost of a more complex multivariate model. Each element of the covariance matrix relates one time point (the row) to another (the column). If you consider that $\rho_{1,1} = \rho_{2,2} = \rho_{3,3} = 1$, you can see the underlying pattern.

---

*A covariance matrix must be square and symmetric, as well as having a property called *positive semi-definiteness*, which is a little more esoteric, but can be checked in a few ways, the simplest of which is that it has no negative eigenvalues. For more details on matrices in statistics, see the book by Gentle [91].

We could also construct such an expression for paired data over time points. Two paired arms at baseline $(t = 0)$ and endpoint $(t = 1)$ would have a mean vector of length four and a four-by-four covariance matrix.

Two independent arms at two time points would also involve a mean vector of length four and a four-by-four covariance matrix, but some of the elements of the covariance matrix would be zero by design because of zero population correlations between arm 1 and arm 2.

$$\begin{pmatrix} \sigma^2_{j10} & \rho\sigma_{j10}\sigma_{j11} & 0 & 0 \\ \rho\sigma_{j10}\sigma_{j11} & \sigma^2_{j11} & 0 & 0 \\ 0 & 0 & \sigma^2_{j20} & \rho\sigma_{j20}\sigma_{j21} \\ 0 & 0 & \rho\sigma_{j20}\sigma_{j21} & \sigma^2_{j21} \end{pmatrix} \quad (8.15)$$

You can consider the covariance matrix in 8.15 as having two submatrices of size two-by-two. The one in the top left describes the bivariate distribution of arm 1 over two time points, and the submatrix in the bottom right does the same for arm 2. If we choose to combine them into a multivariate, matrix representation like this, it will just be a matter of convenience for evaluating probabilities or generating random values.

8.5.3 Beyond multivariate normal

We have spoken so far about multivariate normal distributions for likelihoods, but of course, it is conceivable that some sampling distributions might not be normal. The mathematical formulas immediately become much more complicated as we move away from normality, and although there are some possible options, the simplest approach may be to try transforming variables (and therefore their statistics) so that they approach normality. As above, it is hard to have any assurance about this in the absence of IPD, and an experienced statistician's input will be important.

8.6   Meta-Analysis of Proportions, Incidence or Prevalence

Meta-analysis of proportions is a very commonly procedure used to synthesize data from multiple studies, particularly in domains such as medicine, ecology, psychology, and social sciences. The method focuses on estimating an overall proportion/prevalences and assessing variability across different studies. This subchapter delves into the methodologies involved in the meta-analysis of proportions focusing on current perspective on both classical and Bayesian approaches.

Meta-analysis of proportions involves combining data from various studies to derive a pooled estimate of a proportion and evaluate the heterogeneity among the studies. This technique is highly valuable in prevalence studies, where researchers seek to estimate the proportion of a population exhibiting a particular characteristic, such as the prevalence of a specific disease or behaviour.

Classically, meta-analysis of proportions has employed methods like the inverse variance method, which utilizes weighted averages of transformed proportions and their associated variances. Common transformations include the logit, arcsine, and Freeman-Tukey double arcsine transformations. These transformations are designed to stabilize variances and ensure that the proportions remain within the $[0, 1]$ interval, facilitating more accurate and reliable statistical analysis.

Key classical methods include:

1. Logit transformation: This transformation converts proportions to the log-odds scale, where they can be treated as normally distributed variables. This facilitates the use of standard meta-analytic techniques that assume normality.

2. Arcsine transformation: This method stabilizes the variance of proportions, making it particularly useful for small sample sizes where the variance of raw proportions can be highly unstable.

3. Freeman-Tukey double arcsine transformation: Combining two arcsine transformations, this method offers improved variance stabilization for small proportions and is often preferred in scenarios involving small sample sizes or extreme proportions.

In the last few years many authors have suggested the application of generalized linear mixed models (GLMMs) applied to the logit transformations: GLMMs account for the binary nature of the data and provide a more suitable analysis framework. These models incorporate both common-effect and random effects, allowing for the modelling of within-study and between-study variability simultaneously.

8.6.1 Logit transformation

The logit transformation is one of the most commonly used methods in meta-analysis of proportions. By transforming the proportion to the log-odds, this method stabilizes the variance and allows the transformed proportions to be treated as approximately normally distributed.

$$\text{logit}(p) = \log\left(\frac{p}{1-p}\right) \tag{8.16}$$

Equivalently in R:

```
logitp <- log(p/(1-p))
```

This transformation is particularly useful when the proportions are close to 0 or 1, where the variance of the raw proportions can be highly unstable.

Once the proportions are transformed, the inverse variance method can be applied to pool the logit-transformed proportions from multiple studies. The pooled estimate can then be back-transformed to obtain the overall proportion.

8.6.2 Arcsine transformation

The arcsine transformation is another classic method used to stabilize the variance of proportions. This transformation is particularly beneficial for small sample sizes, where the variance of raw proportions can be highly variable. The arcsine transformation is defined as:

$$\arcsin(\sqrt{p}) \tag{8.17}$$

Equivalently in R:

```
arcsinp <- asin(sqrt(p))
```

The arcsine transformation ensures that the transformed proportions have a finite variance, which remains stable across different values of p. This property makes it an attractive option for meta-analysis, especially when dealing with proportions near 0 or 1.

8.6.3 Freeman-Tukey double arcsine transformation

The Freeman-Tukey double arcsine transformation is a variant of the arcsine transformation that provides even better variance stabilization properties for small proportions. This transformation is defined as:

$$\frac{\arcsin(\sqrt{p}) + \arcsin(\sqrt{1-p})}{2} \tag{8.18}$$

Equivalently in R:

```
ft_p <- 0.5 * (asin(sqrt(p) + asin(sqrt(1-p)))
```

The double arcsine transformation addresses some of the limitations of the single arcsine transformation by combining two arcsine transformations, which helps to stabilize the variance more effectively for small proportions. Arcsine-based transformations do not require continuity corrections for zero event counts, which is advantageous over log and logit transformations.

An essential component of meta-analysis is the estimation of confidence intervals for the pooled proportions. Classical methods typically use asymptotic approximations to calculate confidence intervals for transformed proportions, based on the assumption of normality.

For example, the 95% confidence interval for a logit-transformed proportion is given by:

$$\text{logit}(p) \pm 1.96 \times \text{SE}(\text{logit}(p)) \tag{8.19}$$

where $\text{SE}(\text{logit}(p))$ denotes the standard error of the logit-transformed proportion.

The arcsine and Freeman-Tukey transformations also have their respective methods for calculating confidence intervals. The key is to transform the proportions, calculate the confidence intervals on the transformed scale, and then back-transform the intervals to the original scale.

8.6.4 Generalized linear mixed models (GLMMs)

GLMMs provide a more advanced framework for meta-analysis of proportions, taking into account the binary nature of the data and allowing for the modelling of both fixed and random effects. These models assume a binomial distribution for the observed proportions within each study and a normal distribution for the true proportions across studies.

A typical GLMM for meta-analysis of proportions can be specified as:

$$\begin{aligned} d_j &\sim \text{Binom}(p_j, n_j) \\ \text{logit}(p_j) &= \mu + u_j \\ u_j &\sim \text{N}(0, \tau) \end{aligned} \tag{8.20}$$

where d_j is the observed number of successes in study j, n_j is the total number of observations, p_j is the true proportion, μ is the overall logit-transformed proportion, and u_j is the random effect for study j with standard deviation τ. We would be most interested in reporting $\text{expit}(\mu)$ and τ, where $\text{expit}(\cdot)$ is the inverse logistic function, introduced in Section 1.3.1.

GLMMs offer several advantages over traditional methods, including the ability to model complex data structures and account for within-study and between-study variability more effectively. These models can be estimated using standard statistical software, providing a flexible and powerful tool for meta-analysis of proportions.

The Freeman-Tukey double arcsine transformation was initially developed to stabilize variance in single proportion analyses, facilitating more accurate confidence intervals and hypothesis testing. However, its application in meta-analyses of proportions presents significant challenges. It aims to normalize the distribution of proportions but encounters issues when combining data from studies with differing sample sizes.

Key problems include non-monotonicity, where higher proportions can result in lower transformed values, leading to incorrect rankings [151, 212]. Additionally, invertibility issues arise during back-transformation, requiring an arbitrary specification of sample size that can produce paradoxical results, such as estimates outside the range of observed data. One-stage models like generalized linear mixed models (GLMMs) bypass the need for intermediate transformations, providing more accurate and reliable estimates.

8.6.5   Comparison of Bayesian and non-Bayesian methods

The Bayesian framework is particularly advantageous when dealing with small sample sizes or sparse data, where classical methods may struggle to provide reliable estimates. We can easily implement a binomial-normal hierarchical model. This model assumes that the observed proportions follow a binomial distribution, while the true proportions are modelled with a normal distribution. This methodology provides a more nuanced and accurate estimate of proportions, especially when prior knowledge or previous research findings are available to inform the analysis.

The proposed Bayesian random effect model can be written as Equation 8.20. This is an implementation, at arm level, of the data-generating process in Equation 3.11. We can assume rather vague prior distributions for π and τ such as $\mu \sim N(0, 100)$ and $\tau \sim N^+(0, 5)$. BUGS code would then use `muj[j]` as the transformed shrunken proportion in study j:

```
for(j in 1:m) {
  d[j] ~ dbin(p[j], n[j])
  logit(p[j]) <- muj[j]
  muj[j] ~ dnorm(mu, prec)
}
mu ~ dnorm(0, 1.0E-4)
tau ~ dnorm(0, 0.04)
prec <- pow(tau, -2)
pi <- 1 / (1+exp(-1*mu))
```

9

Network Meta-Analysis

Learning objectives

After reading this chapter, you will be able to:

1. use Bayesian network-meta-analysis to compare more than one intervention

2. compute a Bayesian network meta-analysis for the arm statistics in terms of shared contrasts

3. understand the consistency assumption and how to check it

Often, there are several possible interventions, which we want to help our audience choose from. Some studies may have compared interventions A and B, some may have compared B and C, and so on. Combining all this information is the task of network meta-analysis, also known as indirect treatment comparisons or mixed treatment comparisons meta-analysis. We will refer to it as network meta-analysis (NMA).

NMA has long utilised Bayesian methods and software, as reflected in our scoping reviews [94, 218], which suggest that NMAs now make up more than half of all Bayesian meta-analyses*. It may well be the case that you have approached this book because you are principally interested in NMAs, and Bayesian methods are a means to an end. If that is so, and you have opened the book at this page, then we should warn you that are many valuable ideas in earlier chapters, which underpin the ideas here. As the Cochrane Handbook says: "Do not start here!" [112]

NMA allows us to make comparisons between interventions A, B and C, even when no trial exists that compares A to C. It requires a network of connections (Figure 9.1), where each line shows that a study has compared the intervention option at one end of the line to that at the other end. The numbers alongside the lines show how many studies made that comparison. We will explain how to form the network, and select which studies must be included, in Section 9.1.5.

NMA allows us to compare and rank multiple intervention options in one meta-analysis. This is much more helpful to the decision-maker than a series of unconnected meta-analyses comparing each pair of intervention options. We will call these *pairwise meta-analyses*.

Adopting a Bayesian approach also means that, in addition to the possibilities already mentioned, such as informative priors, we can present the probability of a particular intervention option being the best. We will see how to implement this in Section 9.2.

---

*The reason for this, we suspect, is partly that NMA does not have an easy, point-and-click interface like RevMan, and also because example BUGS code has been recommended for use [57], and is widely used, sometimes carelessly [94]. The popularity of the example code was a major reason for us to write this book.

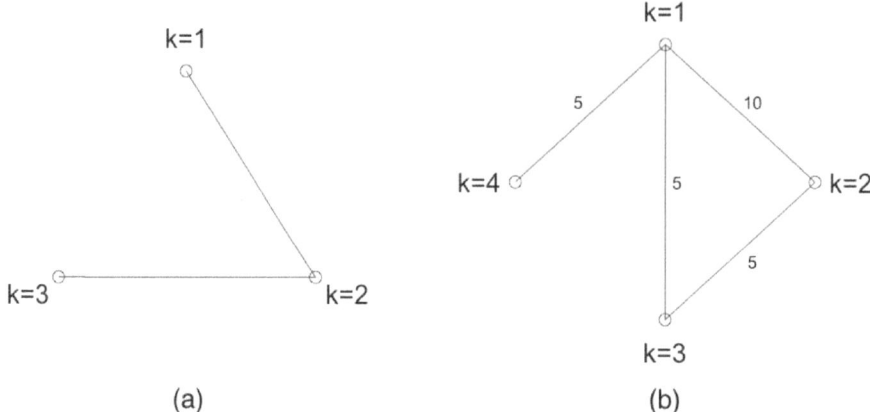

FIGURE 9.1
Two basic networks of studies: (a) a hypothetical basic network of studies on three intervention options, and (b) a simple but real network of four chemotherapy interventions). (Adapted from Dias *et al.*).

NMA is also attractive because it allows us to draw on evidence as widely as possible, given some assumptions. If we are simply interesting in comparing A and B, then studies comparing A and D, and B and D, will also provide information. We call the contribution of the A-B studies *direct evidence* and that of the A-D and B-D studies *indirect evidence*.

The practice of NMA would be quite simple if the direct and indirect evidence always agreed, a condition that is called *consistency*. However, there are reasons why it might not be the same, and we will consider how to detect this and what to do about it in Section 9.3.

Like the rest of this book, this chapter aims to provide you with a practical introduction. NMA is diverse and actively developing field, and to learn more, we recommend the book by Dias and colleagues [56], and we will present the same Bayesian models that they use. However, it is worth clarifying that we differ from them in embracing the many uses of priors. Also, not every NMA expert agrees with their views on modelling, which we will expand on below.

There are several links between NMA and emerging topics, which we address in Chapter 17.

9.1   General Principles

Suppose, as before, that our evidence base contains m studies, but now, study j can have K_j arms, which could be more than two. As before, we will write subscripts like d_{jk}, which would indicate the number of participants with a binary event in arm k of study j. However, to make these comparable between studies, we will use a consistent number in k to index a particular treatment. If $k = 3$ means a group exercise intervention, it will mean that in all studies. A study might then have non-consecutive k subscripts, and we will use K for the total number of interventions in the evidence base.

When we refer to contrasts between arms, we must now use the two k subscripts. In this book, we will only have single-digit k numbers, so to write something like θ_{j23} will hopefully be unambiguous. It means the contrast between arms $k = 2$ and $k = 3$, in study j, and in particular it is $k = 3$ *minus* $k = 2$. We think of this as the effect of moving from $k = 2$ to $k = 3$, though we should be careful not to imply a causal relationship if it is not justified.

To refer to this generally, we will write $\theta_{jkk'}$.

If we are dealing with log odds ratios, for example, it will be:

$$\theta_{j23} = \log(\omega_{j3}) - \log(\omega_{j2}) \tag{9.1}$$

Pairwise meta-analysis is a special case of NMA, where $K = 2$. In fact, if we set out the Bayesian model code the right way, we will find that we can use the same NMA code for pairwise analyses.

As in the arm-based chapter, predicted statistics in each arm must be constructed from unknown population contrasts, plus one of the study's arm stats to reflect inter-study heterogeneity. Here is a simple data-generating process (DGP) for a study of continuous outcomes that contains interventions $k = 1$ and $k = 3$, and reports mean differences (we omit priors for clarity):

Heterogeneity:
$$\theta_{j13} \sim N(\theta_{13}, \tau)$$
Sampling distributions: $\tag{9.2}$
$$\mu_{j3} = \mu_{j1} + \theta_{j13}$$
$$\hat{\mu}_{jk} \sim N(\mu_{jk}, SE(\hat{\mu}_{jk}))$$

Look closely at the first line under "Sampling distributions": one of the arm means (μ_{j1}) is not calculated like the others, but is estimated directly as an unknown in the model. There can be heterogeneity distributions for contrasts, but not for arm-specific unknowns, making them *fixed effects*.

Intervention $k = 1$ thus becomes the baseline intervention for this study. Trial-specific baselines are essentially *nuisance parameters*: we must estimate them in order to complete inference from our model, but they are not useful to us (other than detecting if we have done something wrong, or our sampling software has misbehaved). We do not put heterogeneity distributions on them in case they bias away from the true study-specific value, especially in conditions of few studies—see Chapter 8 for an explanation of how this can happen.

Not every study will contain $k = 1$, and they will have other baselines. In our NMA, we must relate all of these baselines back to one shared *reference intervention*[†], and we will measure all intervention effects relative to that. We will show this in mathematical formulas shortly, and in code in Section 9.2.

First, we must set out the same concept of DGP for binary outcomes, reporting (log) odds ratios:

Heterogeneity:
$$\theta_{j13} \sim N(\theta_{13}, \tau)$$
Sampling distributions: $\tag{9.3}$
$$\log(\omega_{j3}) = \log(\omega_{j1}) + \theta_{j13}$$
$$\log(\hat{\omega}_{jk}) \sim N(\log(\omega_{jk}), SE(\log(\hat{\omega}_{jk})))$$

The last line assumes a normal sampling distribution of the log odds, which depends on reasonable sample size, but if we cannot rely on this, we can use the binomial likelihood instead:

$$d_{jk} \sim \text{Binom}(\text{expit}(\omega_{jk}), n_{jk}) \tag{9.4}$$

[†]Reference interventions are sometimes called anchors, and occasionally pivots.

Note that there is only one shared heterogeneity standard deviation, τ, for all contrasts. This is a simplification to the model that many NMAs make, largely because there can be very low numbers of studies in any combination of two interventions. However, empirical priors can help (see Section 9.1.4).

Heterogeneity affects the contrasts, and we will be interested in quantifying and perhaps explaining it. There could also be inter-study differences that affect all arms equally, but such a difference will not affect contrasts. The assumption here is that such inter-study differences, affecting all arms in a study, can be assessed by looking at any one of the arms, and it is sensible to make that the fixed effect of the baseline intervention arm.

9.1.1   A dissenting view

Constructing contrasts, and arm-specific expected statistics, from basic contrasts is the method recommended by several NMA experts, and it is the one that we advocate too. However, an argument has also been made to view NMA as a missing data problem, where information is available on some interventions in some studies. The interventions that each study did *not* include are regarded as missing [115], and then the unknowns in the model are arm-specific, not contrasts.

This is an attractive theoretical framework but the counter-argument makes a strong case that the arm-based unknowns have a high risk of biasing results [55]. This debate is most likely not over, nor are these two standpoints the last word in NMA theory. The rejoinder by the missing data proponents makes a strong case too, and includes this thought-provoking sentence—perhaps we are all swayed by custom and culture, especially when working in a relative paucity of information:

> "As researchers steeped not in the work of the Cochrane Collaboration but instead in hierarchical Bayesian theory, methods, and computing, we naturally prefer to model *all* correlations we think might be present in *all* data sources we use" [116]

9.1.2   Multiple interventions and references

If we take $k = 1$ as the reference intervention, then any study including a $k = 1$ arm can simply have it set as the baseline, and the DGP above holds.

Those that do not contain a $k = 1$ arm will have a different baseline arm. A study with $k = 2$ and $k = 3$, for example, might use $k = 2$ as baseline. So, we need to set up the model so that the population unknown intervention effects $\theta_{kk'}$ draw on information from all studies.

Set $k = 1$ as the reference. Then, by definition, $\theta_{11} = \theta_{j11} = \hat{\theta}_{j11}0$. That means that there is no sampling distribution for it. However any other contrast relative to $k = 1$ is of interest to us and will have a prior and a likelihood based on the sampling distribution.

In a study with $k = 2$ and $k = 3$, we will be able to estimate θ_{j23}. We must form it out of the underlying contrasts with the reference:

$$\theta_{23} = \theta_{13} - \theta_{12}$$

Heterogeneity:

$$\theta_{j23} \sim N(\theta_{23}, \tau) \tag{9.5}$$

Sampling distribution:

$$\hat{\theta}_{j23} \sim N(\theta_{j23}, SE(\hat{\theta}_{j23}))$$

This implies that, if we can just infer all the contrasts with the reference ($\theta_{1k'}$), as well as τ and the nuisance parameters for the baseline arms, then everything else will follow.

The choice of which intervention to make the reference is often made for ease of interpretation: placebo, or standard care, a well-known and established intervention, or no intervention, might be chosen if it is present in the network. Otherwise, it would be sensible to choose an intervention that is connected directly in the network to the most alternatives [56].

9.1.3 Consistency assumption

In the DGPs above, we have adopted the assumption of *consistency*: that contrasts are stable across trials. This allowed us to have the first line in Equation 9.5, which stated: $\theta_{23} = \theta_{13} - \theta_{12}$. This means that the direct and the indirect evidence agree (plus-minus heterogeneity and sampling error, but no systemic bias).

In the network on the left of Figure 9.1, there would be no way check this assumption. The only information linking $k = 1$ and $k = 3$ would be the indirect evidence. In any network with a loop, however, there is both direct and indirect evidence, and they can be compared.

The network on the right side of Figure 9.1 would allow consistency to be checked among $k = 1$, $k = 2$, and $k = 3$, but not for any comparison with $k = 4$. We will discuss ways to do this checking in Section 9.3.

9.1.4 Heterogeneity

We have only described a simple heterogeneity model so far, where there is one shared standard deviation, τ, for all contrasts, and those study-specific random effects are all independent of one another. That implies that the values of, say, θ_{j12} and θ_{j13} tell us nothing about what θ_{j14} will turn out to be.

If you have reason to doubt this, you could model multiple heterogeneities. We feel it is unlikely in most settings that independence of random effects holds. Turner and colleagues describe two ways of modelling this (both are adequate), and suggest empirical priors for various types of outcomes [263].

Whether there is one τ or more than one, we expect correlation between study-specific contrasts that involve a common intervention. As we are building our model out of contrasts with the reference intervention, this will always be the case, for example between θ_{j12} and θ_{j13}, because both involve the reference $k = 1$. To capture this in our code, we could use a multivariate distribution, as shown in Section 8.5, but under some reasonable assumptions, it is easier to include it in the code as a *conditional distribution*—conditional on all the other contrasts' random effects in the study.

The simple heterogeneity model implies a covariance matrix for the multivariate distribution with no off-diagonal elements, because all the correlations are zero:

$$\begin{bmatrix} \tau^2 & 0 & 0 & \cdots & 0 \\ 0 & \tau^2 & 0 & \cdots & 0 \\ \vdots & & \ddots & & \vdots \\ 0 & 0 & \cdots & \tau^2 & 0 \\ 0 & 0 & \cdots & 0 & \tau^2 \end{bmatrix} \tag{9.6}$$

The conditional specification of heterogeneity aims at a covariance matrix with a single τ, hence a diagonal of τ^2, as above, but with all correlations set to a common value, say 0.5

[113]. This gives the following *exchangeable* covariance matrix:

$$\begin{bmatrix} \tau^2 & \tau^2/2 & \tau^2/2 & \dots & \tau^2/2 \\ \tau^2/2 & \tau^2 & \tau^2/2 & \dots & \tau^2/2 \\ \vdots & & \ddots & & \vdots \\ \tau^2/2 & \tau^2/2 & \dots & \tau^2 & \tau^2/2 \\ \tau^2/2 & \tau^2/2 & \dots & \tau^2/2 & \tau^2 \end{bmatrix} \tag{9.7}$$

While it's possible to supply such a matrix to BUGS, JAGS, Stan or Stata, and to request a multivariate distribution, the conditional specification is easier, and works like this. $\theta_{j11} = 0$ by definition. Then, from $k = 2$ onward, we have more and more information to pin down the expected random effect. As there is correlation among all the contrast random effects, by the time we get to $k = K_j$, we will know a lot about study j, and in particular, whether it has higher or lower contrasts to the reference than average. It is not guaranteed that a high θ_{j12} means a high θ_{j14}, for example, but it is more likely.

The mean of the heterogeneity distribution for θ_{j1k} will be:

$$\theta_{1k} + \frac{1}{k-1} \left((\theta_{j12} - \theta_{12}) + (\theta_{j13} - \theta_{13}) + \dots (\theta_{j1(k-1)} - \theta_{1(k-1)}) \right) \tag{9.8}$$

The series on the right of this formula is the sum of all the previous (1 to $k-1$) differences between the study's random effect and the unknown population contrast. Every time one of the previous study random effects was higher, for example, the mean of the kth random effect will go up a little too. If you prefer summation notation, you can write it like this:

$$\theta_{1k} + \frac{1}{k-1} \sum_{i=1}^{k-1} \theta_{j1i} - \theta_{1i} \tag{9.9}$$

Consider what happens in these formulas when $i = 1$: because $\theta_{j11} = \theta_{11} = 0$, that term simply disappears from the sum (it is equal to zero). So, you can think of this as a sum from 1 to $k - 1$, or from 2 to $k - 1$, the end result will be the same.

This formula will work for any study that contains *all* the interventions, but in reality, we must alter it a little. The logic will stay the same.

When study j does not contain intervention $k = 1$, it will have a different baseline intervention, and we need to elaborate the formula a little. Let's call the baseline $k = \ddot{k}$, and instead of adding terms built from every consecutive value of k, we will write "$< k$" under the summation, as a casual shorthand* for all the interventions in study j which come before the current intervention of interest, k. The formula here may help your understanding, but what really matters is the computer implementation, which is to follow.

$$(\theta_{1k} - \theta_{1\ddot{k}}) + \frac{1}{k-1} \sum_{<k} \left((\theta_{j1i} - \theta_{j1\ddot{k}}) - (\theta_{1i} - \theta_{1\ddot{k}}) \right) \tag{9.10}$$

This formula describes a heterogeneity distribution for the contrast $\theta_{j\ddot{k}k}$, which has the same role as θ_{j23} in Equation 9.5.

The heterogeneity standard deviation for θ_{j1k} is simpler:

$$\tau \sqrt{\frac{k}{2(k-1)}} \tag{9.11}$$

---

*This is one of only two places in this book where we give in to casual shorthands in the mathematics, because to spell it out (with an intersection of sets or some doubly subscript symbol) would probably be unhelpfully obscure for most of our intended readers. We hope that you do not feel patronised by this!

As k increases, more information becomes available. The formula above steadily shrinks the heterogeneity variance from τ^2 toward $\frac{\tau^2}{2}$. It may feel strange that we arbitrarily assign k and shrink some of the conditional heterogeneity distributions, but remember that these are the contrasts to the reference intervention, which combine to make up the totality of observed contrasts and arm statistics in the network. In combination, the effect is the same as a multivariate normal distribution.

To try correlations between random effects other than 0.5, it is probably easier to use the multivariate normal distribution, because the conditional specification is especially simple for 0.5. The general formula is explained in Appendix C.4 of *The BUGS Book* [156], though it requires some matrix calculations. We show a multivariate implementation in Stan in Section 9.2.3.

More flexible models, and advice on choosing log-normal priors, is given in an open-access paper by Turner and colleagues [263]. It is also possible to extend the heterogeneity analysis in NMA to meta-regression and subgroups [56, 213].

Heterogeneity in NMA is a serious concern, because inter-study differences, which we do not fully understand, and which affect contrasts, may undermine the consistency assumption. This is an ongoing area of methodological research [3].

9.1.5   Forming the network

The network structure is critical to everything that follows, and the classification of interventions in individual studies into classes that will be treated as alike in NMA needs to be agreed and signed off by the whole project team.

A particular concern in many settings is deciding when study variations in intervention justify inclusion as a different k. Sometimes, the boundary between one class and another can be very blurred, and studies can implement multiple interventions together.

Forming a network starts with the identification of all the classes of intervention that you may be interested in comparing, if they are present in the evidence base. This list ought to be reflected in your search strategy. Next, draw the lines connecting all the classes where there are studies making those comparisons.

At this stage, you may find that the network is not entirely connected, but has two or more islands. If this is the case, you need to extend your search to other interventions, which may not be of much interest, but will connect all the network together.

Suppose you are researching exercise compared to anti-inflammatory drugs for osteoarthritis symptoms. You find studies comparing some exercise methods to one another (tai chi to aquarobics, for example). You also find drug-to-drug studies, but no study that compares drug(s) to exercise(s)[†]. However, if you included steroid injections, you might locate a study comparing steroid injections to exercise, and another comparing steroid injections to other drugs. This would connect up your network (Figure 9.2).

To ensure that there is no cherry-picking of connecting interventions or studies involving them, *any* connecting intervention should be included, thus obtaining as much information as possible (shown as "other?" in Figure 9.2, and a search should be run for any relevant studies connecting the network to that new intervention.

[†]This is not entirely surprising. Drug companies likely sponsored most of the drug studies, and were preoccupied with proving their product better than the competitor. Exercise studies are done by clinical physiotherapy teams and academics, focused on their profession's choices, and without the resources for drug studies. It can be a very valuable part of your NMA output to call for new research that might connect a network and shed light on comparative efficacy of the "islands".

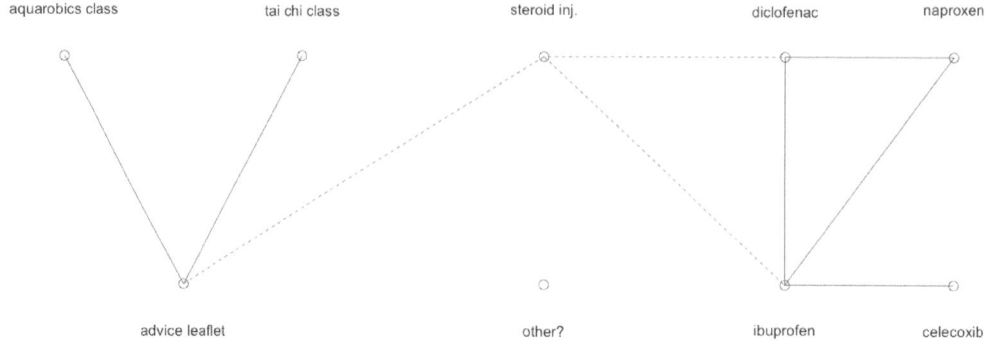

FIGURE 9.2
Hypothetical network of treatments in osteoarthritis, informed by work on the 2008 NICE Guideline [75]. Dashed lines are potentially added to connect the "islands".

9.2   Software Implementation

NMA is such a common use of Bayesian methods in meta-analysis that we give examples with BUGS but also show some differences with Stan in this chapter, and we comment briefly on JAGS and Stata.

Implementation of these models in a probabilistic programming language is not too hard. The unknowns of principal interest are the contrasts with the reference, because we can use them to directly compare and rank the intervention options. Ranking is best done after obtaining the posterior sample, by acting on each posterior draw. It is possible to do it inside your Bayesian software, but it is less clear for beginners.

The three aspects that will look new are: multiple interventions, nested indexing, and study-specific fixed effects, and, in the random effects models, the conditional heterogeneity standard deviation.

By nested indexing, we mean that the data includes a column recording the intervention used in each arm, called `tx[]`. This contains integers from 1 to 7, and we can use them to look up the relevant unknowns. For example, `theta[tx[i]]` will first get `tx[i]`, which is the intervention number in the current arm (row `i`). If this is 3, for example, then `theta[3]` is obtained and used in our calculations. We can apply this nested indexing to study numbers, baseline interventions and so on.

Remember that we should expect study baseline arm statistics (μ_{jk}) and the study-specific contrasts ($\theta_{jkk'}$) to be correlated in sampling distributions and posteriors, especially for small n_j. This is just the same as we might see between an intercept and a slope in a regression.

We will use a well-known example of randomised controlled trials comparing six thrombolytic ("clot-buster") drugs after heart attack with a stent to open the artery (percutaneous transluminal coronary angioplasty, PTCA). The binary outcome is 35-day mortality. The network is shown in typical fashion in Figure 9.3, using Stata (see below). The size of the circles indicates the number of participants in each study, and the thickness of the lines indicates the number of studies linking two intervention options.

 The code in this section is adapted from Dias and colleagues [56], and the full versions for WinBUGS and Stan are online.

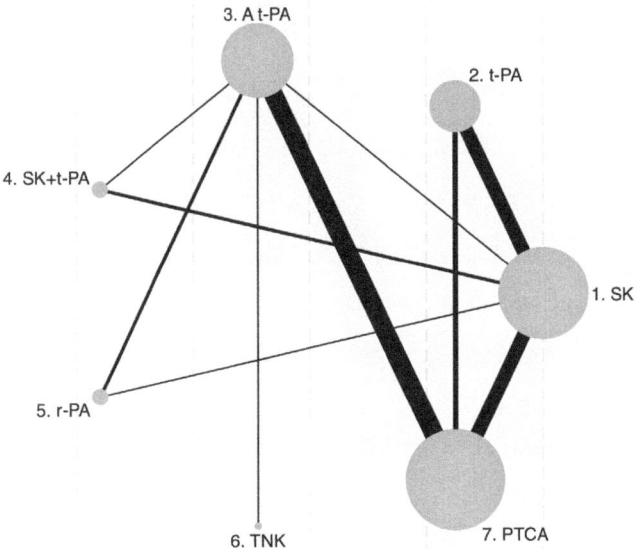

FIGURE 9.3
Network of studies comparing thrombolytic drugs and stenting (PTCA). Streptokinase (SK) is $k = 1$, and k numbers cycle from it anti-clockwise, ending at $k = 7$ for PTCA.

9.2.1 BUGS and JAGS

We have a "tall" dataset with one row for each combination of study and arm. There are columns for the study and intervention ID, and for the baseline intervention ID for that study. For the first of these three versions of the model, we provide WinBUGS with data as a list of scalars and then a tab-delimited format, which begins like this:

```
list(N=73, m=36, K=7)

study[] tx[] baseline[] d[]    n[]
1       1    1          1472   20251
1       3    1          652    10396
1       4    1          723    10374
2       1    1          3      65
2       2    1          3      64
3       1    1          12     159
3       2    1          7      157
4       1    1          7      85
4       2    1          4      86
5       1    1          10     135
5       2    1          5      135
[... 62 more lines ...]
```

For JAGS via the R package rjags, or BUGS via R packages, we can send the objects directly from R.

In the data, the `study[]` column contains the j number of the study, the `tx[]` column contains the k number of that intervention, while `baseline[]` corresponds to $\ddot{k}$.

The common effect code is:

```
model{
  # prior:
  theta[1]<-0
  for (k in 2:K){
    theta[k] ~ dnorm(0, 0.25)
  }
  for(j in 1:m){
    mu[j] ~ dnorm(0,.0001)
  }

  # likelihood:
  for(i in 1:N){
    logit(p[i]) <- mu[study[i]] +
                   theta[tx[i]] -
                   theta[baseline[i]]
    d[i] ~ dbin(p[i],n[i])
  }
}
```

The `theta[]` posteriors are shown in Figure 9.4. `theta[1]` is omitted as it is fixed at zero. We can see that `theta[7]`, the effect of stenting (PTCA) is clearly shifted into negative values and has a much lower mean than the others. This suggests that no thrombolytic drug

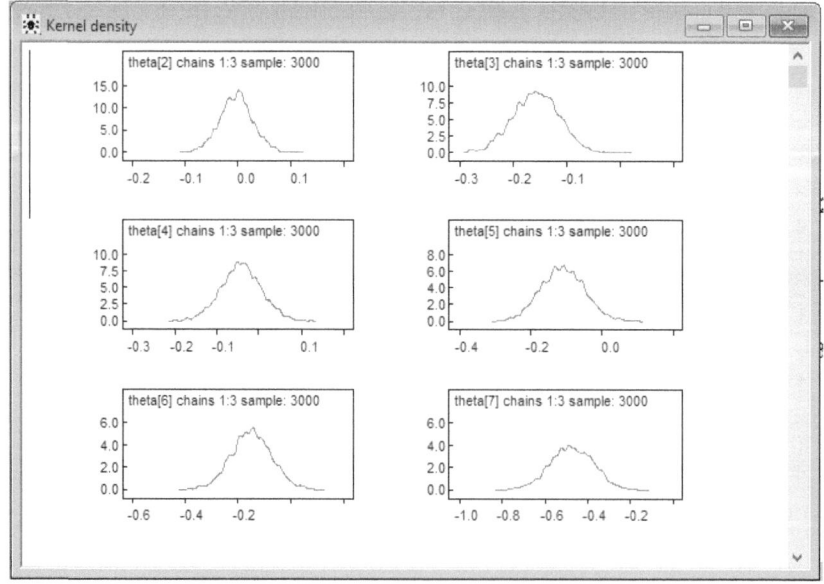

FIGURE 9.4
Marginal posterior densities of θ_{1k}, from WinBUGS.

can compete with stenting, on average, to reduce 35-day mortality. This meta-analysis can tell us nothing about combinations of interventions, or sequencing one after another, or which patients will not benefit from stenting—those were not the questions it set out to answer.

The following code is used (with the same data) for the simple heterogeneity model with no correlations:

```
model{
  # prior:
  tau ~ dnorm(0,2)I(0,)
  theta[1]<-0
  for (k in 2:K){
    theta[k] ~ dnorm(0, 0.25)
  }
  for(j in 1:m){
    mu[j] ~ dnorm(0,.0001)
  }

  # heterogeneity:
  tau_prec <- pow(tau,-2)
  for(j in 1:m){
    theta_j[j,1] <- 0
    for(k in 2:K) {
      theta_j[j,k] ~ dnorm(theta[k],tau_prec)
    }
  }

  # likelihood:
  for(i in 1:N){
    logit(p[i]) <- mu[study[i]] +
                   theta_j[study[i],tx[i]] -
                   theta_j[study[i],baseline[i]]
    d[i] ~ dbin(p[i],n[i])
  }
}
```

Note that we have applied a half-normal prior to the heterogeneity standard deviation. If yuou are using JAGS, you will have to switch I(0,) for T(0,).

Mixing of the chains is slow and they are strongly autocorrelated. The traceplot for `tau` appears in Section 2.5 after 20,000 iterations, thinning to every tenth (Dias and colleagues ran it for 150,000 iterations, which is not unusual in BUGS and JAGS.) Results are similar to those from the common effect model. The heterogeneity standard deviation, `tau` is probably close to zero, as seen in Figure 9.5.

The code for the conditional heterogeneity model deserves careful attention. It requires data that is wider, with a column for each arm, up to 3. Note the WinBUGS trick of calling the columns something like a matrix so that it can then be called as such inside the code:

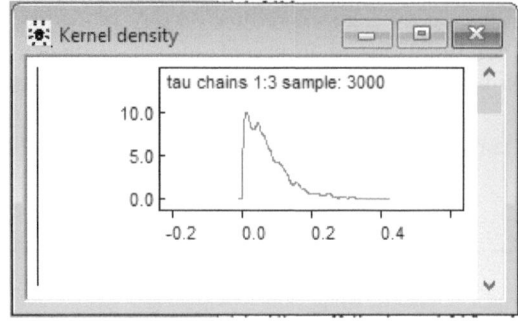

FIGURE 9.5

Marginal posterior density for the heterogeneity standard deviation in the common hetero-geneity random effects model with no correlations, from WinBUGS.

```
list(m=36, K=7)

k_j[] tx[,1] tx[,2] tx[,3] d[,1] n[,1] d[,2] n[,2] d[,3] n[,3]
3     1      3      4      1472  20251 652   10396  723   10374
2     1      2      NA     3     65    3     64     NA    NA
2     1      2      NA     12    159   7     157    NA    NA
2     1      2      NA     7     85    4     86     NA    NA
2     1      2      NA     10    135   5     135    NA    NA
2     1      2      NA     887   10396 929   10372  NA    NA
2     1      2      NA     5     63    2     59     NA    NA
2     1      2      NA     1455  13780 1418  13746  NA    NA
2     1      2      NA     9     130   6     123    NA    NA
[... 27 more lines ...]
```

NA means missing values. These do not cause a problem because the looping in the code never accesses them.

```
model{
  # prior:
  tau ~ dnorm(0,2)I(0,)
  theta[1]<-0
  for (k in 2:K){
    theta[k] ~ dnorm(0, 0.25)
  }
  for(j in 1:m){
    mu[j] ~ dnorm(0,.0001)
  }

  # heterogeneity:
  tau_prec <- pow(tau,-2)
  for(j in 1:m){
    theta_j[j,1] <- 0
```

```
    cond_adj[j,1] <- 0
    for(k in 2:k_j[j]) {
      cond_adj[j,k] <- theta_j[j,k] -
                       (theta[tx[j,k]]-theta[tx[j,1]])
      het_mean[j,k] <- theta[tx[j,k]]-theta[tx[j,1]] +
                       sum(cond_adj[j,1:k-1])/(k-1)
      het_prec[j,k] <- tau_prec*2*(k-1)/k
      theta_j[j,k] ~ dnorm(het_mean[j,k],het_prec[j,k])
    }
  }

  # likelihood:
  for(j in 1:m){
    for(k in 1:k_j[j]){
      logit(p[j,k]) <- mu[j] +
                       theta_j[j,k] -
                       theta_j[j,1]
      d[j,k] ~ dbin(p[j,k],n[j,k])
    }
  }
}
```

This calculates each term of the sum from Equation 9.10 as `cond_adj`, then adds these up and divides by $(k-1)$ for each arm k. Note that in the code, k indexes the arm *within the study*, so they are consecutive numbers, and not the same as the k in our mathematical notation. This requirement for loops limits our choices of how we can send the data, and this is the least bad of a few unpalatable options for setting out the code and data. In Section 9.2.3, we consider how it can be set up in Stan.

We ran three chains for 10,000 iterations after 1000 warm-up, and thinned it to every tenth. Results are similar to the other two models: there is no strong evidence to support a particular heterogeneity model, and `tau` appears to be small but not negligible. However, there are a small number of more extreme posterior draws for all the values of `theta[]`, as seen in Figure 9.6. If interest were focused on the tails of these marginal distributions, then because of the high autocorrelation in the MCMC chains, it would be sensible to obtain many more draws. With the Gibbs sampler, it is not uncommon to require millions of iterations, perhaps thinned to every hundred if available memory is a concern. Dias and colleagues ran it for 150,000 iterations [56].

In order to accommodate correlations other than 0.5, or more complex correlation structures, it is easier to model all the elements of `theta`, except the first, as arising from a multivariate heterogeneity distribution. We see an example of this in BUGS code, in a somewhat different setting, in Section 12.2.

9.2.2 R interfaces to JAGS

R packages `bnma` and `gemtc` are high-level interfaces that call JAGS to run preset NMA models in the background. Although we recommend working directly with the probabilistic programming language of JAGS, or alternatives, you may be interested in these R packages. Chen and Peace give a detailed example of using `gemtc` for NMA of a continuous outcome [41].

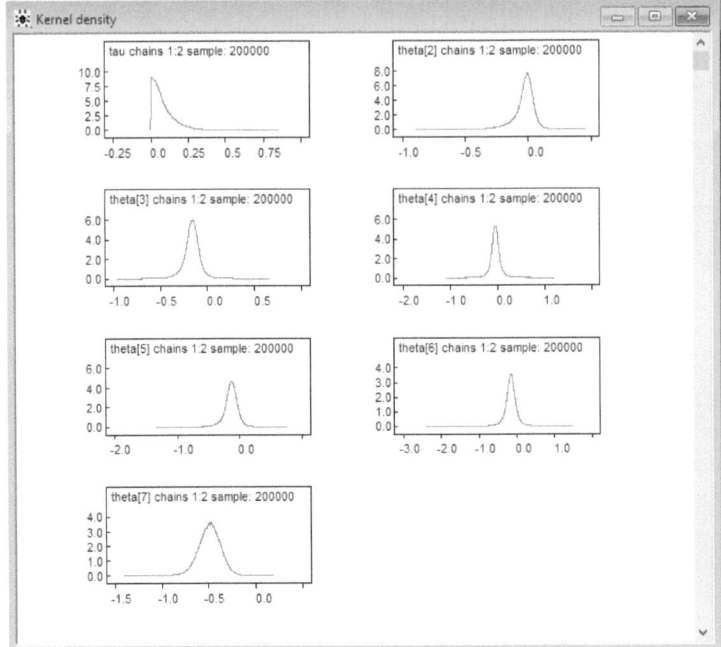

FIGURE 9.6
Marginal posterior densities of θ_{1k} in the conditional heterogeneity random effects model with exchangeable correlations of 0.5, from WinBUGS.

9.2.3   Stan

There are a few important differences between BUGS/JAGS and Stan, which we should discuss here. If NMA is a large part of your meta-analytic practice, then the differences in programming syntax are important, and you might prefer to work with Stan. Some differences are illustrated here, but the translations of all the models to Stan are available online.

Any software using the Gibbs sampler algorithm or random walk Metropolis-Hastings will be able to deal with the quasi-degenerate trick of setting `theta[1]` to a very small standard deviation around zero. The benefit of this is that you can then treat every element of `theta` as having a normal prior distribution. In Stan, which uses Hamiltonian Monte Carlo (see Section 2.4.4), it is possible but not usually a good idea.

This is because Stan has to take small steps from one iteration to the next, and the size of the step is limited by the unknown with the smallest range of values. `theta[1]`, if it has a standard deviation of 0.0001 or similar, will force a similarly small step size, and slow Stan down accordingly.

The answer to this problem is to sample from a $(K-1)$-vector of standard normal distributions, and then insert these into the K-vector to use in any of the heterogeneity models. This is the code for the random effect model with common heterogeneity:

```
data {
    int N;      // total number of study-arms (73)
    int m;      // number of studies (36)
    int K;      // number of treatments (7)
```

```
  array[N] int baseline;      // baseline id
  array[N] int study;         // study id
  array[N] int tx;            // treatment id
  array[N] int d;    // number of deaths
  array[N] int n;    // number of participants
}
parameters {
  array[m] real mu;
  array[K-1] real theta; // omit the reference intervention
  real<lower=0> tau;
  array[m,(K-1)] real theta_j_norm;
}
transformed parameters {
  array[m,K] real theta_j;
  for(j in 1:m) {
    theta_j[j,1] = 0.0;
    for(k in 2:K) {
        theta_j[j,k] = theta[k-1] + theta_j_norm[j,k-1]*tau;
    }
  }
}
model {
  // priors:
  mu ~ normal(0,100);
  for(k in 1:(K-1)) {
    theta[k] ~ normal(0,0.707);
  }
  tau ~ normal(0,2);

  // heterogeneity:
  for(j in 1:m) {
    for(k in 2:K) {
        theta_j_norm[j,k-1] ~ std_normal();
    }
  }

  // likelihood:
  for(i in 1:N) {
    d[i] ~ binomial_logit(n[i],
                  mu[study[i]] +
                  theta_j[study[i],tx[i]] -
                  theta_j[study[i],baseline[i]]);
  }
}
,
```

We have kept the usual formulation of `theta_j` as a matrix with m rows and K columns, but the `theta` vector has only K-1 elements, as we omit the reference intervention.

The first column of `theta_j`, relating to the reference intervention, is set to exactly zero in the `transformed parameters` block. Then, the remaining columns are filled with the random effects, with means `theta[k]` and standard deviation `tau`. We achieve this by sampling a `m` by `K` matrix of standard normal distributed values (mean 0, standard deviation 1), called `theta_j_norm`, multiply them by `tau` and add `theta[k-1]`.

The standard deviation of $0.707 = \frac{1}{\sqrt{2}}$ on the prior for `tau` matches the precision of 2 in the BUGS code.

This model mixes well compared to the same model in BUGS, partly thanks to Stan's algorithm, and partly because the parameter (unknown) space uses the standard normal distribution, rather than shrinking and expanding as `tau` tries different values.

Another difference is that, in the conditional specification in BUGS, we sent a matrix containing some `NA` missing values, to capture the fact that studies had different numbers of arms. Stan does not permit missing values, so a different approach is needed. However, Stan allows more flexibility in coding, which helps. We do not have to use a new meaning of `k` like in BUGS (the number of the intervention within each study), in order to add all the previous interventions' values of `cond_adj` together. This keeps the code a little easier to read. The code is available online.

9.2.4   Stata

Stata has historically been ahead of most software in developing meta-analysis capabilities. This was often developed first by expert users, and much of that is now adopted into core Stata. Network meta-analysis is now available through the `network` commands developed by Ian White [280], which in turn call on the `network_graphs` package of commands by Anna Chaimani and Georgia Salanti. There is also work ongoing to develop commands for Bayesian network meta-analysis. We hope that there will be Bayesian NMA capability within a few years of this book's publication.

We should also note that the `bayesmh evaluators` syntax, though not simple for beginners to grasp, gives great flexibility for model specification.

9.3   Dealing with Inconsistency

Inconsistency and heterogeneity are difficult to distinguish from one another in NMA, unless there are very many studies. If there is a loop in the network, and within that loop, we find a difference between direct and indirect evidence, then that suggests inconsistency. However, the direct and indirect evidence will come from different studies, so is it inconsistency or just heterogeneity between those studies?

Heterogeneity estimates, especially with fairly vague priors on τ and few trials, will be large and can mask inconsistency [58]. To tell them apart, we need many studies. This remains a difficult challenge in NMA [3].

In the same way that we can try to explain heterogeneity (see Section 4.7) as arising from study characteristics which impact on the contrasts. Using the term "effect modifiers" from causal inference for this [110], Dias and colleagues explain it precisely this way:

> "[...] inconsistency is caused by [...] an imbalance in the distribution of effect modifiers in the direct and indirect evidence" [56]

The more we know about these study differences, the better equipped we are to disentangle the heterogeneity-inconsistency phenomenon; painstaking extraction of data and metadata from the studies will be extremely important.

There are a number of ways to try to detect or quantify inconsistency within a network, that are not necessarily Bayesian. One of these, inconsistency degrees of freedom, gives us an idea of the scope for testing consistency assumptions: how many pairwise comparisons minus how many θ_{1k} there are in the consistency model.

There are also hypothesis tests (proposed by Bucher) where the null hypothesis is of no difference between direct and indirect evidence within loops, which may be a step too far from a Bayesian explanation of inference for most practitioners. A more Bayesian approach, though somewhat heuristic, is the concept of splitting studies (nodes in the network), with particular application in the Gibbs sampler, proposed by O'Hagan [58].

Our preference is to approach the problem through multiple models and model comparison. A simple way of specifying an *inconsistency model* is to remove the notion that the expected value of any contrast can be constructed from the "basic" θ_{1k} contrasts. Instead, for every combination of interventions k and k' that appears as an observed contrast in the evidence base, $\hat{\theta}_{jkk'}$, we include a study-specific random effect $\hat{\theta}_{jkk'}$, which comes from a heterogeneity distribution:

Heterogeneity:
$$\theta_{jkk'} \sim \mathrm{N}(\theta_{kk'}, \tau)$$

Sampling distribution:
$$\hat{\theta}_{jkk'} \sim \mathrm{N}(\theta_{jkk'}, \mathrm{SE}(\hat{\theta}_{jkk'}))$$

(9.12)

While the consistency model requires inference on $K - 1$ unknowns of the form θ_{1k}, the inconsistency model could have as many as $\frac{K(K-1)}{2}$. To compare the ability of these two models to explain the data, we could use the posterior predictive methods described in Section 2.5.4. Alternatives that are more reductive include leave-one-out cross-validation and information criteria [88, 156, 242]. Dias and colleagues give worked examples [56].

9.4 Challenges in Network Meta-Analysis

NMA allows us to compare and rank multiple intervention options in one meta-analysis, which is more helpful to decision makers than a series of unconnected pairwise meta-analyses. However, NMA faces several methodological and practical challenges that can affect the validity and applicability of its findings.

One of the foremost concerns is the presence of heterogeneity and inconsistency within a network of studies. Substantial variability among study results and discrepancies between direct and indirect evidence can compromise the reliability of NMA outcomes [3]. Addressing these issues requires appropriate methodological strategies to minimise their influence, such as employing advanced statistical models that account for heterogeneity and testing for inconsistencies within the network.

The complexity inherent in NMAs—particularly those involving datasets with numerous treatments and outcomes, and more sophisticated models for heterogeneity—increases the risk of misinterpretation. Effectively communicating NMA results needs to focus on helping decision makers to identify the most appropriate interventions, particularly when balancing various benefits and risks [175].

Various ranking methods exist, including Bayesian approaches such as the surface under the cumulative ranking curve (SUCRA) and frequentist methods such as the P-score. Critics have argued that these methods often fail to consider the limitations of the evidence base, such as the risk of bias, and may provide a false sense of precision.

Over-reliance on treatment rankings, such as those presented in league tables, has been criticised for not adequately reflecting the uncertainty associated with each position. Rankings may misleadingly suggest superiority among treatments when the differences are not clinically meaningful. Research indicates that ranking treatments based solely on SUCRA or P-scores offers no real advantage over ranking them based on point estimates [49].

Another critical concern is the identification and management of trial-level outliers. Although heterogeneity and inconsistency have been extensively discussed, there is limited guidance on effectively detecting and handling studies that significantly deviate from the rest of the network [286].

9.5   Writing Up

In addition to the general advice of Chapter 7, when presenting NMA results, you should explain:

1. motivation for NMA rather than pairwise meta-analysis

2. decisions to combine or separate interventions

3. justification of priors

4. sensitivity analysis for priors

5. choice of heterogeneity model and correlation matrix, if applicable

6. assessment of inconsistency

7. choice of reference intervention

8. extension of network in order to connect islands

9. method to find studies using interventions that connect islands

10. ranking method

The network structure should be shown. There are several software tools for this in R and Stata. Other visualisations are a subject of ongoing proposals and evaluation [175, 270].

Reporting guidelines / checklist have been proposed, including a PRISMA extension for NMAs [60, 120].

It is quite common to see NMA publications that begin with pairwise comparisons and then show the NMA [94]. This is appropriate for a technical audience that are familiar with NMA, but presents a challenge to less statistically trained decision-makers. How are they to reconcile the pairwise and the NMA? Without understanding of the relationships, they may cherry-pick the statistic that best fits their expectations or that pleases their stakeholders.

Worse yet is the practice of casual eclecticism, where the pairwise meta-analyses are frequentist and the NMA is Bayesian. Three irreconcilable differences can arise, in addition to simple differences in the numbers and conclusions. Firstly, a frequentist interpretation of probability usually precludes any meaning other than an asymptotic proportion "in the long-run"*, while the Bayesian admits a wider range of meanings. They are describing different things. Secondly, if there is anything other than a flat or diffuse prior in the Bayesian NMA, the methods are attempting to estimate different targets (estimands). Thirdly, the frequentist meta-analysis may provide p-values, while the Bayesian NMA will not, and in the other direction, the frequentist meta-analyses will not provide probabilities of A being a superior choice to B. If you must do both, make them compatible in methods.

---

*"in the long run" is itself a misleading phrase: there is no need, in the frequentist concept of probability, to be physically able to nearly replicate the NMA indefinitely, nor do those near-replicates have to take place sequentially—but philosophical considerations are beyond the scope of this book.

10

Individual Participant Data

Learning objectives

After reading this chapter, you will be able to:

1. understand the difference between individual participant data (IPD) and "aggregate data" meta-analyses

2. choose and justify a one-stage or two-stage method for IPD meta-analysis

3. contribute to the systematic review process so that any IPD meta-analysis from the studies that arise is accurate and unbiased

4. identify potential sources of bias or threats to external validity that can be addressed through IPD meta-analysis

Meta-analyses traditionally rely on study statistics extracted from published studies. However, there is a growing interest in using individual participant data (IPD) for meta-analyses. IPD refers to the raw data collected for each participant in a research study, such as baseline characteristics, prognostic factors, treatments received, various outcomes, and follow-up details. This data is typically represented in a dataset where each row corresponds to a participant and each column to a variable.

The use of IPD in meta-analyses introduces several additional steps compared to traditional meta-analyses, which IPD literature refers to as *aggregate data* (AD) meta-analyses. These steps primarily include the collection, verification, harmonization, and pooling of IPD from all relevant studies to answer specific research questions. It is crucial to emphasize that a meta-analysis must be comprehensive. Researchers need to gather all available evidence rather than selectively pooling studies based on accessibility. An additional source of bias affecting IPD meta-analysis is *availability bias*, when the studies offering IPD are unlike those that do not.

One of the key advantages of IPD meta-analyses is their ability to evaluate participant-level characteristics in relation to various outcomes more robustly. AD meta-analyses rely on summary statistics reported in publications, which may not capture the nuances that the meta-analyst is interested in.

IPD opens the possibility of exploring interactions between participant characteristics and treatment effects. Also, by analysing the data inside each study, we can obtain correlations and other rarely-reported statistics. We can also assess (in)consistency for NMAs.

The ability to standardise outcomes and covariate definitions across studies is another relevant benefit of IPD meta-analyses. This standardisation ensures consistency in how outcomes and covariates are measured and reported, which is essential for reliable comparisons across studies. This process involves thorough checks for data validity, range, and

DOI: 10.1201/9781003375821-10

consistency of variables, which can identify and correct errors or inconsistencies that might otherwise compromise the analysis. For example, researchers can ensure that the same definitions and measurement methods are used for key variables, which facilitates more accurate and meaningful comparisons.

IPD meta-analyses also offer greater flexibility in statistical analysis. Researchers are not constrained by the original study methods and can employ different statistical methods better suited to the specific research question. For example, IPD meta-analysis has been proposed for studies reporting survival analyses with restricted mean survival time [278].

While IPD meta-analyses have numerous advantages, it is essential to assess the added value they bring before embarking on such an endeavour. When outcome definitions are consistent across studies, both AD and IPD meta-analyses will yield similar results.

Given the substantial efforts required for IPD meta-analyses, researchers must carefully consider whether the potential benefits justify the additional complexity and resources. This assessment involves evaluating whether the detailed participant-level analysis, the inclusion of unpublished data, and the enhanced flexibility in statistical methods will provide significant improvements over traditional aggregate data approaches.

10.1   Two-Stage vs One-Stage Approach

There are two primary approaches to conducting an IPD meta-analysis: the two-stage approach and the one-stage approach. In the two-stage approach, the first stage is to analyse each study separately, making any necessary amendments to synchronise study statistics. In the second stage, these individual study results are combined in an AD meta-analysis, to produce a pooled estimate along with its uncertainty, such as confidence or credible intervals.

This approach is often preferred because it allows the use of standard meta-analytic models (common effect or random effects) in the second stage, making it particularly accessible to a wider range of professionals, especially non-statisticians. Of course Bayesian models can be used in this approach. The first stage can employ any consistent method across all included studies, though if both stages are Bayesian, they should not both have informative priors on θ, or this will make an unintentionally double-strength prior.

The one-stage approach, on the other hand, involves analysing the IPD from all studies simultaneously using an appropriate multilevel model, also known as a hierarchical or mixed effects model. This model needs to be tailored to the specific type of outcome data and include appropriate assumptions about whether each parameter of the model (e.g., intercept, treatment effect) is common, stratified, or random across trials. These three choices relate directly to the common effect, fixed effects, and random effects models described in Part 1 of this book. For example, in the case of a continuous outcome variable that we are confident is normally distributed in the population, it will make use of all the parts of the data-generating process in Section 3.5.1.

The one-stage approach has been recommended when trials are small in terms of the number of participants or events [202]. This is because it avoids synthesizing trial-specific estimates that are assumed to be normally distributed with known variances and instead produces meta-analysis results by modelling the underlying distribution of the outcome data directly, for example using binomial likelihood for proportions and Poisson for counts. However, as we have described, likelihoods can be chosen flexibly in Bayesian modeling, so this is not a compelling rationale to prefer one-stage IPD in Bayesian meta-analysis.

Additionally, one-stage models offer greater flexibility, allowing researchers to consider a broader set of assumptions linking studies, such as whether residual variances are the same in each study or whether baseline hazard functions are distinct or proportional across trials.

The practical choice between these approaches often depends on the specifics of the data and the research question, as well as the experience of the systematic review team. For instance, in situations where the studies are highly heterogeneous or have few participants, a one-stage approach might be preferable. Conversely, when the studies are more homogeneous and the focus is on transparency and simplicity, a two-stage approach might be more suitable. Ultimately, the choice should be guided by the research objectives, the nature of the data, and the available resources.

In the context of meta-analysis, it is important to consider the statistical properties of the different approaches. One-stage approaches are often more flexible because they allow for the fitting of a wider range of models [172]. This flexibility can be particularly advantageous when dealing with complex data structures or when more sophisticated modelling is required. However, the two-stage approach is often seen as simpler and more transparent, which can be beneficial for ensuring that the analysis is understood and can be replicated by other researchers.

The precision of the estimates obtained from one-stage and two-stage approaches has been a topic of considerable debate. While some argue that one-stage approaches can lead to more precise estimates, this is not always the case. For example, in situations where the studies included in the meta-analysis are relatively small, the precision of the estimates from one-stage and two-stage approaches can be quite similar. This is because, in such cases, the variability between studies is relatively low, and the additional flexibility offered by the one-stage approach does not necessarily translate into more precise estimates.

The two-stage approach also allows for practical adaptations, such as tailoring models to different study designs in the first stage, which can be more challenging in a one-stage framework.

Both approaches can accommodate missing data, but the methods for handling it may differ. In the two-stage approach, missing data can be addressed using study-specific models in the first stage [35], which can be convenient when different studies have different patterns of missingness, as well as different potential predictor variables for missing values. In contrast, a one-stage approach might be preferable for systematically missing covariates, as it allows for borrowing information across studies. Regardless of the approach, it is crucial to ensure that the methods for handling missing data are compatible with the overall meta-analysis model.

Riley and colleagues recommended that researchers carefully consider the specifics of their data and research questions when choosing between one-stage and two-stage approaches [203]. Additionally, conducting both one-stage and two-stage analyses and comparing the results can provide valuable insights and help identify any discrepancies due to different modelling assumptions or estimation methods.

In terms of the practical implications of these different approaches, it is important to consider the specific context in which the meta-analysis is being conducted. For example, if the studies included in the meta-analysis are highly heterogeneous, the additional flexibility offered by the one-stage approach can be beneficial for accounting for this heterogeneity. On the other hand, if the studies are relatively homogeneous and the focus is on ensuring the transparency and reproducibility of the analysis, the two-stage approach may be more appropriate.

10.2   One-Stage Models

When all the studies provide IPD, the one-stage analysis is a multilevel model [87]. There is extensive advice on fitting Bayesian multilevel models to your data, for example for BUGS and JAGS [156], brms [33], or Stan [242]. The only software option in this book that does not accommodate these models is bayesmeta. We will illustrate this with simulated data that imitate the green tea meta-analysis. Here, all studies report the same single outcome, which is normally distributed, with common standard deviation across arms, but this is just one of the many data-generating processes that you are free to fit in IPD, and you should choose an appropriate one:

```r
# simulating IPD in R:

m <- 10    # number of studies
n_arm <- 20    # number of participants per arm
true_theta <- (-0.5)
true_mu_ctl <- (-0.1)

true_tau <- 0.5
true_bmi_sd <- 3

u <- rnorm(m, true_theta, true_tau)
study <- rep(1:m, each=(n_arm*2))
tx <- rep(rep(c(0,1), each=n_arm), m)

true_bmi_mean <- true_mu_ctl +
                (true_theta + u[study]) * tx

bmi <- rnorm(400, true_bmi_mean, true_bmi_sd)

data <- data.frame(bmi, study, tx)
```

The code below is a standard multilevel model in BUGS:

```
model{
# priors:

theta ~ dnorm(0, 0.1)
mu_ctl ~ dnorm(0, 0.25)

tau ~ dnorm(0,1)I(0,)
tau_prec <- 1 / (tau * tau)

bmi_sd ~ dnorm(0,0.1)I(0,)
bmi_prec <- 1 / (bmi_sd * bmi_sd)
```

```
# random effect / heterogeneity:

for(j in 1:10) {
  u[j] ~ dnorm(0, tau_prec)
}


# likelihood:
for(i in 1:400) {
  mu_bmi[i] <- mu_ctl +
              (theta + u[study[i]]) * tx[i]
  bmi[i] ~ dnorm(mu_bmi[i], bmi_prec)
}
}
```

This is a random effects model; the stratified version described earlier is the term used in IPD literature for a fixed effects analysis, where each θ_j has either no prior (flat) or a suitably wide uniform prior. The common effect enforces $\theta_j = \theta\ ;\forall j$. Riley and colleagues argue against the common effect approach, a view which we share [202].

The disadvantage of a one-stage approach is clear here, in that all studies must be to some extent compatible with the same DGP and model. If some studies were cluster randomised, for example, then a two-stage approach would be advisable.

In survival or time-to-event data, studies are linked by a *frailty model* with random effects on, for example, log hazard ratios. Bear in mind that survival analyses can be very different in nature, for example those leading to hazard ratios, restricted mean survival time, or competing risks analysis, and must be handled with suitable statistical expertise in the team.

10.3 Integrating Individual Participant Data and Aggregate Data in Bayesian Meta-Analyses

Bayesian methods accommodate ways to combine some aggregate data studies (those reporting statistics) with IPD studies. The simplest way to think of this is that the AD studies have likelihood contributions as shown in Chapters 3 and 4, while the IPD studies and their shared θ and τ are as shown above [202].

As before, we can simulate a mixture of IPD and AD studies and show how the likelihood changes in a simple BUGS model. We will do this by summarising half of the studies simulated in the previous section, using the R package `dplyr` for convenience.

```
# simulation of IPD+AD

library(dplyr)

m_ad <- 5   # number of studies with AD
```

```
data_ad <- filter(data, study<=m_ad)
data_ipd <- filter(data, study>m_ad)

stats_bmi <- summarise(group_by(data_ad, study, tx),
                       mean_bmi = mean(bmi),
                       sd_bmi = sd(bmi),
                       n = n(),
                       se_mean = sd_bmi / sqrt(n))
stats_bmi_int = filter(stats_bmi, tx==1)
stats_bmi_ctl = filter(stats_bmi, tx==0)

md_bmi <- stats_bmi_int$mean_bmi - stats_bmi_ctl$mean_bmi
se_md_bmi <- sqrt((stats_bmi_int$se_mean)^2 + (stats_bmi_ctl$se_mean)^2)
prec_md_bmi <- 1 / (se_md_bmi^2)
```

The BUGS likelihood now splits into two parts, and the data are supplied separately for AD and IPD. We just show the likelihood lines:

```
# IPD likelihood:
for(i in 1:200) {
  mu_bmi[i] <- mu_ctl + (theta + u[study[i]]) * tx[i]
  bmi[i] ~ dnorm(mu_bmi[i], bmi_prec)
}

# AD likelihood:
for(j in 1:5) {
  md_bmi ~ dnorm(theta + u[j], prec_md_bmi[j])
}
```

Both parts of the u vector can be associated with the heterogeneity prior in a single line of code. In Stan we would use a `target+=` syntax to accumulate both AD and IPD likelihoods into the (log) posterior.

This approach of simulating data is useful when you are experimenting with bespoke models and want to check that their outputs are sensible and what you intended, before you run them on real data.

Statistics from aggregate data studies can be used to inform prior distributions for the effect size in a Bayesian meta-analysis of the IPD studies. These priors, often referred to as *meta-analytic priors*, represent the posterior distributions of the unknowns from the aggregate data studies.

This methodology was recently employed in a meta-analysis of intensive glucose control in critically ill adults [4]. In this study, IPD was available for 20 trials, while 14 trials provided only aggregate data (statistics). The aggregate data studies contributed to a meta-analytic prior for the treatment effect, which was integrated with hierarchical Bayesian models for the IPD studies. This combined approach ensured that all relevant data informed the posterior estimates of the intervention's efficacy and safety.

10.4   Intervention-Covariate Interactions in IPD Meta-Analysis

Understanding which participants benefit the most from particular interventions is a potentially useful output of meta-analysis, but will typically require IPD. We can assess differences between subpopulations by estimating intervention-covariate interactions. This shows whether different participant characteristics influence treatment effects.

Fisher and colleagues have discussed three approaches commonly used to analyse these interactions in IPD meta-analyses [73]. An estimate of purely between-study interaction, using study-level summaries of covariates, such as the proportion of participants with a specific characteristic, we are very unlikely to obtain an accurate estimate of the causal relationship. This could be attempted even in the absence of IPD. This is an example of what has been called *aggregation bias* or the *ecological fallacy* in more general multilevel data modelling settings.

Another flawed approach involves splitting participants into subgroups or strata based on the covariates, analysing each subgroup, then meta-analysing the subgroup statistics. This is conceptually similar to methods for adjusting for confounders from the mid 20th century, such as the Mantel-Haenszel method in epidemiology. Fisher and colleagues recommend analysing interactions within each study's IPD, then running a random effects meta-analysis on those statistics.

10.5   Deciding on the Approach

The IPD meta-analyses offer significant advantages over traditional aggregate data meta-analyses, including improved data quality, increased statistical power, and greater flexibility in statistical methods. Although the process is more complex and resource-intensive than traditional aggregate data meta-analyses, the potential benefits in terms of data quality, analytical flexibility, and the ability to draw more precise and personalized conclusions make IPD meta-analyses an invaluable approach in evidence-based research.

Researchers must carefully weigh the added value and potential insights gained from IPD meta-analyses against the additional efforts required, ensuring that the chosen approach aligns with the research objectives and available resources. In terms of the discourse around one-stage vs two-stage IPD meta-analyses we have acknowledged how both have their merits, and the choice between them should be guided by the specifics of the data, research questions, and available resources.

Researchers must also weigh the added complexity and resource requirements of the one-stage approach against its potential for more precise and flexible modelling. Conversely, the two-stage approach's simplicity and transparency can be advantageous, especially when dealing with larger, more homogeneous studies or when transparency and reproducibility are paramount. By carefully considering these factors, researchers can select the most appropriate approach for their IPD meta-analysis projects.

11

Unreported Statistics

Learning objectives

After reading this chapter, you will be able to:

1. describe unreported study statistics in terms of missing data theory

2. choose between different methods to represent unreported statistics with a prior distribution

3. program a meta-analysis in Bayesian software to capture the relationships among reported and unreported statistics

One of the most common problems that meta-analysts encounter, which might inspire them to find out about Bayesian methods, is that of missing statistics. Usually, clinical trials are very assiduous in reporting baseline characteristics in the classic "Table One" of a paper. Statistics at the end of treatment, or at follow-up, are sometimes much more limited, which is a nuisance to systematic reviewers and meta-analysts.

Trials usually have primary outcomes (those declared beforehand to be of principal interest) and secondary outcomes (anything they thought would also be of interest). The secondary outcomes are generally reported with less detail than the primary ones.

Another cause of missing detail is that the time point that you, the meta-analyst, are interested in might not be the one that the trialists focused their attention on.

By far the best solution to any of these problems is to get the information you need directly from the authors of the original trial paper, but we recognise that all too often, they do not respond, or no longer have the data, or are otherwise unable to help. This chapter gives some advice on what to try next, in the Bayesian paradigm.

We ought to ask ourselves two questions: what values are possible for the unreported statistic, and are some values more probable than others?

The unknown statistic can be treated like any other unknown, and be represented by a prior distribution. The term *imputation* is used of inferring a number that was calculated or measured, but is just not known to us. If there is enough information to guide this Bayesian approach, then we believe it is always preferable to impute, rather than omitting the entire study from your meta-analysis.

In this chapter, we assume a worst case scenario where there are no individual participant data (IPD) to inform imputation, but of course, when IPD is available for one or more comparable studies in the evidence base, it should be analysed to provide extra information.

The structure of the chapter is determined by some specific problems, each of which casts light on some aspects of choosing a prior distribution, modelling and coding:

1. missing post-intervention standard deviations

2. ambiguous post-intervention sample size

3. a mixture of post-intervention statistics and change from baseline statistics

4. there is a missing contrast statistic but (non)significance is stated

5. only a p-value and sample size is provided

We recommend reading all parts of this chapter, because some of the lessons that arise as we discuss different problems are widely applicable.

11.1   Missing Data Theory

It is common to have a dataset which requires analysis, but has some missing data. Many of the ideas about this came from an influential Bayesian statistician, Don Rubin [208]. He suggested the following taxonomy for such problems:

1. Missing Completely At Random (MCAR): the fact that the value is missing has nothing to do with the value itself, or any other information; in other words, the probability of being missing is the same for all observations.

2. Missing At Random (MAR): some other, known, variable can be used to predict the missing value; the probability of being missing differs according to some other, known, variable.

3. Missing Not At Random (MNAR)*: some variable can be used to predict the missing value, but unfortunately, that variable is not known—it might, in fact, be the missing value itself.

Broadly speaking, these three categories appear above in the order of increasing difficulty for the analyst.

A lot of work on missing values in recent years has used a method called multiple imputation, which is quietly Bayesian in that it uses probability to describe uncertainty in missing data (an epistemic unknown—see Chapter 2). It is a two-step process, modelling the missing data and imputing them in multiple pseudo-datasets, then analysing all those datasets separately and combining the results.

There is also the possibility of including both the model for the missing data and the meta-analysis model of substantive interest in a one-step Bayesian model, which estimates both the missing data and the other parameters of interest at the same time, and that is what we consider in this chapter. We must also consider the broader question of whether it will be useful; the alternatives might be simply plugging in an informed guess and treating it as though it is known, or excluding the study in question entirely.

This chapter considers studies where aggregate data (statistics) are missing. A different problem, also common, arises where the individual studies are fully reported but you suspect they may be biased by missing data within their own analyses. Including these in meta-analysis calls for some form of bias adjustment using expert opinion or external empirical evidence [162].

In Bayesian meta-analysis, any unreported statistics that we want to include should be represented by a probability distribution, because they are epistemic unknowns. It is a quite

---

*Occasionally, and very confusingly, we have seen this written as Not Missing At Random. If you see NMAR mentioned, be assured that it is simply a mangled synonym for MNAR.

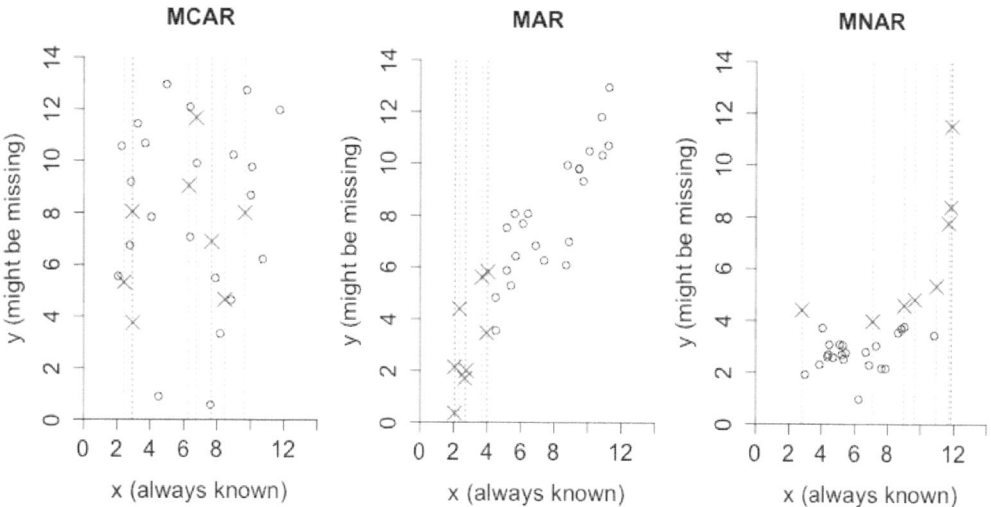

FIGURE 11.1

Illustration of Rubin's taxonomy of missingness; the vertical dotted lines show the known horizontal position for observations where the vertical location is missing, while the true vertical position is marked ×. MCAR missing y data can be estimated without bias by just using the distribution of the known y-values (vertical positions). MAR data cannot be estimated the same way without bias, but can be estimated if we take the relationship between x (which is always known) and y into account. MNAR data cannot be accurately estimated in any way, unless we have exogenous information about why and how it is different to the known data.

different situation to missing *data*, because we usually know a lot about each study and how comparable it is to other studies.

We will now consider different ways of including unreported stat, considering the most common problem of unreported statistics, in our experience.

11.2 A Common Problem: Missing Standard Deviations

In trials with a continuous outcome, assessing mean differences, sometimes post-intervention means (or just a mean difference between arms) are reported, without standard deviations. As detailed in Chapter 5, we can often calculate the standard deviation from other related statistics, such as the standard error of the mean, confidence intervals, t-statistics and so on. However, there are times when these other statistics are also absent. This is such a common problem that it is useful to explore it as our first example.

Imputing the missing standard deviation is not just a matter of curiosity. It will be needed for the standard error of the mean difference, hence the intra-study variance, which is central to meta-analysis [244].

Non-Bayesian methods have to fall back on plugging in an estimate and acting as though it were known, or at best doing some sensitivity analysis with a few different guesses. The Cochrane Handbook itself advises meta-analysts "to borrow the SD [standard deviation] from one or more other studies" by choosing one, averaging them, or choosing the largest [112]. They cite a study that shows this was approximately correct in two case studies [81].

This suggested process is single imputation: plugging in a single number. In Section 13.4 of their book, Sutton and colleagues describe using a similar approach [248]. Although it might be possible to do this with an unbiased estimate, whatever we plug in will underestimate the total uncertainty, because the actual missing standard deviation could be somewhat lower or higher than our guess. This is why using a probability distribution is better suited to the problem[†].

The challenge is to find a probability distribution that we can justify. Four approaches are outlined below. They all share one underlying concept: we use some information that we *do* know to set a prior for the values that we *do not* know.

The ideas in this section, for unreported standard deviations, can be implemented in a wide variety of the software we have considered so far: BUGS, JAGS, Stan, Stata, and `brms`. Examples are given on the website.

11.2.1   Choosing the target statistic for imputation

For a standard meta-analysis of intervention versus control, contrast statistics and their standard errors are needed, and it makes sense to impute the standard errors directly. What follows in this chapter refers to standard deviations but can be applied to standard errors of contrast statistics, unless we suggest otherwise.

When considering continuous outcomes, the standard error will often be based on a pooled standard deviation (see Equation 3.1), and imputation can target that instead. This has the advantage that we can use the theoretical sampling distribution (see Section 11.2.4). However, if you are using other studies' pooled standard deviations to tell you about a study that has not reported it, you will need to rely on at least one of the following assumptions being correct:

1. the standard deviation is the same in both arms

2. the ratio of sample sizes in arms is the same in all studies

If neither of these can be trusted, after examining the other studies, then it will be more reliable to impute separate standard deviations in the individual arms.

If your project is a network meta-analysis, and you are using an arm-based model, then you should impute standard deviations for each arm.

11.2.2   Use the known standard deviations (MCAR)

If you adopt the MCAR assumption, you are asserting that the fact that a certain study has an unreported standard deviation tells us nothing about any other aspect of the study, known or unknown—it is a purely random process, uninfluenced by anything else. That means that you can simply use the observed distribution of the known standard deviations as the prior for the unreported one.

You can visualise the distribution of the observed standard deviations by a histogram or density plot. You must then choose a distribution which adequately represents that shape,

---

[†]The reason we are unconvinced by the Furukawa study[81] is that they took two meta-analyses and deleted each study's standard deviation in turn, imputing with the doubly pooled (over arms and then over studies) known standard deviations. Their single imputation is assessed with the average performance over all studies, but in practice we are not imputing over all studies: we have a particular study to hand, with particular characteristics. In the same way that a treatment may be beneficial at a population average, yet a physician chooses an alternative for a particular patient, we must sometimes tailor our methods to the study at hand rather than the average of all possible studies.

but you should allow some extra spread above and below the observed values. One way to do this is visually, though the question of how much extra spread to add is then a subjective judgement.

Another choice would be to use maximum likelihood estimation to find a population distribution from which the observed statistics were drawn. Because they are statistics rather than data, this will be a sampling distribution.

If the standard deviations do not fit any off-the-shelf distribution well, you could try the variances instead. These are the same procedures that you might use for elicited prior opinions, and they are explained in Chapter 6. Because standard deviations and variances must be positive numbers, we would expect the distribution to be skewed with a longer tail to the right*. The exact theoretical form of the sampling distribution is actually in terms of a function of the variance, given below in Section 11.2.4.

With only one observed pooled standard deviation per study, you will probably not have much information to go on to prefer one distribution over any other reasonable candidate. You could opt for a simple distribution that is quite forgiving of values a little different to those observed, and that likely means not ruling out any positive number. Remember, though, that this prior should be informative and empirically justified, not diffuse.

Another option is to extract more standard deviations from the studies. Adding baseline standard deviations will double the information you have to define your prior distribution, and there may also be interim or longer follow-up statistics. These might all be regarded as arising from the same sampling distribution, though that is an assumption.

11.2.3   Heterogeneity on the variances? (MAR)

If you extract multiple standard deviations from each study (baseline, post-intervention, and perhaps others), you may be in a position to consider whether the study with the missing statistic would be correctly represented by the distribution of the other studies.

If it has unusual baseline standard deviations, then it may be sensible to adjust the prior for the unreported post-intervention standard deviation up or down from those observed in the other studies. It is perhaps tempting at this stage to think of it as a new form of heterogeneity, applying to the variances rather than the mean difference.

However, the added value of making your model more complicated in that way is not clear. Specifically, you are unlikely to have enough information to guide the choice of such a heterogeneity distribution—there is no reason why it would be normal or any other particular shape. Also, between-study variation is most likely driven by inclusion/exclusion criteria in the studies, which are usually well-documented, or floor and ceiling effects in bounded outcome scales (see Chapter 17).

Using information about individual studies to predict the unreported statistic would be more informative than a random heterogeneity process. So, we do not recommend this approach unless there is a compelling reason. Instead, we would apply a manually chosen prior to each study's unreported standard deviation that reflects the distribution of all known standard deviations, but is moved to prefer somewhat higher or lower values, depending on what is known about the study to hand, including baseline standard deviations and inclusion/exclusion criteria.

11.2.4   Sampling distribution of the variance (MCAR or MAR)

We found in Chapter 1 that observed means and mean differences have normal sampling distributions except in very small sample sizes. The pooled standard deviation, $s_{j\bullet}$, must be

---

*However, large sample sizes will make this less pronounced because of the Central Limit Theorem.

a positive number, and so tends to have a skewed, rather than symmetric, distribution. In a slightly more complicated way, we can use the study observed variances $s_{j\bullet}^2$ and relate them to the population variance, σ^2, using a chi-squared distribution (Figure 8.1) with $n_j - 1$ degrees of freedom:

$$\frac{s_{j\bullet}^2(n_j - 1)}{\sigma^2} \sim \chi^2(n_j - 1) \tag{11.1}$$

In the pseudocode below, this chi-squared distributed variable is called `variance_x2`. Suppose that studies 1 to 9 provide pooled standard deviations, but not study 10. The sampling distribution of the variables `variance_x2[1]` to `variance_x2[9]` define the likelihood of σ, which can then be used in the likelihood of the 10th study's other statistics of interest. The chi-squared distribution is shown in Figure 8.1.

```
sigma ~ uniform(0.01,10)    # prior
for(j in 1:9) {
  variance_x2[j] = s[j]^2 * (n[j]-1) / sigma^2
  variance_x2[j] ~ chi_sq(n[j]-1)
}
```

This code can then be followed by the usual meta-analytic likelihood. Depending on your choice of software, the imputed study 10 might have to be included in its own line of code, using `sigma` and `n[j]` to calculate its standard error. We provide full code for this example online. It is an example of including a vector of study statistics where some elements are knowns and some are unknowns.

As with other sampling distributions, this is simply a formula that enables you to find the probability of a certain $s_{j\bullet}$, σ and n_j co-existing, and can contribute to the likelihood of a model.

If you add this to your model, you will infer the true value of the population standard deviation, σ, based on the studies that reported standard deviations. Then, this sampling distribution is used to impute the unreported standard deviations. This is a formalised version of what we proposed in Section 11.2.2 above.

So far, there is one population σ for all studies. On the other hand, if you suspect that there are important inter-study differences, then you can build this into your sampling distribution in a simple way. If you have reason to believe the study with omitted post-intervention standard deviations will have 20% larger standard deviation than the rest of the evidence base, you can simply multiply σ by that scaling factor, for use in the standard error of the tenth study.

Any assumptions like this 20% increase should be documented, signed off by stakeholders in the project, and justified. In most situations, it should also be checked with sensitivity analysis: if it were 10% or 30%, would that make notable changes to the results, or even qualitative changes to the conclusion of the meta-analysis?

This section's approach to imputation targets variances specifically, therefore standard deviations too, and those imputed values can then afterwards be converted to standard errors for use in the meta-analysis likelihood.

11.2.5 Use other information correlated with the SDs (MAR)

We now introduce an additional complication to our notation. $s_{j\bullet1}$ has three subscripts: it comes from study j, is pooled across both arms (shown by the bullet $\bullet$), and relates to the 1st time point (the baseline). We will show the related post-intervention standard deviation as $s_{j\bullet2}$ here, though in practice there may be interim (mid-intervention) statistics. In general, the subscripts are s_{jkt}.

In some situations, you might find that studies' post-intervention pooled standard deviations ($s_{j\bullet2}$) are correlated with other statistics or study-level facts. The baseline pooled standard deviation, $s_{j\bullet1}$ is likely to be most informative, and if a correlation is evident between these time points, then the baseline should be used to make the imputation at post-intervention more accurate and narrower in distribution.

In Chapter 17, we discuss bounded outcome scales, where low or high means can induce artificial changes in standard deviation, so with floor and ceiling effects, the mean can also be informative of unreported standard deviations.

One way to do this is by a regression line, predicting $s_{j\bullet2}$ from $s_{j\bullet1}$. The imputation for $s_{j\bullet2}$ will then use a prior distribution centred on the prediction given $s_{j\bullet1}$, with the observed residual distribution. It is difficult to make any general recommendations for such a regression, other than that many statisticians find distributions of log standard deviations to be more symmetric (hence amenable to simple linear regression)†. A regression formula might be:

$$\log s_{j\bullet2} = \alpha + \beta \log s_{j\bullet1} + \epsilon_j$$
$$\epsilon_j \sim \mathrm{N}(0, \sigma_\epsilon) \tag{11.2}$$

Once you have α, β and σ_ϵ, you can impute: $\log s_{j\bullet2} \sim \mathrm{N}(\alpha + \beta \log s_{j\bullet1}, \sigma_\epsilon)$.

Alternatively, you can simply divide the evidence base into those studies which have $s_{j\bullet1}$ similar* to that in the study that is missing $s_{j\bullet2}$, and base your prior on them alone.

Whenever you draw on other information to refine your distribution for imputing unreported statistics, it is at the cost of additional assumptions. In this problem of missing post-intervention standard deviations, the assumption is that there is one shared population standard deviation (or some easily understood relationship defining it), so information on other studies or time points can be informative about the one you are missing.

The most likely impediment to this approach is a lack of studies. Meta-analyses often have to pool only a small numbers of studies, and there may be too few that are similar to the study in question to allow any reliable prediction. For this reason, some other methods used for missing *data*, such as hot deck imputation [6], are not useful in the meta-analysis context.

---

†You can regress each study's post-intervention and baseline log standard deviations together, or their log variances. (If you do not object to doing some secondary school algebra, you will likely get some extra insight from proving, with basic properties of logarithms and the linear regression formula, that these two options will always yield the same slope.)

*The decision of what "similar" means is for you to justify and document in your own circumstances.

11.2.6   Use expert opinion (MNAR)

In the MNAR situation, the unreported standard deviation is lower or higher than might be expected, given all other available information. In this case, we are reduced to sensitivity analysis, but we can use expert opinion priors (see Chapter 6) to provide a distribution for the unknown statistic, $s_{j\bullet 2}$, or for how much higher or lower it is than the σ suggested by the rest of the studies.

For further reading on MNAR imputation, we recommend Chapter 14 of Congdon's book [45] and Chapter 10 of the second edition of "Multiple Imputation and its Applications" [35], which are both very thorough and authoritative, although they do not specifically explore meta-analysis.

11.3   Is Imputation Adding Any Value?

Although there are ways to impute unreported statistics and include studies that would otherwise be excluded, it may not actually make much difference to the meta-analysis. Before spending time and energy on a more complicated model, or eliciting priors, you could consider what proportion of studies will be brought back into the meta-analysis, and how large those studies are.

If only a few studies would be saved, or if they are small in sample size, then you could discuss with stakeholders whether this is a priority. An approximate sensitivity analysis, where you plug in some different simple priors as shown in Section 11.2.2, and also run the meta-analysis without the affected studies, would inform this discussion. You can invent the priors to be roughly representative of an empirical MCAR model and a variety of MAR/MNAR models that vary from the empirical distribution of the other studies' standard deviations.

If results (point estimate and credible interval) do not change in any noteworthy way, you might decide to exclude those studies with unreported statistics. If the credible intervals narrow appreciably, but the point estimate is hardly changed, you might use a MCAR empirical prior on the basis that this is simple.

11.4   Unreported Sample Sizes

A quite different problem of unreported statistics occurs when the sample size, n_{jkt}, in study j, arm k, and time point t is not given, yet it is needed to calculate a standard error.

For example, we might know that, in study 4, 212 participants were randomised to the intervention arm ($n_{4\mathbf{Int}1} = 212$), and this provides an upper limit. Perhaps we are told that 60% of participants completed *all* the outcome assessments, which provides a lower limit[†]. Some R functions to obtain plausible ranges of numerators or denominators are provided online.

In this example, all we know is that n_{jkt} is a natural number (0, 1, 2, 3 ...) and that $127 \leq n_{jkt} \leq 212$.

If a study is lacking its sample size, there will be uncertainty in the standard error, which any meta-analysis will require, for any statistic. As for unreported standard deviations

---

[†]However, you should always check what values would lead to the reported value where a statistic (60%) has been rounded off. Both 127/212 and 128/212, rounded to percentages, would match 60%.

above, we should use the information we do have to make a prior distribution for the sample size.

An unknown sample size requires a discrete prior distribution, in that it can only take certain values. This is possible in BUGS and JAGS, but not in Stan, because of the algorithms that are used*.

You can choose to give different prior probabilities to different possible values of n_{jkt}. In the example above, where $127 \leq n_{jkt} \leq 212$, there are $212 - 126 = 86$ possible values. BUGS and JAGS support a generic "categorical" distribution, where the user provides a vector of probabilities, one for each possible value. To make this uniform, allocate the same probability to each:

```
for(i in 1:86) { prob[i] = 1/86 }
n ~ dcat(prob[n-126])
```

JAGS allows any positive value to be entered as the probability, and it adjusts them so that they add to one. BUGS requires them to be proper probabilities (See Appendix C.5 of *The BUGS Book* [156]).

If you decide that the higher end of the range is twice as probable as the lower end, you can specify this too. The calculation of `prob[i]` proceeds thus (and can be amended for different prior patterns): suppose that `prob[1]` (which relates to $n_{jkt} = 127$) is p, while `prob[86]` (which relates to $n_{jkt} = 212$) will be $2p$. The intervening probabilities rise in a straight line, so `prob[i]` will be:

$$\left(1 + \frac{i-1}{85}\right) p \tag{11.3}$$

We can then code this in JAGS without worrying about whether they add to one, by just setting $p = 1$ for simplicity:

```
for(i in 1:86) { prob[i] = 1+(i-1)/85 }
n ~ dcat(prob[n-126])
```

For BUGS, we must find the sum of all 86 possible values and divide by that, to make them add to one. In R, for example, we could type:

```
> i <- 1:86
> sum(1+(i-1)/85)
[1] 129
```

If we set $p = \frac{1}{129}$, then we can use this in BUGS:

```
for(i in 1:86) { prob[i] = (1+(i-1)/85)/129 }
n ~ dcat(prob[n-126])
```

---

*See the Stan guidance on integrating out discrete nuisance parameters at `https://mc-stan.org/docs/stan-users-guide/latent-discrete.html`

It is also possible to use one of the preset discrete distributions in BUGS or JAGS, such as the binomial.

11.4.1   Two possible values

In a related problem, we have seen papers where it is not clear whether reported statistics are based on all the randomised participants, or those who completed assessment at a given time point. Sometimes studies report both per protocol and intention to treat statistics, and there can be ambiguities between them. This means that there are two distinct values that n_{jkt} might take.

This can be coded in a similar way to the previous example, using pp as a binary variable which indicates whether the results are per protocol:

```
for(i in 1:2) { prob[i] = 0.5 }
pp ~ dcat(prob[pp+1])
n = 127 + 85*pp
```

However, a simpler approach is to calculate the uncertain standard error under the two possible sample sizes, and include a discrete prior for that instead. Sensitivity analysis, like in Section 11.3, might show that it makes little difference, justifying a single imputation like the midpoint between the two values.

There is more discussion of per protocol and intention to treat statistics in Chapter 16.

11.5   Application to Other Situations

11.5.1   A mixture of post-intervention and change from baseline statistics

Another common problem is when some studies report change from baseline and others report outcomes at the end of intervention. In the case of continuous outcomes with means and standard deviations, the means can be readily converted, but not so the standard deviations. This is because the change from baseline is a difference between two correlated random variables: a participant who is healthier than average at baseline is likely to be healthier at end of intervention too (see Section 1.4.2 and Equation 1.15).

To convert the studies into the same statistics, and have standard errors on those statistics, we need to know the correlation between baseline and post-intervention outcomes, yet this is extremely rare in published studies. The impact of different values is generally not strong, and so a simple prior is all that is needed.

The study-specific correlation, r_j will be a number between -1 and 1, but almost certainly in the positive half of this range. If there are any studies reporting the same outcome on the same timescale, and providing standard deviations for baseline, post-intervention, and change, you could use Equation 1.15 to obtain r_j in those studies, and this could guide your choice of prior. You should also guide the computer away from 0 and 1, which might cause computational problems.

We will show two examples of priors, but we are not recommending them for general use: you should consider such priors on a case-by-case basis. One option is a uniform prior such as:

$$r_j \sim \mathrm{U}(0.2, 0.8) \tag{11.4}$$

which is zero outside (for example) $[0.2, 0.8]$. Another option is a beta distribution, which is naturally defined between 0 and 1, so you can rescale your unknown value from $[0.2, 0.8]$ to $[0, 1]$:

$$\frac{r_j - 0.2}{0.8 - 0.2} \sim \mathrm{Beta}(3, 3) \tag{11.5}$$

These two examples above have zero probability outside $[0.2, 0.8]$. As with any constrained prior distribution, you should take care not to impose limits which distort the posterior.

With moderate sample size, $\sinh(r_j)$ (sinh is the hyperbolic sine, a function available on all relevant software) has a normal sampling distribution and is sometimes called Fisher's z-transformation. Some analysts are more familiar with using it than the raw r_j.

11.5.2   An unreported contrast statistic, and also significance

Above, we describe a situation where a contrast statistic is reported but not its standard error (or when means are given but not standard deviations). In these situations, you will often have access to some other statistic that gives partial information about the missing value.

The simplest and most useful instance of this is where a contrast statistic is noted to be significant or not. Studies will usually also report the direction of effect. If you know the hypothesis test that was used, this will provide a lower or upper limit on the missing standard error.

In the simple case of a t-test, where you know the sample size n_j, the study statistic $\hat{\theta}$ and its standard error $\widehat{SE}(\hat{\theta})$ must combine to give a p-value:

$$t\left(\frac{\hat{\theta}}{\widehat{SE}(\hat{\theta})}, \mathrm{df} = n_j - 2\right) = p \tag{11.6}$$

Suppose that you are told that $\hat{\theta}$ is significantly different to zero (the null hypothesis is rejected). This means that $p < 0.05$ (unless a different threshold is being used). You can find the threshold value of the t statistic at $p = 0.05$, and what value of $\frac{\hat{\theta}}{\widehat{SE}(\hat{\theta})}$ would relate to that, so you know that the study must have found a value greater than that. This sets an upper limit on $\widehat{SE}(\hat{\theta})$.

If the study reported non-significance, then $p \geq 0.05$ and you could set a lower limit on $\widehat{SE}(\hat{\theta})$.

11.5.3   Nothing but a p-value

Studies might sometimes only provide a p-value, especially for secondary outcomes and secondary time points. In general, you could work with this, and although it is interesting to think through the problem, it is most likely too uncertain to be of much use.

You would have to impute both the contrast (or arm) statistic and its standard error. They would be constrained together to provide the p-value in question, so they have a bivariate distribution.

Referring to Equation 11.6, we can see that p and n_j are known. This implies that $\frac{\hat{\theta}}{\widehat{SE}(\hat{\theta})}$ is a constant[†]. If you look up one combination that would provide the desired p-value, then you know the constant[*]. Suppose, for example, that it is 2.8. Now, $\hat{\theta} = 2.8\,\widehat{SE}(\hat{\theta})$ and so you only have to impute $\widehat{SE}(\hat{\theta})$ in order to include the study. You then proceed to choose a MCAR, MAR or MNAR prior as detailed above.

If no sample size were reported either, the challenge would be much greater, and perhaps involves too much uncertainty to make any meaningful improvement on omitting the study from your meta-analysis. In theory, though, you could impute the sample size as described above, and then compute the corresponding value of $\frac{\hat{\theta}}{\widehat{SE}(\hat{\theta})}$. In some tests, as the sample size grows, the test statistic's sampling distribution rapidly stabilises as normal. If this is the case, and the sample size is definitely large, you could adopt a normal distribution and ignore the impact of the sample size.

[†] As in the previous section, we assume that the study reports the direction of effect, so we know what side of the t-distribution to evaluate; any study that does not even report direction of effect is probably best left out of meta-analysis.

[*] In the spirit of the footnote in Section 11.4, a p-value reported to only 2 decimal places is likely to be compatible with a range of different constants. It seems quite reasonable to us to pick the midpoint rather than elaborate the imputation further.

12

Living Systematic Reviews and Bayesian Updating

Learning objectives

After reading this chapter, you will be able to:

1. recognise the value of living systematic reviews and prospective meta-analysis, and decide whether they are relevant to your work

2. understand and explain the principle of Bayesian updating

3. weigh up the speed, yet statistical complexity, of updating with only likelihoods from new studies, against the precise estimates of using all studies

This chapter presents the Bayesian approach as a coherent framework for continuous evidence monitoring and updating, which is implemented in the form of living systematic reviews and prospective meta-analyses. Such an approach is invaluable for rapid updates to evidence synthesis to make informed decisions.

We then elaborate on the concept of Bayesian updating, where the posterior distribution from a previous meta-analysis can be used as the prior for a new analysis, and the likelihood only needs to be calculated for the latest batch of data. This is more difficult than it seems at first, and we show a simple example to give you some intuition about the problem.

12.1 Living Systematic Reviews and Prospective Meta-Analyses

A living systematic review (LSR) is an ongoing, continuously updated systematic review that provides the current state of knowledge from the evidence base on a specific topic [66, 230]. Unlike traditional systematic reviews conducted at a single point in time, LSRs are regularly updated as new research emerges. They are particularly valuable in fields characterized by rapidly evolving research, uncertain evidence bases, and significant potential impacts on policy or practice decisions [65].

In contrast, in a prospective meta-analysis (PMA), studies are identified and included before their results are available or published [223, 285]. This approach minimises selective reporting and publication bias, thereby enhancing the credibility of the research. Together, LSRs and PMAs address the limitations of traditional systematic reviews and retrospective meta-analyses, offering a more effective means of promptly informing decision-makers.

The use of LSRs and PMAs has grown in recent years, particularly accelerated by the COVID-19 pandemic, when rapid evidence synthesis was critical [25, 137]. There are a

DOI: 10.1201/9781003375821-12

number of motivations for choosing these approaches, and frameworks for understanding their utility and applications as a meta-research design are emerging [158].

There might be situations where researchers have in-house access to trials (or other study designs) previously conducted within the same organisation, such as a pharmaceutical or medical devices manufacturer. They might be able to integrate their new data with the existing evidence base even before the new results are formally published. This approach is akin to a prospective meta-analysis but is distinguished by the immediacy with which new data are pooled and therefore we might call it *real-time meta-analysis**.

From a commercial perspective, this method leverages the competitive advantage of early data access to update the evidence base in almost real-time. From the perspective of decision makers, it is undoubtedly useful to be able to access the full analysis of a new study, while also seeing it in the context of all available evidence. This could be especially helpful when the decision maker must consider the possibility of intervention-covariate interactions.

In applying Bayesian meta-analysis to such scenarios, we need to supply prior distributions that in some sense precede both existing evidence and new, unpublished data. Weakly informative priors can be employed to focus on the construction of the model while acknowledging the equipoise inherent in experimental studies. The incorporation of real-time data necessitates careful consideration of heterogeneity and selection of appropriate prior distributions for unknown parameters. We expand on some of these issues in this chapter.

LSRs also present challenges for various aspects of the systematic review process, including: scoping, conducting searches, selecting studies, abstracting data, assessing risk of bias, performing meta-analyses, conducting narrative syntheses, assessing the strength of evidence, and formulating conclusions [165].

Frequentist methods, including significance testing as a quantification of decision-making, are often unsuitable for the LSRs and PMAs. Repeated updates and analyses inherent in LSRs and PMAs increase the risk of falsely (non-)significant findings, and errors of magnitude and sign, due to multiple testing [65, 230]. Some methods, such as Trial Sequential Analysis [26], and Sequential Meta-Analysis [114] have been developed to control for these errors.

To us, the Bayesian approach is well-suited for analysing LSRs and PMAs [65, 283], as it reflects the learning process intrinsic to these designs, where new evidence updates previous knowledge. A common concern among researchers schooled in frequentist methods is how to adjust for repeated testing, but in the Bayesian context this is not a problem [86].

Firstly, incorporating prior knowledge into the analysis can improve estimate precision, especially during the initial phases of evidence synthesis when new studies are few or effect size estimates are unstable [238]. In the context of LSRs and PMAs, where data constantly evolve, estimates from Bayesian analyses converge over successive iterations, with the posterior from one analysis serving as the prior for the next, thus forming a continuous chain of updates [181]. We expand on the concept of Bayesian updating in Section 12.2.

Secondly, Bayesian meta-analysis offers flexibility in modelling heterogeneity and complex relationships within data, explicitly accounting for variations between studies and allowing information sharing across studies [262]. This flexibility is crucial for LSRs and PMAs, where studies may vary significantly in design, population, and setting, thereby introducing considerable uncertainties [65, 283].

Finally, Bayesian meta-analysis naturally quantifies uncertainty around pooled effect estimates and other parameters of interest by examining the posterior distribution [283]. This approach facilitates straightforward result interpretation and seamlessly integrates

---

*For instance, Gian Luca worked on a systematic review and meta-analysis of this nature, published by Hammond and colleagues [101]. The objective was to compare balanced crystalloids and saline in critically ill adults. This allowed publication of an evidence synthesis almost simultaneously with the publication of the new trial results [72].

with informed decision-making processes, well suited to the evolving nature of evidence synthesis in LSRs and PMAs.

LSRs and PMAs offer opportunities to reduce the persistent gap between research findings and healthcare practice, known as the evidence-practice gap. While systematic reviews and meta-analyses have been instrumental in bridging this gap, their effectiveness is compromised by challenges in maintaining currency and accuracy. Research indicates that the time lag from primary study publication to systematic review publication ranges from 2.5 to 6.5 years, resulting in significant inaccuracies as new evidence is often not incorporated into existing reviews and from there to best practice clinical guidelines [66].

Efficiency is crucial for the success of LSRs, and advances in technology, such as artificial intelligence for study identification and data extraction, have the potential to revolutionise practice [66, 165]. It will also be important, though less glamorous, to make use of structured data formats, shared ontologies, and linked open data or synthetic open data (see Section 17.10).

Seidler and colleagues offer a comprehensive guide on conducting PMAs [223]. Key aspects of planning any PMA include: implementing thorough search methods to identify ongoing studies, defining priority of outcomes, managing collaborations, and establishing publication policies. Conducting PMAs presents challenges such as database completeness and timeliness, and delays in study completion.

The use of PRISMA and GRADE is recommended for reporting and assessing the quality of evidence in PMAs. However, there is a pressing need for comprehensive reporting guidelines and evidence-based rating tools specific to PMAs, to enhance their quality.

12.2 Bayesian Updating

We discussed several meanings that prior distributions can take in Chapter 2. One of those is the posterior of a previous analysis. This is called *Bayesian updating*. The idea is that we only need to include the latest studies in order to update a previous meta-analysis, so long as we can include the previous results as our prior distribution. It is important to realise that the time saving will come from not screening and reviewing the older studies, rather than the time to run the Bayesian model[†].

This is often mentioned in introductory Bayesian teaching, but is rarely practiced, because it is harder than it sounds. To emphasise the dual role of the posterior from a previous analysis as the prior of the next, we sometimes write it as "prior/posterior".

We will set out the idea mathematically first, but if you prefer, you can take the method on trust and skip the formulas.

You may recall from Chapter 2 that Bayes' theorem says that the posterior probability density is the product of the likelihood and the prior probability density, multiplied by a constant. We first saw this in Equation 2.1, but here we will explicitly add the constant C_1 and show that we are analysing a first batch of data, $\boldsymbol{Y}_1$. Remember that $\boldsymbol{\theta}$ indicates some collection of *all* the unknowns.

$$P(\boldsymbol{\theta}|\boldsymbol{Y}_1) = C_1 P(\boldsymbol{Y}_1|\boldsymbol{\theta})P(\boldsymbol{\theta}) \tag{12.1}$$

[†]In truly "big data" settings, Bayesian updating has a more compelling justification in terms of computation time, but meta-analysis usually has rather small numbers of observations that contribute to likelihood, even in IPD.

If we get a second batch of data, $\boldsymbol{Y}_2$, and use the above posterior as the new prior, we will obtain:

$$
\begin{aligned}
P(\boldsymbol{\theta}|\boldsymbol{Y}_1, \boldsymbol{Y}_2) &= C_2 P(\boldsymbol{Y}_2|\boldsymbol{\theta})P(\boldsymbol{\theta}|\boldsymbol{Y}_1) \\
&= C_1 C_2 P(\boldsymbol{Y}_2|\boldsymbol{\theta})P(\boldsymbol{Y}_1|\boldsymbol{\theta})P(\boldsymbol{\theta}) \\
&\propto P(\boldsymbol{Y}_1, \boldsymbol{Y}_2|\boldsymbol{\theta})P(\boldsymbol{\theta})
\end{aligned}
\tag{12.2}
$$

In this, $C_1 C_2$ is a constant and can be ignored in the algorithms we use. Also, recall that the likelihood of the unknowns, given independent studies, is just the product of all the probabilities of the individual studies. So, $P(\boldsymbol{Y}_2|\boldsymbol{\theta})P(\boldsymbol{Y}_1|\boldsymbol{\theta})$ is just the likelihood given both the first and second batches of data.

In theory at least, this could continue indefinitely. In practice, the posterior density each time is an estimate, and repeated updating accumulates distortion[*].

This means that the batch processing should lead to the same result that we would have obtained if we had started with the same original prior and analysed both batches together.

12.2.1   Practicalities

In an ideal world, the previous meta-analysis would have been done with Bayesian methods—it probably was not, unless it was a network meta-analysis (NMA)—and you would have access to the posterior draws. Then, you might fit a density estimate to those draws and use that as a prior for your new meta-analysis, including only the new studies that have emerged since the search for the previous meta-analysis. Remember that the prior and posterior are joint distribution over as many dimensions as there are unknowns, so simply fitting shapes one by one to the histograms or kernel densities is not sufficient—unless the only unknowns are one θ and one τ.

In reality, it is very unlikely that you could obtain the posterior draws, unless you either were the previous studies' authors, or had all the input statistics and all the code, and were able to replicate their work exactly—but if that were the case, you could simply analyse all the studies together.

The parameters (unknowns) that you will be interested in are the θs and τ. There is no need to obtain previous random effects θ_j, because the same studies will not appear in the new analysis.

When the previous meta-analysis was non-Bayesian, you may still be able to use the joint sampling distribution of all the parameters as a prior. This is equivalent to using a flat prior and then meta-analysing all the studies.

However, without the posterior draws themselves, you will have to start from the published estimates for the parameters, and their standard errors. No meta-analysis that we have ever seen has published the correlations among those parameters, and that would be required to make a joint distribution. Nevertheless, you can adopt some reasonable assumptions: τ should be uncorrelated with any θ, but there will be moderate correlations among the θs in the case of NMA. We do not expect correlations among the θs in subgroups. Sensitivity analysis can help to determine whether there is scope for Bayesian updating without injecting unacceptable uncertainty into your work. If there is just too much uncertainty, you should review the situation with collaborators and consider stopping and embarking on a re-analysis of all the old study statistics.

Another complicating factor is that new studies may require new unknowns: not just new random effects but new subgroups or interventions in a NMA. These unknowns will need

---

[*]Older readers might have once made copies of their friends' copies of other people's cassette tapes, with the same effect.

new prior distributions to be chosen, according to whatever interpretation you prefer, so long as they can be justified as compatible with the previous meta-analysis. If the classification of new studies into subgroups, or their arms into interventions, would suggest changing the classification of studies or arms in the previous meta-analysis, then it will invalidate the old posterior, and a complete re-analysis would be justified.

12.2.2 A worked example

We will revisit the thrombolytics network meta-analysis (NMA) from Section 9.2.1 as an example, which highlights the need for care in estimating the posterior distribution. We will imagine that all the 20th century studies were previously analysed, and then updated with the 21st century ones only.

We will use the conditional specification of heterogeneity. In this example, there are six unknowns in the `theta` vector, and one `tau`. The individual studies' `mu` random effects are not relevant to updating.

The prior part of the original BUGS model code is:

```
tau ~ dnorm(0,2)I(0,)
theta[1] <- 0
for (k in 2:K){
  theta[k] ~ dnorm(0, 0.25)
}
for(j in 1:m){
  mu[j] ~ dnorm(0,.0001)
}
```

After running the model on the 26 arms from 20th century studies, for 100,000 iterations of two chains in WinBUGS, thinned to every tenth, we obtain the following statistics (among others):

node	mean	sd	MC error
theta[2]	-0.06365	0.1225	0.002024
theta[3]	-0.1352	0.1263	0.001144
theta[4]	-0.02004	0.1537	0.001368
theta[5]	-0.1234	0.1465	0.001283
theta[6]	-0.1301	0.219	0.001877
theta[7]	-0.6114	0.2037	0.004582
tau	0.1247	0.1171	0.002826

Firstly, imagine that the 20th century analysis was published by other researchers. We would likely have access to the posterior means and standard deviations, as above, or maximum likelihood estimates and their standard errors. We would have to make assumptions about correlations, as suggested above.

We might assume zero correlation between `tau` and all elements of `theta`. Also, the first element of `theta` is fixed at zero, so it will also have zero correlation with everything else. All other elements of `theta` might have weak to moderate positive correlations of about 0.3.

In BUGS, we could add this by having a univariate distribution for `tau` and a multivariate normal distribution for `theta[2:7]`, which is then combined with the fixed `theta[1]`. BUGS requires a precision matrix for the multivariate distribution, which is the inverse of the covariance matrix, which we encountered in Section 8.5.

We can assemble the covariance matrix from the standard deviations and correlations, and invert it to obtain the precision matrix. This is possible inside BUGS or Stan, but we prefer to do this sort of preparatory work in general statistical software so that we can check it before sending it into the model. The code below is for R:

```
# standard deviations and variances:
sd_vector <- c(0.1225, 0.1263, 0.1537, 0.1465, 0.219, 0.2037)
variance_vector <- sd_vector * sd_vector

# assumed correlation matrix:
corr_matrix <- matrix(0.3, nrow=6, ncol=6)
diag(corr_matrix) <- 1.0

# assemble covariance vector by matrix multiplication:
cov_matrix <- (variance_vector %*% t(variance_vector)) * corr_matrix

# invert to get the precision matrix
prec_matrix <- solve(cov_matrix)
```

This can then be copied back into WinBUGS for the update with 21st century studies. We add `mean_vector` and `prec_matrix` to the data:

```
list(m=10,
     mean_vector=c(-0.06365, -0.1352, -0.02004, -0.1234, -0.1301, -0.6114),
     prec_matrix=structure(.Data=c(5582.65, -716.15, -483.57, -532.27,
                -238.19, -275.31, -716.15, 4940.50, -454.91, -500.73,
                -224.07, -259.00, -483.57, -454.91, 2252.63, -338.11,
                -151.30, -174.89, -532.27, -500.73, -338.11, 2729.19,
                -166.54, -192.50, -238.19, -224.07, -151.30, -166.54,
                546.52,  -86.14, -275.31, -259.00, -174.89, -192.50,
                -86.14,  730.16),
                .Dim=c(6,6))
```

The prior section of the code then uses these in the multivariate normal distribution. Note that we no longer need to include K = 7 in our data, because we are not looping over the interventions.

Asymptotic normality is a justifiable assumption for the `theta` vector[†], but not for `tau`. We estimated a half-t distribution for `tau` by generating simulated data and comparing mean and standard deviations with those reported by BUGS. We settled on 5 degrees of freedom, mean 0 and standard deviation 0.13:

[†]This is because all unknowns approach a normal posterior as the amount of data grows. However, meta-analysis does not generally involve many studies, so we should be cautious in this setting. In fact, as we will show below, the multivariate normal turns out to be a flawed choice in this instance.

```
x <- 0.13*abs(rt(100000,5));mean(x);sd(x);
```

Remember that the standard deviation of the t distribution is not the same as its scale parameter, but we can simply sample from the standard t and multiply it by 0.13.

```
tau <- tau_st * 0.13
tau_st ~ dt(0,1,5)I(0,)
theta[1] <- 0
theta[2:7] ~ dmnorm(mean_vector[1:6], prec_matrix[1:6,1:6])
for(j in 1:m){
  mu[j] ~ dnorm(0,.0001)
}
```

If we are in a position to replicate the old meta-analysis, we might find more subtle signals in the correlations, which can be obtained from WinBUGS via the `Inference / Correlations` menu, or by extracting posterior draws through `Inference / Samples...` and the `coda` button [156]. However, it is unclear how useful it is to add more complications into the model in pursuit of small patterns in the correlation structure. Broadly speaking, the actual posterior correlations from meta-analysis of the 20th century studies support our assumed 0.3 value, except that `theta[2]` is very weakly correlated with any of the others.

We ran the 21st century meta-analysis for 100,000 iterations in two chains, thinning to every tenth draw. Posterior means are quite close to those previously obtained in Chapter 9 by running the model on all studies in one pass, as shown in Table 12.1. However, the mean of `theta[7]` is further from zero, and in the updating analysis, all the standard deviations are much smaller. This shrinking of the marginal posteriors possibly reflects the fact that the marginal densities in Figure 9.6 were somewhat long-tailed, which a normal distribution did not capture. `tau`, which had a more carefully tailored and t-distributed prior/posterior, does not exhibit this shrinkage.

The notable difference between the marginal posterior densities of `theta[2:7]` in Figure 12.1, and those seen in Figure 9.6, is that the updating analysis produced posterior distributions that are more like normal distributions. This adds evidence that our updating prior has imposed an assumed shape, above and beyond the mean and standard deviation.

TABLE 12.1
Posterior statistics from the updating analysis, compared with the all-in-one conditional heterogeneity model from Section 9.2.1.

Unknown	Updating Analysis		All-In-One Analysis	
	Mean	SD	Mean	SD
tau	0.108	0.084	0.083	0.075
theta[2]	-0.062	0.015	-0.034	0.086
theta[3]	-0.136	0.016	-0.168	0.086
theta[4]	-0.018	0.023	-0.040	0.109
theta[5]	-0.122	0.021	-0.130	0.109
theta[6]	-0.126	0.048	-0.161	0.154
theta[7]	-0.595	0.040	-0.493	0.119

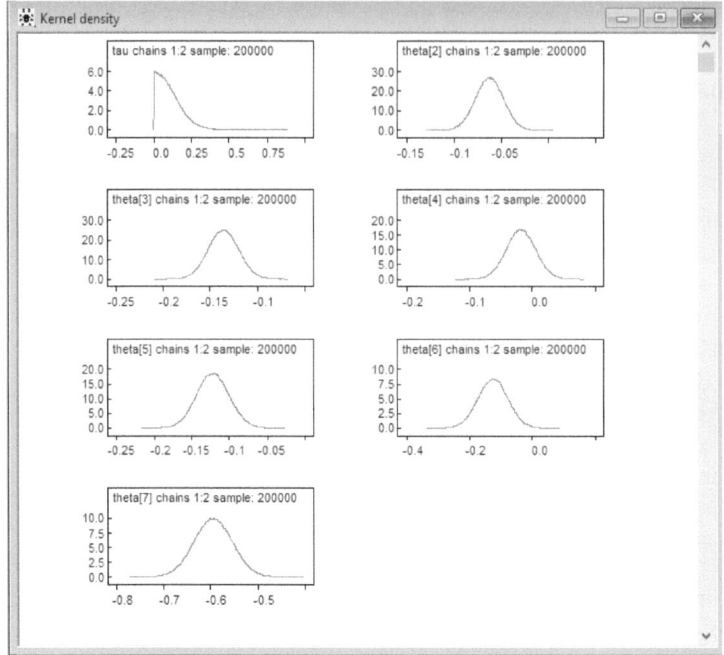

FIGURE 12.1

Marginal posterior densities after updating with multivariate normal prior/posterior, from WinBUGS.

We will leave this example at this point, though it could be enhanced through different multivariate densities. It serves as a reminder that estimating densities is a challenging task, especially in several dimensions, and a statistical methodology in its own right [222]. The choice of the distribution for updating should not be taken lightly, but only after careful examination of plots like these. With more expert statistical input, a non-parametric approach could be attempted, such as kernel or kudzu density function we described in Section 6.4 for elicited priors.

 The full code to run this example is on the website. Remember that it is deliberately flawed, to demonstrate the processes and caveats around updating, and is **not recommended** in general.

13

Publication Bias

Publication bias occurs when the chance of a study's results being published is influenced by the results themselves. This eliminates certain studies—typically those that are smaller or have less exciting results—from the evidence base [54, 204].

To some extent, publication bias should be expected and checked for in every systematic review (unless you are pooling results from in-house studies at a pharmaceutical company or similar sponsor of research). Cross-checking the identified studies against registered protocols and grey literature, such as technical reports, web pages and conference abstracts, may help.

Some meta-analyses request summary statistics from registered trials that have completed but not published, and present them as a subgroup. One example by Axfors and colleagues adopted this approach because the desire to support rapid decision-making on controversial potential treatments in the COVID-19 pandemic was the driver [8]. Related methods are discussed in Chapter 12.

The funnel plot (see Section 3.3), and some related hypothesis tests, are the usual ways to inspect the pattern of study statistics [204]. As m, the number of studies in the meta-analysis, is typically small, the evidence for bias is often inconclusive. The funnel plot is useful but tests create a binary classification (bias or no bias) which hides this uncertainty.

In the situation where everything has been done to track down studies, and yet suspicion remains about publication bias, our task is to try to adjust the meta-analysis in some way, to estimate the unbiased result that might have been.

A well-established method which makes no probabilistic model is called *trim and fill*. This seeks to balance the funnel plot by adding pseudo-studies that might have been published but were not. Some early Bayesian methods took a similar *data augmentation* approach [233]. The Bayesian approach we prefer appeals to the same logic: we must recognise that the sampling distribution under publication bias is not symmetric [152] and may be a mixture of two distributions bolted together or morphing into one another. However,

DOI: 10.1201/9781003375821-13

our preferred method is to build a more complicated model. First, it is worth considering whether adding a simple prior would suffice.

13.1   Elicited Bias Priors

A simple way of adjusting for publication bias is to add an unknown δ to the mean value of θ and then use the model as before, applying an informative prior, $P(\delta)$, on that bias term. For example, in a common effect meta-analysis, where δ is the bias:

$$\delta \sim P(\delta)$$
$$\hat{\theta}_j \sim N(\theta + \delta, \widehat{SE}(\hat{\theta}_j)) \tag{13.1}$$

This does not allow you to estimate the bias in any way, but simply adjusts the results for a plausible prior distribution of biases. The disadvantage is that the shape of the distribution is unchanged, just shifted to one side, and as we will see in the next section, that may not be realistic.

13.2   Selection Models

A *selection model* for publication bias, or other biased data, consists of two parts: the usual model that we would apply to unbiased data, and a model of the probability of being included in the available data.

The second part will contain some selection equation which predicts probability based on characteristics of the study results. Various such models have been suggested, differing according to exactly what aspects of the results influence the probability.

We will now briefly show how it is possible to put these models together and have the software separate their constituent parts. If the probability theory is not in your comfort zone, please feel free to skip ahead.

Suppose that studies exist, published or not, according to some sampling distribution, $P(Y_j|\theta)$. They report Y_j, which includes the point estimate, standard error, sample size and other knowns. Also, if they are published then $a_j = 1$, if not, $a_j = 0$; we observe a_j and Y_j. They are then published or not with probability $P(a_j = 1|Y_j)$, which is determined by the known attributes of the study*, and is implicitly the same as $P(a_j|Y_j, \theta)$. Now, according to basic rules of conditional and joint probabilities:

$$P(a_j = 1|Y_j, \theta)P(Y_j|\theta) = P(a_j = 1, Y_j|\theta) \tag{13.2}$$

So, the likelihood, which is the probability of the knowns given the unknowns, is the selection probability, multiplied by the unselected sampling distribution density (Figure 13.1. If we can set our models out in this way, we will show below that we can separate the two components, and have our software estimate the unbiased unknowns θ.

The model in Figure 13.1 introduces two additional unknowns: the location of the selection threshold, and the size of the drop on the left-hand side.

---

*If you read Chapter 11, consider how this is another kind of missing data model. Think about whether publication-biased studies are Missing At Random or Missing Not At Random.

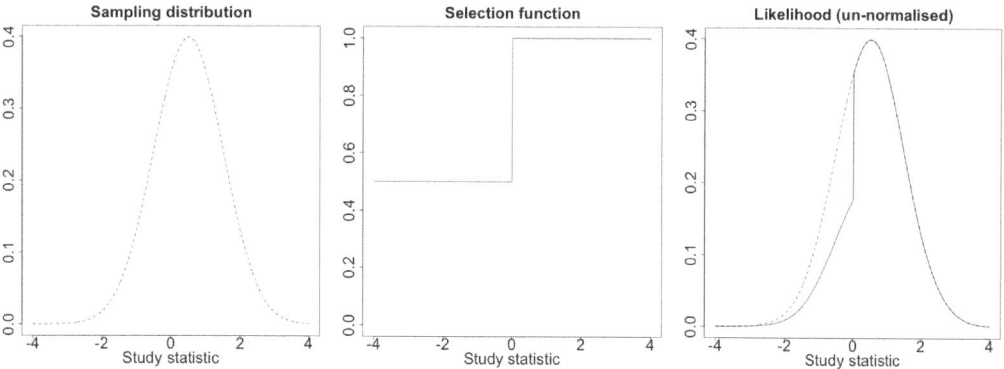

FIGURE 13.1

A simple selection model with a sharp drop in probability of being published; the likelihood is the product of the unbiased sampling distribution and the selection function.

13.2.1 Direction alone influences publication

We will begin with a very simple model and expand from there. In a common effect meta-analysis model, a study's point estimate, $\hat{\theta}_j$, has a normal sampling distribution:

$$\hat{\theta}_j \sim \mathrm{N}(\theta, \widehat{SE}(\hat{\theta}_j)) \tag{13.3}$$

We will write the likelihood contribution of each study j as $\mathrm{P}(\hat{\theta}_j | \theta, \widehat{SE}(\hat{\theta}_j))$, the probability of $\hat{\theta}_j$ given sampling distribution parameters θ and $\widehat{SE}(\hat{\theta}_j)$. The probability density or mass function $\mathrm{P}(\cdot)$ could represent any distribution, but in this case it is the normal distribution. (The dot inside $\mathrm{P}(\cdot)$ is a mathematical placeholder for any inputs to the function.)

Suppose that all studies with point estimates that favour a new intervention (we will write this as $\hat{\theta}_j > 0$) are equally likely to be published with probability $\zeta_j = 1$, and all studies with $\hat{\theta}_j \leq 0$ equally (but less) likely, with probability $\zeta_j = 0.5$. (ζ is the Greek letter zeta.)

It does not matter that we have correctly guessed the absolute values of these probabilities of publication, only that the ratio between them is correct: the chance of being published is cut in half by having $\hat{\theta}_j \leq 0$.

The sampling distribution for study j is then:

$$\begin{aligned}
&\zeta_j\, \mathrm{P}(\hat{\theta}_j | \theta, \widehat{SE}(\hat{\theta}_j)) \\
&\text{If } \hat{\theta}_j \leq 0\text{: } \zeta_j = 1 \\
&\text{If } \hat{\theta}_j > 0\text{: } \zeta_j = 0.5
\end{aligned} \tag{13.4}$$

Figure 13.1 shows the effect of this on the sampling distribution, where $\theta = 0.5$ and $\zeta = 0.5$, of one trial with $\widehat{SE}(\hat{\theta}_j) = 1$. Each study is either in the reduced part of the curve, or not. The mean of data from this distribution will be biased to around 0.71, compared to the true $\theta = 0.5$.

The mean of the curve (θ) is a subject of inference and the software will try different values in posterior draws, but the threshold will be fixed at 0 and ζ will be fixed at 0.5.

Our goal is to line up the assumed sampling distribution shape with the observed data. If there are indeed about half as many studies with $\hat{\theta}_j \leq 0$, then it will provide us with a good estimate of the unbiased θ. However, the difficulty is in justifying the choice of selection model. If we knew the characteristics of all the missing studies, we would have a chance of pinning down the model.

The sampling distribution we have just constructed from two parts stuck together does not integrate to one, and so is not a proper probability density function, unless we normalise it[†]. However, this does not matter for MCMC algorithms, as we only require something proportional to the posterior density.

This most basic model is not entirely meaningless. It is well known that, at least in medical journals, studies with a significant point estimate in favour of a new intervention are called "positive", and otherwise "negative", despite the protests of statisticians, and further, that non-significant point estimates on the favourable side are described with various degrees of spin as "trending towards" significance, and the like. We will next consider a model based on significance at $p < 0.05$.

13.2.2   Significance alone influences publication

We could adapt the model above to significance by imposing the cutpoint on the p-value itself, instead of on $\hat{\theta}_j$. However, this will not help us to estimate θ, unless we link the p-value[*] back to θ.

For a study to be statistically significant with $p < 0.05$, let's begin with a simple case of a hypothesis test where the effect estimate, $\hat{\theta}_j$, is divided by its standard error and compared to a pre-determined threshold, technically known as the *critical value*.

In z-tests, known as Wald tests, the critical value for a two-sided hypothesis is ± 1.96, while in t-tests, it will vary depending on the sample size. The likelihood will be similar to Equation 13.4, for example for a two-sided z-test:

$$\zeta_j \mathrm{P}(\hat{\theta}_j | \theta, \widehat{SE}(\hat{\theta}_j))$$

$$\text{If } \frac{\left|\hat{\theta}_j\right|}{\widehat{SE}(\hat{\theta}_j)} \leq 1.96 : \zeta \, \mathrm{N}(\theta, \widehat{SE}_j) \tag{13.5}$$

$$\text{Otherwise} : \mathrm{N}(\theta, \widehat{SE}_j)$$

In practice, we can classify studies on the basis of the p-values themselves and then estimate the parameters of the sampling distribution. There will no longer be a sharp drop at a given value of $\hat{\theta}_j$, like we saw in Figure 13.1.

This effectively states that both the point estimate and its standard error affect the probability of publication, and that we know exactly the formula for it. There are reasons why we should not be so sure of this idea, which we explore next.

Similarly to the model above, where the intervention effect, divided by its standard error, influences the probability of publication, we could use different effect sizes, such as Cohen's D. In some fields, where these effect sizes are given much credence, this might be better justified.

13.2.3   Selection curves

It seems implausible that all the change in probability of publication happens immediately at the point of the threshold. A smooth ramp up or down is more plausible (Figure 13.2).

[†] . . . in the manner of Section 2.2.1

[*] You may have heard of a very early method of meta-analysis, devised by Fisher, that was based entirely on p-values. That will not help us here, because Bayesian models aim to provide probabilistic insights into the unknown of principal interest, θ.

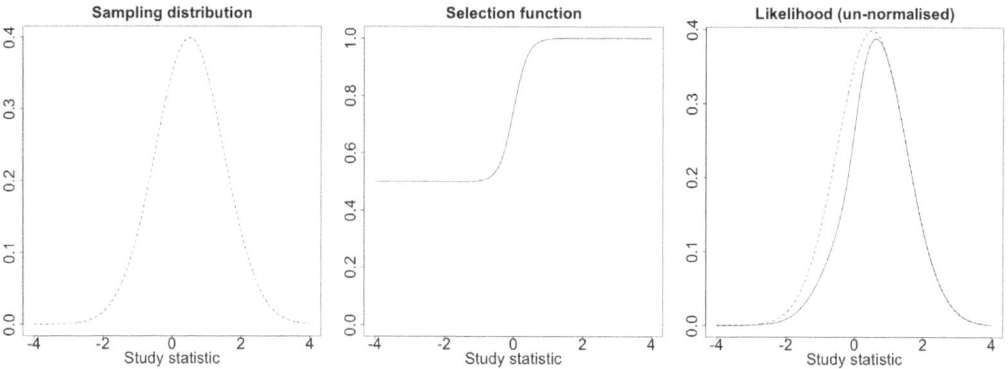

FIGURE 13.2
A simple selection model with an inverse logistic function for the probability of being published.

This model, using an inverse logistic function for the ramp, introduces three additional unknowns: the centre, the height, and the steepness of the ramp.

This will also be helpful for Stan in particular, because the posterior distribution should not have any discontinuous jumps in value [242]. Each study will have its own ζ_j.

The inverse logistic function in Figure 13.2 can be viewed as an extended form of logistic regression model. The probability of publication could be predicted by the observed study statistic, assuming that selection only occurs on one side of the sampling distribution (studies with significant evidence of benefit are more likely to be published):

$$\text{Use Cohen's } D: D_j = \frac{\hat{\theta}_j}{\widehat{SE}(\hat{\theta}_j)}$$

$$\log\left(\frac{\zeta_j}{1 - \zeta_j}\right) = \gamma_0 + \gamma_1 D_j \tag{13.6}$$

$$\cdot \; \zeta_j = \frac{1}{1 + e^{-(\gamma_0 + \gamma_1 D_j)}}$$

but we find it clearer to define the γ parameters differently, introduce the difference in probability between high and low asymptotes as γ_2, and write this as an inverse logistic function that takes a centred and scaled $\frac{D_j - \gamma_0}{\gamma_1}$ as input:

$$\zeta_j = (1 - \gamma_2) + \gamma_2 \frac{1}{1 + e^{-(\frac{D_j - \gamma_0}{\gamma_1})}} \tag{13.7}$$

To use a two-sided selection function instead, we could make the selection function the product of two ramps, or work with the absolute value $|D_j|$.

Here, γ_0 controls the midpoint of the ramp, and γ_1 its steepness. As we estimate these unknowns along with θ and τ, the sampling distribution curve will move and the studies will contribute different values to the likelihood. We should be careful not to ask too much of the software all at once, in case of under-identification (see Section 2.5).

It would be sensible to specify the value of all the γs, make sure the model returns meaningful results, then specify two and estimate the other, and so on. With small collections of studies, it may not be possible to estimate a .

Previously, we fixed the relationship between the point estimate of the intervention effect, $\hat{\theta}_j$, and its standard error, $\widehat{SE}(\hat{\theta}_j)$, by just dividing one by the other. We can treat them separately, which would introduce six unknowns to our model. This is the approach of the Copas selection model [204], which suggests that publication is separately influenced by the size of the estimated intervention effect and its uncertainty. However, as we saw before, asking for too many unknowns to be estimated from a small evidence base may not yield useful results in Bayesian sampling algorithms. Our advice is to keep it simple, build complications slowly, and be careful to justify all the choices.

Similar work in this area has used a *probit* model instead, where the probability of publication is found through the normal cumulative distribution function [204]. In practice, there is likely little difference between this and the logistic.

13.3   Software Implementation

To program a strange sampling distribution into our likelihood, we cannot use the off-the-shelf preset distributions. BUGS/JAGS and Stan take quite different approaches to this, which we will illustrate below, while Stata allows bespoke likelihoods to be programmed using the `bayesmh evaluators` functionality.

We will consider a dataset of 11 RCTs treating stroke with drugs called gangliosides, from an old Cochrane review [34]. This has evidence of asymmetry in the funnel plot (Figure 13.3). Odds ratios over 1 (log OR over 0) favour the gangliosides.

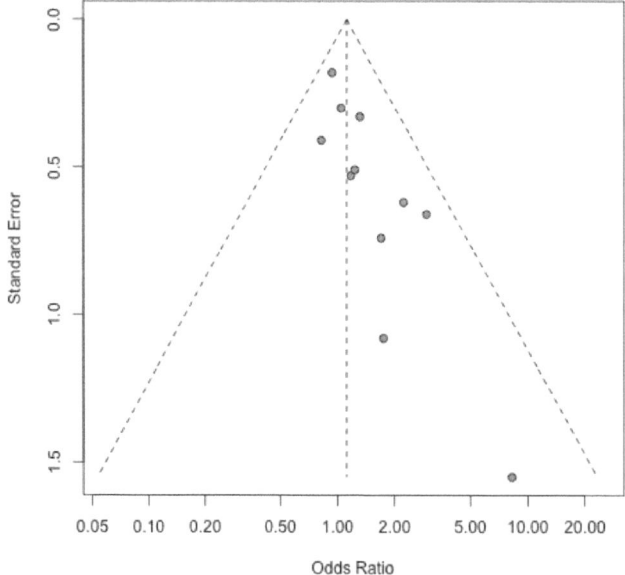

FIGURE 13.3
Funnel plot of 11 studies treating acute stroke with gangliosides.

```
library(readr)
library(meta)
ganglio <- read_csv("ganglio.csv")

# derive new variable for whether or not the logOR favoured gangliosides
ganglio$favoured <- as.numeric(ganglio$logor>0)

# basic generic-inverse-variance (common-effect) meta-analysis

ga_ma <- metagen(TE=ganglio$logor,
                 seTE=ganglio$se,
                 sm="OR",
                 common=TRUE,
                 random=FALSE,
                 method.tau="DL")

summary(ga_ma)
forest(ga_ma,sortvar=ganglio$se)
funnel(ga_ma)
```

The frequentist common effect meta-analysis estimates $\theta = 1.11$ with 95% confidence interval 0.89 to 1.40.

To implement the simple model in Equation 13.4, we need to calculate a likelihood for each study of $\zeta\, P(\hat{\theta}_j|\theta, \widehat{SE}(\hat{\theta}_j))$. In this case, $P(\cdot)$ is the normal distribution. This is a log likelihood of:

$$\log \zeta_j + \log P(\hat{\theta}_j|\theta, \widehat{SE}(\hat{\theta}_j)) \tag{13.8}$$

In BUGS / JAGS, and then in Stan, we will show how to do this by obtaining the usual normal log probability and then adding $\log \zeta_j$ (or any other values).

13.3.1   BUGS / JAGS

The techniques employed in BUGS and JAGS are called the "ones trick" and the "zeros trick". They use the binomial or Poisson distributions to add a value of your choice to the accumulating log posterior [156].

We will use the zeros trick in the code below. We need to create a new column in our data called `z[]`, which contains only zeros. Then, we pretend that `z[j]` is data that has a likelihood contribution, and make the likelihood Poisson with mean equal to `-1 * log(0.5 + 0.5*favoured[j])`, which is $-\log(\zeta_j)$. This is $-\log(1) = 0$ for "favoured" studies and $-\log(0.5) = 0.6931472$ otherwise.

This works because the probability of observing 1 from a Poisson distribution with mean μ is $e^{-\mu}$. In this case, $e^{-(-\log(\zeta_j))} = e^{\log(\zeta_j)} = \zeta_j$, which is what we need.

```
model {
  # prior
  theta ~ dnorm(0,0.25)

  or <- exp(theta)
  for(j in 1:m) {
    prec[j] <- pow(se[j], -2)
    logor[j] ~ dnorm(theta, prec[j])
    logfav[j] <- -1 * log(0.5 + 0.5*favoured[j])
    z[j] ~ dpois(logfav[j])
  }
}
```

The posterior mean was 1.07, slightly reduced from the frequentist 1.11.

13.3.2   Stan

Stan has a more direct way of adding to the accumulating log posterior, using a syntax that is quite different to the usual probability distribution with a ~ tilde.

When we begin a line in Stan with `target +=` we add whatever is on the right-hand side to the log posterior. It can be used for log priors or log likelihoods. Some Stan users prefer its clarity and switch to it for all their work [†].

```
data {
  int m;
  array[m] real logor;
  array[m] real se;
  array[m] real favoured;
}
parameters {
  real theta;
}
transformed parameters {
  real or;      // the odds ratio
  or = exp(theta);
}
model {
  // priors
  theta ~ normal(0,2);

  for(j in 1:m) {
    /*
```

[†] For every distribution that you have accessed via the tilde syntax, such as `normal()`, there is also a function `normal_lpdf()` to be used in the `target +=` syntax. Instead of `x ~ normal(mu, sigma);` for example, we would write `target += normal_lpdf(x | mu, sigma);`. Discrete-valued probability distributions have the same functions but with suffix `_lpmf` for the log probability mass function.

```
    The likelihood is either normal density or half
    normal density, depending on favoured. It will be
    clearer to use the Stan target+= syntax here.
  */
  target+= log(0.5 + 0.5*favoured[j]) +
          normal_lpdf(logor[j] | theta, se[j]);
 }
}
```

In the code above, we can see that ζ_j is represented by the component of the likelihood: `0.5 + 0.5*favoured[j]`. If we had a logistic equation for ζ_j, we could substitute its predicted values in here instead. The γ coefficients could either be estimated at the same time, or separately.

We tend to prefer one-step processes of Bayesian inference, in this case, estimating ζ_j or γ at the same time as the usual meta-analytic unknowns, θ and τ. However, a two-step approach can be helpful when the complete combined model is hard to fit. If it is all done at the same time, then the uncertainty in the γ coefficients will *propagate* through to θ, widening the credible intervals to take into account both parts of the model. If we estimate the γs first, and then feed them in, we lose that uncertainty and make the selection model more like a sensitivity analysis.

13.4 Real-World Complications

We may reasonably anticipate all our studies to be frequentist and hypothesis-testing in nature, though as time passes, Bayesian adaptive designs are more common in biomedical RCTs. Recently, some peer-reviewed journals have started discouraging, or even banning, the publication of p-values, and encouraging confidence intervals instead, or alternative p-value thresholds. These are all additional complications for such a selection model.

The outcome that we meta-analysts are interested in may not be the primary outcome of an individual study. If so, it is more likely to have been the primary outcome that influenced publication. The same applies to different time points. However, there is limited scope for using information from other outcomes, unless we can be confident that there is correlation among them.

No doubt, it is not only the statistics of the study that influences publication but also metadata, notably the fame of the organisation and authors that carried out the research. Even if reviewers do not know these, editors might well do.

In some experimental settings, particularly healthcare RCTs, studies may stop early according to some pre-specified rule. Some stop because the benefit is so compelling that it would be unethical to continue randomising participants to any other intervention. Some stop because one intervention turns out to have compelling evidence of harm. Some stop because interim analysis shows it is highly unlikely that the trial will go on to show significant benefit.

In each of these cases, it is the reduced statistical power that concerns us. At an interim analysis, there will be more uncertainty about the final outcome than if we waited and measured it. The interim analysis itself should take this into account in a number of statistically sound ways, but the goal of that interim analysis is to make a binary decision to continue or not, with a certain error probability. In contrast, the goal of meta-analysis is to estimate and infer the posterior probability of the intervention effect. So, we are not only concerned with the increased uncertainty (that is captured in the standard error), but with the bias that can be induced in these studies if they had stopping rules in only one direction [37]. Notably, those that stop for futility or harm may be less interesting to editors (unless the harm is great).

It is important to carefully examine the studies, and their protocols if available, for the rigour of the stopping rules and the appropriateness of the statistical procedures [272, 15]. Details are beyond the scope of this book; you should consult a statistician experienced in trial conduct if you are uncertain.

A variation on publication bias occurs when the study is published, but not all of its analyses or outcomes appear. If those that are included are selected on the basis of the results themselves, then the problem is called *reporting bias*. Few serious modelling methods have been suggested for reporting bias in meta-analysis [187, 259], meaning that simply adding a bias term with an informative prior is the only simple, tried-and-tested way of adjusting for it at present. There are some distributions of p-values within a study that are plausible, and others might raise suspicion of selective reporting or even *p-hacking* [89], especially if there is a preponderance just below 0.05.

14

Multiple Statistics

Learning objectives
After reading this chapter, you will be able to:

1. convert one statistic to another for inclusion in a meta-analysis, if the approximation is tolerable

2. combine different statistics in one Bayesian meta-analysis, using likelihood with shared unknowns

3. extract additional information from studies required to understand the underlying data distributions

---

A common frustration for meta-analysts occurs when studies in the evidence base are comparable in terms of PICO (participants, intervention, comparison, outcome), but then summarise the outcome variable with different statistics. Clinical trials sometimes dichotomise outcome measures to classify participants as "responders". The odds ratio or risk ratio for being a responder cannot then be combined with mean differences from other trials.

The most common way to deal with this is to make an approximate conversion from odds ratio to standardised mean difference and then include all studies. Approximate conversions were reviewed by Da Costa and colleagues in 2012, who found four comparable formulas [50], one of which is recommended by the Cochrane Handbook [112]. A shortcoming of these formulas is that they make no use of information on means and standard deviations at baseline in dichotomised studies, or means, standard deviations and correlations in comparable studies, or on the criteria for classifying participants as responders. In short, they do not make use of the full information across the evidence base, which is usually very likely to tell us something about the studies.

There have been several contributors to methodology around this problem, though it is disappointing to see that proper statistical modelling, linking different statistics via likelihood and shared unknowns, remains the exception rather than the norm.

The most influential early work on the Bayesian synthesis of diverse evidence sources coined the phrase "Confidence Profile Method" [63], and tackled several problems of evidence base by finding shared underlying unknowns. However, this did not consider multiple statistics of the same outcome variable, though it is an application of the same idea. Other related work includes a more complex Bayesian model for network meta-analysis including multiple statistics *and* multiple outcomes [59], information from different time points [155], and regression models [256]. O'Rourke explored likelihoods combining different statistics in his PhD thesis [184].

A Bayesian approach to this problem allows us to model heterogeneity as part of the data-generating process (DGP), and therefore each study's random effect can be informed

DOI: 10.1201/9781003375821-14

by whatever information is available. It is compatible with all the various interpretation of priors (see Section 2.2.3), as the important aspect is in the likelihood. This also means that you can adopt likelihood formulas for meta-analysis of multiple statistics if they are proposed in a non-Bayesian context.

14.1 Dichotomised Outcome Variables

In this chapter, we will consider one common problem, which we believe will illustrate the approach. We will suppose that there are only two-arm studies, no individual participant data, and no other challenges addressed in other chapters. Where some studies report means and standard deviations, but other report proportions of "responders", we will most likely have the following statistics available from a post-intervention assessment: means and standard deviations in the two arms of some trials, and proportions of "responders" in others.

Our first task will be to decide how the DGP produces the data, and what statistic represents this process. In this problem, we believe that there is a continuous-valued outcome variable which has later been dichotomised by study authors. So, we should relate all the statistics back to the mean and standard deviation of the outcome variable.

We suppose that there is some distribution (probability density function) of participant-level outcome values, and that this has been sliced at some threshold into two parts. The probability of being above or below the threshold, and hence a "responder" or not, will be the area under the curve.

So, if we know the shape of the distribution (for example, normal), and its parameters (mean and standard deviation), then we can calculate the probability of being a "responder". The mean and standard deviation can be used in the normal likelihood for studies reporting means and standard deviations, and the probability can be used in the binomial likelihood for studies reporting number of "responders".

The weak link in this process is likely to be the decision about the shape of the data distribution. If there is any individual participant data available, even if you are not using it in the meta-analysis, this should be the first source of information on the distribution shape. Ask project collaborators and colleagues for histograms of the outcome variable in question. As long as their samples were drawn from a reasonably similar population, this will be very informative. You should keep a record of this investigation and use it to justify your choices.

Do not simply adopt the normal distribution because you are aware of published means and standard deviations: many researchers publish these statistics regardless of the distribution of the variable. Another warning worth repeating is that sometimes researchers have heard that statistics acquire a normal sampling distribution as the sample size rises, and have often been given a heuristic threshold for this ($n = 30$ is a common number that gets mentioned). They might confuse this with the distribution of the data itself, and assume that if $n > 30$, then it must be normal. Do not fall into this trap!

A simple DGP for our example with some dichotomised studies, assuming a normal distribution for the data, is only a combination of those we set out for continuous outcomes (studies report means and standard deviations) and for binary outcomes (studies reporting proportions). Here, y_{ijkt} is the outcome variable recorded for participant i in study j and arm k, at time point t. The outcome post-intervention (y_{ijk1}), and possibly at baseline (y_{ijk0}), are combined with the threshold η_j to give the binary outcome $g_j(y_{ijk1}, y_{ijk0}, \eta_j)$. Note that the threshold, and the dichotomising function $g_j(\cdot)$, can vary between studies.

The baseline data informs the baseline statistics, and these may be useful in some of the forms of dichotomisation, which we set out in Section 14.1.1.

The number of participants in each arm and time point, n_{jkt}, is known, and ideally the correlation r_{jk} between y_{ijk0} and y_{ijk1}. IN the multivariate normal case, this will also be the correlation between the means in their sampling distribution. Where some of these statistics are not published, various approaches to assume and impute them, or use prior distributions for them, can be employed, following Chapter 5.

In this example, where the data are normally distributed, we can set out the data at both baseline and post-intervention as arising from a bivariate normal distribution with a vector of two means and a 2×2 covariance matrix Σ_{jk}. However, as this may be unfamiliar to many readers, we will show it here for each arm and time point in turn.

There is a population mean at baseline, μ_0, which we can assume is the same for all studies, or we can add a heterogeneity distribution to (see the considerations in Chapter 8). Then, the population change from baseline in the control arms is δ, and the population difference between intervention and control arms post-intervention is θ. We will also assume that there is one common standard deviation, σ.

Studies $1 \leq j \leq m_d$ are dichotomised, and studies $(m_d + 1) \leq j \leq m$ are not. We write a common effect version here, where the definition of a responder is left to be defined, and $\mathbb{I}(\cdot)$ is the identity function, which returns a 1 if the condition in the brackets is met, and 0 otherwise.

Data:

$$y_{ijk0} \sim \mathrm{N}(\mu_0, \sigma) \quad , \forall i, j, k$$

$$y_{ij\mathbf{Ctl}1} \sim \mathrm{N}(\mu_0 + \delta, \sigma) \quad , \forall i, j$$

$$y_{ij\mathbf{Int}1} \sim \mathrm{N}(\mu_0 + \delta + \theta, \sigma) \quad , \forall i, j$$

Dichotomisation:

$$g_j(y_{ijk1}, y_{ijk0}, \eta_j) = \mathbb{I}(\cdot) \quad , 1 \leq j \leq m_d$$

Sampling distributions:

$$\bar{y}_{jk0} \sim \mathrm{N}\left(\mu_0, \frac{\sigma}{\sqrt{n_{jk0}}}\right) \quad , \forall i, j, k$$

$$\bar{y}_{j\mathbf{Ctl}1} \sim \mathrm{N}\left(\mu_0 + \delta, \frac{\sigma}{\sqrt{n_{j\mathbf{Ctl}1}}}\right) \quad , \forall i, j$$

$$\bar{y}_{j\mathbf{Int}1} \sim \mathrm{N}\left(\mu_0 + \delta + \theta, \frac{\sigma}{\sqrt{n_{j\mathbf{Int}1}}}\right) \quad , \forall i, j$$

$$g_j(y_{ijk1}, y_{ijk0}, \eta_j) \sim \mathrm{Binom}(n_{jk\bullet}, \mathrm{P}(g_j(\cdot) = 1 | \eta_k, \bar{y}_{jkt}, s_{jkt}, r_{jk}))$$

(14.1)

This shows the connections to the two kinds of reported statistic, but we need to supply a formula for the very general probability $\mathrm{P}(g_j(\cdot) = 1 | \eta_k, \bar{y}_{jkt}, s_{jkt}, r_{jk})$, which is the focus of Section 14.1.1.

You can switch the normal distribution for any other that you like. All that is needed is a cumulative probability function for the binomial likelihoods (the probability of being below or above a threshold), and the sampling distribution of the mean, which can be found online or in a good standard inference textbook [38]. In Section 5.3.2, we showed a simulation approach to estimating the sampling distribution of a statistic from a distribution, and if there is no off-the-shelf formula, you could try this as a Plan B for your sampling distribution.

A "fully Bayesian" model (see Section 8.4) will require the sampling distributions of both the mean *and* standard deviation or variance. This is an extension of the method for the mean, but we must bear in mind that, although means and standard deviations are uncorrelated in the sampling distribution arising from normally distributed data, that does not hold in general, in particular for bounded outcome variables with floor and ceiling effects (see Chapter 17). More detail on this is really beyond the scope of this book, so you should be prepared to seek expert advice if it arises.

14.1.1 A taxonomy of dichotomisations

The most common forms of $g_j(\cdot)$ for some threshold η_k (the inequalities can be reversed depending on context) are:

$$\text{Absolute thresholds: } g_j(y_{ij\text{Int}1}, y_{ij\text{Int}0}, \eta_j) = \mathbb{I}(y_{ij\text{Int}1} < \eta_j)$$
$$\text{Relative-difference thresholds: } g_j(y_{ij\text{Int}1}, y_{ij\text{Int}0}, \eta_j) = \mathbb{I}(y_{ij\text{Int}1} - y_{ij\text{Int}0} < \eta_j) \qquad (14.2)$$
$$\text{Relative-ratio thresholds: } g_j(y_{ij\text{Int}1}, y_{ij\text{Int}0}, \eta_j) = \mathbb{I}(y_{ij\text{Int}1}/y_{ij\text{Int}0} < \eta_j)$$

$\mathbb{I}$ is the indicator function: if the condition inside the brackets is true, it will return 1, otherwise 0. In our experience, studies are usually thorough in reporting $g_j(\cdot)$ and η_j, although ambiguities do occur, as we will see in Section 14.2.

It will help to imagine these three types of threshold in the context of a hypothetical clinical trial to lower systolic blood pressure (Figure 14.1). Here, we see the two time points visualised as a bivariate normal distribution.

1. For absolute thresholds, such as post-intervention (endpoint) systolic blood pressure below 130mmHg ($\eta_j = 130$), only the marginal distribution of y_{ijk1} matters.

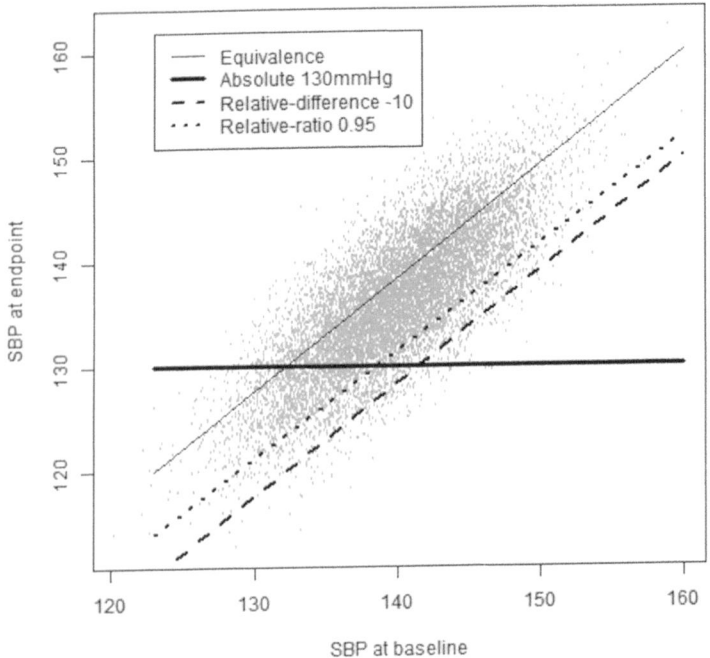

FIGURE 14.1
Three forms of dichotomisation in a hypothetical trial to lower blood pressure.

For normally distributed outcomes, this is:

$$P(g_j(\eta_j, \bar{y}_{jk1}, s_{jk1}) = 1) = \Phi\left(\frac{\eta_j - \bar{y}_{jk1}}{s_{jk1}}\right) \tag{14.3}$$

where Φ is the normal cumulative distribution function.

2. A relative-difference threshold, such as a reduction of 10mmHg or more from baseline ($\eta_j = -10$), divides the joint distribution parallel to the line of equality $y_{ijk1} = y_{ijk0}$. The bivariate distribution only matters in terms of a distribution perpendicular to the line of equality. This represents the difference between the endpoint and baseline variates, and will be normally distributed if both marginal distributions are assumed to be normal (another application of Equation 1.13). $\phi_j = \text{atan}(-\eta_j)$ is the angle of rotation; $\text{atan}(\cdot)$ is the inverse tangent function, which takes a real number and returns an angle in radians, between 0 and 2π.

$$P(g_j(\eta_j, \bar{y}_{jkt}, s_{jkt}, r_{jk}) = 1) = \Phi\left(\frac{\eta_j - (\bar{y}_{jk1} - \bar{y}_{jk0})}{\sqrt{s_{jk1}^2 + s_{jk0}^2 - 2r_{jk}s_{jk1}s_{jk0}}}\right) \tag{14.4}$$

3. For a relative-ratio threshold, such as a reduction of 10% or more from baseline ($\eta_k = 0.9$), we can rotate the joint distribution to a new pair of axes so that one is parallel to the threshold as seen in Figure 14.1[*] The relative ratio is again a random variate which is a linear combination of the two time points.

$$P(g_j(\eta_j, \bar{y}_{jkt}, s_{jkt}, r_{jk}) = 1) =$$
$$\Phi\left(\frac{-\cos\phi_j\bar{y}_{jk1} - \sin\phi_j\bar{y}_{jk0}}{\sqrt{\cos^2\phi_j s_{jk1}^2 + \sin^2\phi_i s_{jk0}^2 - 2\sin\phi_j\cos\phi_j r_{jk}s_{jk1}s_{jk0}}}\right) \tag{14.5}$$

Working out a formula like this, for other bivariate distributions, requires confidence in basic probability theory and secondary school algebra. No matter how confident or experienced you are, always get a colleague to check it, and consider checking it against simulated data.

The relative-difference and relative-ratio thresholds model have to include baseline information, while many standard meta-analytic procedures do not. However, because of the widespread practice of thoroughly reporting participants' characteristics at baseline, in our experience, the great majority of trials provide enough detail to support this. Where these are missing, it is better to include priors informed by other similar studies rather than impute a single assumed value.

---

[*]For readers with more mathematical backgrounds:
Rotation through an angle of $\phi_j = \text{atan}(-\eta_j)$ (negative because it is a clockwise rotation) implies postmul-

tiplication of the data matrix $Y = \begin{pmatrix} y_{1jk0} & y_{1jk1} \\ y_{2jk0} & y_{2jk1} \\ \vdots & \vdots \\ y_{n_{jk0}jk0} & y_{n_{jk1}jk1} \end{pmatrix}$

by a rotation matrix $\mathbf{R} = \begin{pmatrix} \cos\phi_j & -\sin\phi_j \\ \sin\phi_j & \cos\phi_j \end{pmatrix}$.

14.1.2   Software implementation

We provide an example of Stan code below for the absolute threshold model, and then the relevant lines to change in the `model` block, to use the relative-difference or relative-ratio thresholds. We prefer Stan in this model because of the clarity in passing a wide range of vectors and integers to the software (the `data` block).

We assume here that all studies provide standard deviations, and we calculate standard errors from those, but this can also be programmed the other way round, and in practice we are likely to supply Stan with both.

```
data {
  real threshold; // absolute threshold
  int<lower=0> t; // total number of trials (tk+td)
  int<lower=0> tk; // number of studies with means
  int<lower=0> td; // number without means
  array[t] int<lower=0> nt; // participants in treatment arm
  array[t] int<lower=0> nc; // participants in control arm
  array[t] real mc0; // baseline means in control
  array[t] real mt0; // baseline means in treatment
  array[t] real<lower=0> sc0; // SDs in control baseline
  array[t] real<lower=0> st0; // SDs in treatment baseline
  array[tk] real mt1; // treatment means where known
  array[t] real<lower=0> st1; // treatment SD known for all
  array[td] int<lower=0> rt1; // number normotensive in tx group
  array[tk] real mc1; // control means where known
  array[t] real<lower=0> sc1; // SDs in control known for all
  array[td] int<lower=0> rc1; // number normotensive in control
}
transformed data {
  array[t] real<lower=0> sec0;
  array[t] real<lower=0> set0;
  array[t] real<lower=0> set1;
  array[t] real<lower=0> sec1;
  // standard errors:
  for (j in 1:t) sec0[j] = sc0[j]/sqrt(nc[j]);
  for (j in 1:t) set0[j] = st0[j]/sqrt(nt[j]);
  for (j in 1:t) set1[j] = st1[j]/sqrt(nt[j]);
  for (j in 1:t) sec1[j] = sc1[j]/sqrt(nc[j]);
}
parameters {
  real mu0; // global mean for both groups at baseline
  real<lower=0> tau; // heterogeneity SD
  array[t] real u; // random effect
  real delta; // global mean of time difference
  real theta; // global mean of treatment effect
}
transformed parameters {
  real<lower=0, upper=1> riskt1[td]; // risk of responder in treatment arm
  real<lower=0, upper=1> riskc1[td]; // risk of responder in control arm
  for (j in 1:td) {
```

```
      riskt1[j] = Phi_approx((threshold-(mu0+u[tk+j]+theta+delta))/st1[tk+j]);
  }
  for (j in 1:td) {
    riskc1[j] = Phi_approx((threshold-(mu0+delta))/sc1[tk+j]);
  }
}
model {
  for (j in 1:t) u[j] ~ normal(0,tau);
  for (j in 1:t) mc0[j] ~ normal(mu0,sec0[j]);
  for (j in 1:t) mt0[j] ~ normal(mu0,set0[j]);
  for (j in 1:tk) mc1[j] ~ normal(mu0+delta,sec1[j]);
  for (j in 1:tk) mt1[j] ~ normal(mu0+theta,set1[j]);
  for (j in 1:td) rc1[j] ~ binomial(nc[j],riskc1[j]);
  for (j in 1:td) rt1[j] ~ binomial(nt[j],riskt1[j]);
  mu0 ~ normal(45,9);
  delta ~ normal(-5,10);
  theta ~ normal(-13,10);
  tau ~ cauchy(0,5);
}
```

The `Phi_approx` function in Stan provides the cumulative probability function for the normal distribution.

The relative-difference lines for the cumulative probability function, where `corr` is the correlation, are:

```
for (i in 1:td) {
  riskt1[j] = Phi_approx((threshold-dt)/
                          (sqrt((st0[tk+j]*st0[tk+j])+
                                (st1[tk+j]*st1[tk+j])-
                                (2*corr*st0[tk+j]*st1[tk+j])))) ;
  riskc1[j] = Phi_approx((threshold-dc)/
                          (sqrt((sc0[tk+j]*sc0[tk+j])+
                                (sc1[tk+j]*sc1[tk+j])-
                                (2*corr*sc0[tk+j]*sc1[tk+j])))) ;
}
```

The relative-ratio lines for the cumulative probability function follow, with sines and cosines pre-calculated for a 10% reduction threshold, shared across all studies. These are:

$$\eta = -0.9$$
$$\phi = \mathrm{atan}(\eta) = -41.99°$$
$$\cos(\phi) = 0.743294$$
$$\sin(\phi) = -0.668965 \tag{14.6}$$
$$\cos^2(\phi) = 0.552486$$
$$\sin^2(\phi) = 0.447514$$

```
for (i in 1:td) {
  riskt1[j] = Phi_approx((-(((-0.668965)*(mu0))+
                            (0.743294*(mu0+u[nk+j]+delta+theta)))))/
                  sqrt(((0.447514*st0[nk+j]*st0[nk+j])+
                        (2*(-0.668965)*0.743294*0.7*st0[nk+j]*st1[nk+j])+
                        (0.552486*st1[nk+j]*st1[nk+j])));
  riskc1[j] = Phi_approx((-(((-0.668965)*(mu0))+
                            (0.743294*(mu0+delta)))))/
                  sqrt(((0.447514*sc0[nk+j]*sc0[nk+j])+
                        (2*(-0.668965)*0.743294*0.7*sc0[nk+j]*sc1[nk+j])+
                        (0.552486*sc1[nk+j]*sc1[nk+j])));
}
```

Full code is available at the book's website. A simulation study of these models, presented at the Joint Statistical Meetings conference in 2014, is also online [95].

14.2   Case Study and Real-World Complications

A Cochrane review and meta-analysis of tricyclic anti-depressants for children and adolescents was chosen as an example application because of the varied and ambiguous ways in which the trials defined responders to treatment [108]. The review published a meta-analysis of all studies reporting means, which showed a significant benefit of treatment, and then a meta-analysis of all studies reporting proportions of responders, which was not significant (see Table 14.2). Eight trials appeared in both meta-analyses. The aim of this feasibility case study is to explore challenges in real-life implementation.

Details of the 14 trials are in Table 14.1, varying in total sample size from 6 to 173, and published between 1981 and 2001. They used a variety of outcome scales, which capture aspects of depression, anxiety, and other aspects of behaviour that would not be considered an indication for medication in this day and age. We do not cite the papers here, as the Cochrane review is open-access. We obtained the original full-text papers and extracted detailed statistics and metadata from them.

One of the trials (Hughes) reported only the number of responders (a 50% or greater reduction from their baseline CDRS score). There were eight other studies that reported both mean differences and numbers of responders. This analysis used only the statistics available to the Cochrane review in order to allow meaningful comparison with it; re-analysis of at least one included paper was subsequently published [178].

The trials reporting numbers of responders use the following definitions (see Table 14.1 for abbreviations):

1. Birmaher : "Absence of major depressive disorder" at end of treatment, BDI ≤ 9, HDRS ≤ 7, or at least a 50% decrease in HDRS (This mirrors the ambiguous wording in the paper with regards to combining these four conditions.)

2. Geller I : CDRS < 20 and various K-SADS-P items < 3

3. Geller II : CDRS < 20 and various K-SADS-P items < 3 and one K-SADS-P item < 4

4. Hughes : CDRS decrease $\geq 50\%$

5. Keller : HDRS ≤ 8 or $\geq 50\%$ decrease in HDRS

TABLE 14.1

Studies in the Cochrane review of tricyclic antidepressants for children. § - numbers used in means differ from those used in risks.

Study	Outcome	Arm	n_{jk}	$\bar{y}_{jk0}$	s_{jk0}	$\bar{y}_{jk1}$	s_{jk1}	d_{jk}/n_{jk}
Bernstein (1990)	CDRS	Ctl	7	36.5	3.4	30.1		
	CDRS	Int	9	41	12.2	29.5		
Bernstein (2000)	CDRS	Ctl	32	52.5	10.8	45.7	16.5	
	CDRS	Int	31	46.8	9.5	34.6	8.9	
Birmaher (1998)	BDI	Ctl	14	24.1	9.8	10.1	11.1	5/14
	BDI	Int	13	29.3	12.6	10.1	11.8	5/13
Birmaher (1998)	HDRS	Ctl	14	21.9	9.11	8.6	11.5	5/14
	HDRS	Int	13	22.9	5.11	7.7	8.0	5/13
Geller I (1989 & 92)	CDRS	Ctl	24	49.6	4.6	32.0	9.8	4/24
	CDRS	Int	26	49.9	4.2	32.9	11.4	8/26
Geller I (1989 & 92)	K-SADS-P	Ctl	24	3.89	0.5	2.2	0.78	
	K-SADS-P	Int	26	3.98	0.42	2.41	0.81	
Geller II (1990)	CDRS	Ctl	19	51.4	3.7	37.8	9.1	4/19
	CDRS	Int	12§	51.3	4.4	34.7	7.8	1/11
Hughes (1990)	CDRS	Ctl	14					7/14
	CDRS	Int	13					6/13
Kashani (1984)	BID	Ctl	4	27.75	4.35	23.75	5.56	
	BID	Int	5	25.60	2.41	18.40	3.29	
Keller (2001)	HDRS	Ctl	85§	18.97	4.1	9.88	7.74	40/87
	HDRS	Int	88§	18.11	4.17	9.20	7.85	47/94
Klein (1998)	HDRS	Ctl	18	21.33	5.2	14.61	2.1	9/18
	HDRS	Int	18	21.44	3.7	10.83	2.1	13/18
Kramer (1981)	DACL	Ctl	10	25.2	0.8	22.7	0.7	
	DACL	Int	10	16.2	1.2	10.3	0.4	
Kutcher (1994)	HDRS	Ctl	25	23.77	5.31	13.42	8.43	9/25
	HDRS	Int	17	22.63	5.17	12.68	8.68	8/17
Kye (1996)	HDRS	Ctl	10	15.3	6.0	7.8	5.5	9/10
	HDRS	Int	12	12.3	5.6	4.7	6.3	11/12
Petti (1982)	BID	Ctl	3	20.67	22.3	15.33	15.04	
	BID	Int	3	41.33	19.3	7	8.19	
Puig Antich (1987)	K-SADS-P	Ctl	22	3.0	0.66	1.9	0.86	
	K-SADS-P	Int	16	3.1	0.43	1.9	0.68	

Abbreviations: Pla, placebo; Tri, tricyclics; CDRS, Children's Depression Rating Scale; HDRS (also known as Ham-D), Hamilton Depression Rating Scale; BID, Bellevue Index of Depression; BDI, Beck Depression Inventory; K-SADS-P, Kiddie Schedule for Affective Disorders and Schizophrenia - Present symptoms; DACL, Depression Adjective Check List.

Note: Empty cells indicate statistics not reported in the papers. Some values have been derived from what was published. Decimal places are as published.

6. Klein : Psychiatrist's global assessment "improved" or better.

7. Kutcher : HDRS decrease $\geq 50\%$

8. Kye : HDRS decrease $\geq 50\%$

9. Puig-Antich : Two K-SADS-P items < 3

Only three trials had simple thresholds defined on one reported outcome measure (Hughes, Kutcher, Kye), and their responder results could be included as binomial likelihoods via equation (14.5). The Hughes trial, which reported no means or standard deviations, required estimates of its means and standard deviations for Equation 14.5. At each iteration in Stan, $\bar{y}_{jk0}$ and $\bar{y}_{jk1}$ are computed from the current proposed parameter values for μ_0, δ and θ, while s_{jk0} and s_{jk1} are drawn from an empirical $\chi^2(8)$ prior distribution, chosen by comparison to the observed standard deviations. Ideally, we would include this uncertainty in the variances in the Bayesian model, but with small numbers of heterogeneous trials, this seems unlikely to yield much information, and is not the purpose of this analysis. The likelihood for Hughes will remain relatively flat as a result, compared to the other studies, and will have a weak influence on the results.

We used a 50% relative-ratio threshold for the Hughes study, and an absolute threshold of CDRS < 20 for the Geller studies, and computed the following meta-analyses (results shown in Table 2):

1. Frequentist DerSimonian-Laird on standarised mean differences for all studies except Hughes

2. Frequentist DerSimonian-Laird on log odds ratios for responder statistics from Birmaher, Geller I, Geller II, Hughes, Keller, Klein, Kutcher, and Kye

3. Bayesian model on all studies, including means and standard deviations from all studies except Hughes, using the likelihood contributions in Equation 14.1, and responder statistics assuming a relative-ratio threshold from Hughes, using the likelihood contribution in Equation 14.5

4. The same Bayesian model from point 3 above, but using responder statistics rather than mean and standard deviations from Geller I, assuming an absolute threshold, to compare inferred and reported means for Geller I

5. The same Bayesian model from point 3 above, but using responder statistics rather than mean and standard deviations from Geller II, assuming an absolute threshold, to compare inferred and reported means for Geller II

The Geller studies were chosen for model testing because the CDRS scale was reported often enough to provide reasonable information for the prediction. All outcome scales other than CDRS (the most common) were related to it by multiplicative factors ($\gamma_{HDRS}, \gamma_{BDI}$, *etc.*), which were estimated in the analysis, essentially forming a standardised mean difference analysis, and yielding a treatment effect estimate in terms of CDRS points.

Correlations between baseline and endpoint were generally not reported but two trials provided individual patient data (Kashani and Petti), and approximate values could be derived from t-tests in the Kramer paper, and from the responder definition in the two Geller studies. These correlations were -0.36, 0.11, 0.15, 0.19 and 0.24 in ascending order, with a further approximately 0.8 that could not be estimated more precisely. Some are based on very small sample sizes, and we found the negative correlation implausible (in the population). In these analyses, a Beta(4, 4) prior distribution was used for the correlation, which is constrained to between 0 and 1 and is centred on 0.5. We used weakly informative priors on all other parameters, including a half-Cauchy for the heterogeneity standard deviation, which was fashionable at the time (2014):

$$\mu \sim \mathrm{N}(45, 9)$$
$$\delta \sim \mathrm{N}(-5, 10)$$
$$\theta \sim \mathrm{N}(-13, 10) \tag{14.7}$$
$$\tau \sim \mathrm{Cauchy}^+(0, 5)$$
$$\gamma_{\mathrm{SCALE}} \sim \mathrm{U}(0, 5) \quad, \ \forall\, \mathrm{SCALE}$$

The code and data are available online from the book website. The aim of this analysis is to learn about the feasibility of the method and to inform recommendations for practical

TABLE 14.2
Bayesian antidepressants meta-analysis, compared to Cochrane. Estimates in the Bayesian model are posterior means. § - on the scale of standardised mean differences, taken from the meta-analysis of means; DerSimonian-Laird meta-analyses assume no uncertainty in τ so there is no confidence interval.

Model	Estimate	95% CI
Cochrane: standardised mean differences	-0.32	-0.04 to -0.59
Cochrane: risk ratio for being a 'responder'	1.07	0.91 to 1.26
Cochrane: heterogeneity standard deviation §	0.33	N/A to N/A
Bayesian model: baseline mean on CDRS scale, μ_0	40.81	35.80 to 45.99
Bayesian model: time effect on CRDS scale, δ	-3.34	-4.18 to -2.56
Bayesian model: treatment effect on CDRS scale, θ	-14.15	-15.64 to -12.65
Bayesian model: scaling factor for HDRS, γ_{HDRS}	0.50	0.43 to 0.57
Bayesian model: scaling factor for BDI, γ_{BDI}	0.53	0.42 to 0.67
Bayesian model: scaling factor for BID, γ_{BID}	0.54	0.41 to 0.68
Bayesian model: scaling factor for K-SADS-P, γ_{KSADSP}	0.08	0.07 to 0.08
Bayesian model: scaling factor for DACL, γ_{HDRS}	0.76	0.68 to 0.85
Bayesian model: heterogeneity SD on CDRS scale, τ	8.56	5.51 to 13.53
Bayesian model: baseline-endpoint correlation, ρ	0.54	0.21 to 0.83

implementation. Potential aspects of the analysis unrelated to the dichotomisation, such as imputation of endpoint standard deviations, were kept as simple as possible to focus on learning from the proposed method.

The Stan models were fitted to the data in about 10 seconds, generating 5000 draws from the posterior in each of three chains, and discarding the first 1000 of each as warm-up. The results are shown in Table 14.2.

The Cochrane review found a significant benefit of tricyclic antidepressants when considering trials reporting means, and a non-significant benefit when considering trials reporting responders. The Bayesian model finds a benefit[†] (θ) of 14.2 points on the CDRS scale, with a more definitive 95% credible interval (12.6 to 15.6 CDRS points) than Cochrane's confidence interval (0.04 to 0.59 on the scale of standardised mean differences). The mean improvement of -14.2 CDRS points is not immediately comparable to the standardised mean difference of -0.32 from the Cochrane review, because the latter is in units of standard deviations of the between-groups differences between within-groups changes. Other differences between the analyses are: the inclusion of a baseline mean parameter, the multiplicative scaling of the outcome scales rather than standardising each study's estimated effect size, the inclusion of the Hughes paper, the K-SADS-P outcomes from the Geller I paper, and the BDI outcomes from the Birmaher paper

The Bayesian model also provides an estimate of the time effect (δ), comparing endpoint to baseline in the control groups, which might reflect a modest placebo effect or regression to the mean. The posterior mean was a reduction of 3.3 CDRS points, with 95% credible interval of 2.6 to 4.2.

The posterior mean probability of being a responder in the control arm of the Hughes study was 27%, and in the treatment arm 52%. This reflects the mean differences seen in other studies, though Hughes had 7/14 (50%) responders in the control arm and 6/13 (46%) in treatment.

For Geller I, the model predicted: baseline mean of 40.2 (95% CI 31.6 to 49.6; the observed means of 49.6 and 49.9 corresponded to the 97th and 98th posterior centiles

---

[†]There are plenty of other reasons why giving children these drugs is a very bad idea. Remember, this is just a statistics textbook!

respectively), endpoint mean in the control group of 38.0 (95% CI 29.6 to 47.2; observed mean 32.0 was at the 9th posterior centile), and endpoint mean in the treatment group of 25.7 (95% CI 19.0 to 33.4; observed mean 32.9 was at the 97th centile).

For Geller II, the model predicted: baseline mean of 40.1 (95% CI 27.2 to 55.4, observed means 51.4 and 51.3, both at the 93rd posterior centile), endpoint mean in the control group of 37.8 (95% CI 25.1 to 53.0; observed mean 37.8 was at the 52nd posterior centile), and endpoint mean in the treatment group of 25.5 (95% CI 13.4 to 40.4; observed mean 34.7 was at the 90th posterior centile).

As a feasibility case study, this application shows that it is possible for a researcher with some expertise in Bayesian software to fit and check the model. The main challenge will be in deciding how to include studies with ambiguous or complex responder definitions. Also, when a study reports both means and responders, the analyst must choose one statistic to add to the meta-analysis. The presence of uncertainties about the reported statistics may be the most important factor driving this decision.

In the application to the Cochrane review of antidepressants in children, ambiguous or complex definitions of responders were a recurring problem, giving a useful insight into how methods like the models in this paper might be implemented. Any of the threshold types set out in this paper might fail to fit statistics from such studies.

The Cochrane review allows us a limited opportunity to evaluate the model's ability to predict individual study results. The two Geller studies which could be investigated have unusually high changes over time even in the control group (Table 1), perhaps reflecting regression to the mean, and although seven of the eight reported means were inside the 95% credible intervals of the predicted means, they were mostly at high or low quantiles of the posterior. In the case of Geller II, a contributing problem may be that responders were defined with a mixture of CDRS and selected items from K-SADS-P, without reporting individual items of K-SADS-P.

We have considered a simple meta-analysis, to focus on the problem of dichotomisation. Dichotomised studies give us very little information to infer random effects, as they have thrown away information. However, multivariate models including other outcomes that are not dichotomised may help (see Chapter 15). Extension to network meta-analysis is described by Dias and colleagues in a section of their book called "Shared parameter models" [56].

15

Multiple Outcomes or Study Designs

This chapter considers the problem—and opportunity—of an evidence base comprising studies done in various different ways. We class these into two large themes. There may be multiple outcome variables that aim to quantify the same construct, including in particular, outcome scales derived from a collection of individual items. There might also be multiple study designs, such as randomised controlled trials, case-control studies, and so on.

15.1 Multiple Outcome Scales for the Same Construct

There are some topics of research where it is quite common to have various studies report different outcome scales. When the focus is prevention of cardiovascular events, the variables that are measured are almost certainly time at risk and a binary event / no event outcome. In contrast, studies of interventions that target concepts such as self-efficacy, quality of life, or depression could draw on a wide range of possible *outcome scales*.

Scales like these can be combined in a meta-analysis, provided that we are confident that they all make some measurement of the same underlying construct. We should not, for example, throw in a patient awareness questionnaire along with the self-efficacy scales, because they do not even attempt to measure the same construct.

In Chapter 14, we introduced a meta-analysis combining 14 studies that assessed depression with six different scales. The most typical way of dealing with this is to standardise the study statistics, as we saw in Section 3.2.1, so that they are all on the same scale.

DOI: 10.1201/9781003375821-15

The most common standardisation process will equalise the means and standard deviations of outcome scales, but might not address floor and ceiling effects, or differences of sensitivity [174]. It is possible to relate multiple variables to one another and standardise to a common scale at the same time [2]. Sometimes, it may be preferable to break the scales apart (if the data / statistics are available) and work with sub-scales or even individual questions, to avoid this problem of comparing apples and oranges.

We should expect different scales to be correlated, and we may even have some *a priori* indication of which pairs of scales will more strongly correlated than others. This can be based on the constituent questions or measurements that go into the scale. Where there is shared content, we expect higher correlation, but if one scale includes some components that are outside the central construct then that will reduce the correlation.

When researchers develop scales, they typically carry out and publish some psychometric validation [122], and this may give you another *a priori* source of justification for expecting some scales to be inherently closer to the true construct. Sometimes, they identify specific sub-scales which are comprised of a subset of questions (items) and which identify a more specific construct (feelings of hopelessness, for example).

The various depression scales in Chapter 14's example are quite an informative example, although some of them are regarded as antiquated now. If you are new to the topic of multiple outcomes, it is worth looking into them; the actual lists of questions, or the questionnaires, can be found online. It is striking how different they can be, despite all claiming to be scientifically objective quantifications of "depression".

15.1.1   Surrogate and composite outcomes

Surrogate outcomes are those variables which are easier, cheaper or quicker to assess than an ideal outcome. A dietary intervention to prevent cardiovascular events such as heart attacks and stroke might measure blood pressure after a few weeks, rather than wait for years to see what the long-term outcomes are. Nevertheless, it is the long-term outcomes that matter, and the surrogate only informs decision-making because it is correlated with the long-term outcome.

We can make use of the techniques for multiple outcome scales in this setting too, because whenever we measure the objective of the study in multiple ways, and we know that they are correlated, then the same statistical model can apply.

A very common problem in the medical evidence base is the reporting of composite outcomes. A participant in a study of hip replacements might be counted as having had an "event" in a study if they died *or* had another fracture *or* required revision surgery. If other studies report purely one of these binary events, then we expect there to be some correlation between the composite and the pure outcome, but not for them to be the same. We might also constrain the composite to always have a higher population incidence than any of its constituent parts, by definition.

15.2   Multivariate Meta-Analysis

The principal alternative to standardisation is a multivariate meta-analysis, with a multivariate likelihood, including a covariance matrix. See Section 8.5 for the basic definitions. As we explained there, it is unlikely that statistics from the available studies will provide enough information to identify all the correlations among the outcome scales.

One particular problem arises when few studies report each outcome and few report more than one. This creates a sparse network of connections among the studies, and it is those connections that inform correlations. However, it may be possible to estimate correlations in a first step using similar IPD from outside the evidence base, even if this is observational data, as long as multiple outcomes are assessed on the same participants [30], and then run the meta-analysis as a second step. A general inferential technique called bootstrapping can be useful to identify a sampling distribution for the inter-study correlation [29].

The reason to consider the multivariate approach is to capitalise on *borrowing of strength*: reducing uncertainty in our inferences by combining all available information from studies and outcomes that we deem likely to be correlated *a priori*. There has been some effort to identify the characteristics of evidence bases where borrowing of strength may exist, noting the underuse in the medical setting at present [106].

Suppose that we have some studies reporting outcome scale A, which, meta-analysed together, show promise but are not quite compelling evidence. Likewise for outcomes B, C, D, which all target the same underlying construct as A, and all meta-analysed separately. Surely it is clear that the evidence is accumulating for the utility of the intervention, because A, B, C and D are all manifestations of the construct.

Bringing all the evidence together, either by multivariate likelihood, or by standardisation, will be preferable to running several separate meta-analyses on different outcome measures and leaving overall synthesis to the reader.

15.2.1 Model specification

There is extensive advice on Bayesian models, priors and BUGS code for multivariate meta-analysis in the NICE DSU technical support document [29], and we encourage you to use this as a source of detailed advice for these models. Typically, the multivariate heterogeneity, for example here for three outcomes (A, B and C) has the following form.

$$
\begin{bmatrix} \theta_{Aj} \\ \theta_{Bj} \\ \theta_{Cj} \end{bmatrix} \sim \text{MVN} \left(\begin{bmatrix} \theta_A \\ \theta_B \\ \theta_C \end{bmatrix}, \begin{bmatrix} \tau_A^2 & \rho_{AB}\tau_A\tau_B & \rho_{AC}\tau_A\tau_C \\ \rho_{AB}\tau_A\tau_B & \tau_B^2 & \rho_{BC}\tau_B\tau_C \\ \rho_{AC}\tau_A\tau_C & \rho_{BC}\tau_B\tau_C & \tau_C^2 \end{bmatrix} \right) \tag{15.1}
$$

However, we must recognise that there is also intra-study correlation—which we will write as ρ_{wAB}, *etc.*—simply because these outcomes are measured on the same participants. That intra-study correlation alone will induce some part of the inter-study correlation in the study statistics, and if we ignore it, we will conclude that the observed ρs in the covariance matrix above are evidence of large correlation in the likelihood. This can have a strong biasing effect as a strongly correlated multivariate normal likelihood allocates very low—too low—likelihood to studies that do not adhere to the central part of the diagonal, correlated distribution. To compensate for this, our software may end up inflating the heterogeneity standard deviations τs instead.

The sampling distribution will have a similar multivariate normal distribution. In theory, if both sampling distribution and IPD are MVN, then the ρ_{wAB} and other correlations in the sampling distribution will be equal to the correlations among the IPD. The exact form of this relationship depends on the distribution of the IPD. If the IPD is MVN too, then the IPD correlation and sampling distribution correlations will be the same (and hence we can use IPD to inform our ρ_{wAB}s and set strong, empirical priors for them).

When the IPD is not MVN, you should seek expert statistical input, as it is possible to choose priors based on the bootstrap method. Sensitivity analysis for a range of plausible ρ_{wAB} values is a fallback.

$$\begin{bmatrix} \hat{\theta}_{Aj} \\ \hat{\theta}_{Bj} \\ \hat{\theta}_{Cj} \end{bmatrix} \sim \text{MVN} \left(\begin{bmatrix} \theta_{Aj} \\ \theta_{Bj} \\ \theta_{Cj} \end{bmatrix}, \begin{bmatrix} \sigma_A^2 & \rho_{wAB}\sigma_A\sigma_B & \rho_{wAC}\sigma_A\sigma_C \\ \rho_{wAB}\sigma_A\sigma_B & \sigma_B^2 & \rho_{wBC}\sigma_B\sigma_C \\ \rho_{wAC}\sigma_A\sigma_C & \rho_{wBC}\sigma_B\sigma_C & \sigma_C^2 \end{bmatrix} \right) \quad (15.2)$$

Remember that we expect there to be some study or studies reporting more than one outcome scale, and in this case, the same random effect might be employed for all the outcomes in one study.

It is also worth bearing in mind that multivariate models do not capture any strong beliefs about how outcomes should correspond to one another in individual participants, or studies. They only describe the distributions. In cases where we are very confident that the outcomes are all close matches to the same underlying construct (the concept that you hope to quantify and study), we would expect the same qualitative conclusions for all outcomes. Yet the basic normal model does not enforce this, which Dias and colleagues expand on in Section 11.5 of their book [56].

15.2.2 Binary and other outcomes

With a binary outcome variable, or a count or other statistic, we can work with the same multivariate normal models, as the sampling distributions of the study statistics will be asymptotically normal. However, we should justify this approximation. We must feel confident that the studies have sufficient sample size, and that the statistics are sufficiently far from any floor or ceiling effects, for an asymptotic normal sampling distribution to be a reasonable assumption (see Chapter 1).

15.2.3 Software implementation

It is important to be clear about what arguments your software requires for the multivariate normal distribution. Some expect a covariance matrix, others a precision matrix, which is the inverse. You can compute the inverse of a covariance / precision matrix with the functions: `inverse()` in BUGS, `solve()` in R, `inverse_spd()` in Stan, and `invsym()` in Stata.

The following BUGS code is for a bivariate normal likelihood (two outcomes), adapted from the NICE technical support document [29]. We supply a single correlation `corr_w`, which will have a prior unless you are doing repeated sensitivity analysis.

```
rho_w ~ INSERT YOUR PRIOR HERE! # sampling distribution corr.
rho_het ~ INSERT YOUR PRIOR HERE! # heterogeneity corr.

for(j in 1:m) {
  # assemble sampling distribution covariance matrix for study j
  sigma[i,1,1] <- pow(se[i,1],2)
  sigma[i,2,2] <- pow(se[i,2],2)
  sigma[i,1,2] <- sqrt(sigma[i,1,1])*sqrt(sigma[i,2,2])*rho_w
  sigma[i,2,1] <- sqrt(sigma[i,1,1])*sqrt(sigma[i,2,2])*rho_w

  # invert covariance matrix to get precision matrix
  prec_w[i,1:2,1:2] <- inverse(sigma[i,1:2,1:2])
}
```

```
# assemble heterogeneity covariance matrix
for (k in 1:2) {
  tau[k] ~ dunif(0,2) # prior
  tau.sq[k] <- pow(tau[k],2)
  Cov_het[k,k] <- tau.sq[k]
}
Cov_het[1,2] <- rho_het*tau[1]*tau[2]
Cov_het[2,1] <- Cov_het[1,2]

# invert covariance matrix to get precision matrix
prec_het[1:2,1:2] <- inverse(Cov_het[,])

# priors for intervention effects
for (k in 1:2) {
  theta[k] ~ INSERT YOUR PRIOR HERE!
}

# bivariate normal likelihood & heterogeneity:
for(j in 1:m) {
  theta_hat[j,1:2] ~ dmnorm(theta_j[j,1:2], prec_w[i,1:2,1:2])
  theta_j[j,1:2] ~ dmnorm(theta[1:2], prec_het[1:2,1:2])
}
```

In BUGS, `dmnorm()` is the MVN probability density function. There are also functions like this in Stata, Stan, JAGS and `brms`.

More complicated versions of this BUGS code appears in the NICE technical support document [29].

15.2.4 Correlation matrix versus latent variables

Multiple correlated outcome variables can also be conceived of as manifestations of a shared underlying value, which we cannot directly obtain and call a *latent variable*. This is the preferred method in some fields, and is called a *latent variable model*. Because the latent variable is not observed, it is an unknown vector with an element for each of the observations in the data. It could take different values for each of the observations / participants. The observed variables are called *manifest variables*.

In frequentist statistics, inference for the latent variable's individual elements is not possible*, but in Bayesian statistics, we can use priors and posteriors for the elements, as though they were missing data (Missing At Random, informed by the observed data).

Each manifest variable (for example, the depression scales in the previous example) is determined by a function of the latent variable, ± some noise. Usually, we make the function linear and the noise normal (often called Gaussian in this context), which reduces it to a linear regression model.

It is possible to create a multivariate model, with a correlation matrix that defines the relationships among the variables, and an exactly equivalent latent variable model with path

---

*This is because, if we "ran the experiment again", as it is commonly expressed, we would not obtain different values from the sampling distribution of the latent variable elements, but rather completely different elements relating to completely different observations / participants.

coefficients. This is just the same as describing a bivariate dataset either with its means, standard deviations, and correlation, or with its independent variable mean and variance, regression coefficients and residual standard deviation. Song and Lee offer a variety of Bayesian implementations in BUGS in their book [236].

The advantage is purely in the extent to which the mathematical formulation helps us and our collaborators to think about defining the model *a priori*. If we are able to agree on assumptions, justified by theory and previous evidence, that constrain the options for the model, cutting off some paths or setting correlations to zero, then we may be able to simplify our model to the extent that it can be determined by the data to a single, well-behaved posterior distribution.

Latent variable models, and their more complicated superset, structural equation models, are described among emerging topics in Chapter 17.

15.3   Multiple Study Designs

One of the earliest proposed innovative applications of Bayesian meta-analysis was the idea of pooling information from a mixture of randomised controlled trials and non-randomised, observational studies in health interventions or risk factors. This was promoted by Spiegelhalter and colleagues [239, 240] in the early 2000s, though they trace its origin to ten years earlier.

Despite this, it remains rarely used. One reason for this may be the lack of clarity about a pragmatic way to consider building a Bayesian model for such a mixture of studies, and deciding whether it is feasible to proceed. In this chapter, we will summarise the various proposals that have been made, and highlight potential areas for growth and new methodological development.

We consider not just mixtures of randomised and non-randomised studies but also studies with high or low risk of bias, various adjustments for covariates or baseline outcome variables. The goal of most meta-analyses is a causal estimate of the effect of an intervention or a risk factor, and the reason for concern about non-randomised studies is specifically the reduced ability to identify an unbiased causal estimate.

15.3.1   Randomised and non-randomised studies

From the start of Bayesian statisticians considering this problem, the idea of fitting studies into a more detailed hierarchical structure was popular [239]. This would essentially require one heterogeneity distribution for randomised controlled trials, another for case-control studies, and so on. Meta-analysts must consider, on a case-by-case basis, whether these subgroup hetereogeneity distributions would then require bias modelling [254, 265], or if their means would be combined in one overarching hyper-heterogeneity, or via fixed effects, or simply be regarded as a mixture of (probably normal) distributions [59].

Bias modelling is, in some ways, a more pressing concern, since it is likely to be the "deal breaker" that puts a stop to a multi-study-design meta-analysis, rather than selection of heterogeneity structure.

Randomised controlled trials are subject to their own bias relative to population effectiveness: the recruitment process draws from a population that often does not represent the eventual target audience for an intervention, which is how such studies tend to be interpreted by decision-makers [227].

A meta-analysis comparing the two designs shows differences, but no systematic pattern that could clearly guide modelling [216]. A small study of both potential biases in the econometric literature provides a potential template for future methodology to estimate both biases and to make a de-biased inference [84].

A recent review of methods used in 132 published papers with meta-analyses combining randomised and non-randomised studies showed a surprising lack of detailed reporting around the combination [42]. Only 33% of the studies reported pooled results subgrouped by study design, and 10% reported potential confounding factors in the observational studies. It may be that these matters were investigated and found not to be newsworthy enough to report, but that is in itself a failure of responsible reporting.

At the same time, concern was raised about inadequate reporting in observation studies themselves, in order to inform and support potential meta-analyses [258]. A particular concern was under-reporting of potential confounding variables which an observational study might have considered for adjustment and then not used, perhaps through some selection process.

Further, our view is that randomised non-comparative trials (RNCTs) should be excluded from meta-analyses that include randomised controlled comparative trials and/or observational studies. Their inherent methodological limitations — lack of interpretability, absence of prespecified relative effect measures, and reliance on post-hoc comparative analyses — violate core statistical assumptions that fundamentally compromise the validity of pooled estimates. As demonstrated by Sherry and colleagues, RNCTs primarily generate group-specific inferences rather than comparative effect estimates, making them methodologically incompatible with study designs explicitly structured to produce relative treatment effects through either randomisation or appropriate adjustment strategies [226].

In writing a meta-analysis with a mixture of study designs, you should always present an exploration of the differences between study designs. Heterogeneity should be explored with reference to the study characteristics.

15.3.2   Power priors

When meta-analysis is used to inform clinical trial designs, the proper balancing of RCTs and observational studies is of vital importance [177]. These meta-analyses are used solely to obtain an empirical, *meta-analytic prior*, and a method that has become quite widespread in recent years is called the *power prior* [217].

This method adjusts the likelihood, to down-weight the observational studies, by raising them to the power of an unknown α, where $0 \le \alpha \le 1$. Suppose studies $j = 1$ to $j = q$ are RCTs, while $j = (q + 1)$ to $j = m$ are observational:

$$\mathrm{P}(\boldsymbol{\theta}|\boldsymbol{Y}) \propto \mathrm{P}(\boldsymbol{\theta}) \prod_{j=1}^{q} \mathrm{P}(\boldsymbol{Y}_j|\boldsymbol{\theta}) \prod_{j=q+1}^{m} \mathrm{P}(\boldsymbol{Y}_j|\boldsymbol{\theta})^{\alpha} \tag{15.3}$$

Typically, a Beta prior is applied to α and it is inferred as another unknown. This essentially has the effect that the computer prioritises fitting the unknowns $\boldsymbol{\theta} = \{\theta, \tau, \ldots\}$ to the RCT statistics, rather than the observational studies.

We recognise that you might not necessarily be interested in producing a meta-analytic prior, yet you cannot use the same adjustment on the likelihood in your Bayesian meta-analysis without altering the result [188]—this method is restricted to the meta-analytic prior setting, and even then, only when we definitely want to down-weight the historic data / study statistics. It remains an area under active research.

15.3.3   Variance inflation

There are two ways in which observational, non-randomised studies may not provide adequate inference for a causal estimand. Firstly, the additional influence of many confounding factors may add together and inflate the uncertainty around our estimates. This means inflating the standard deviation of the posterior, but in this context, people usually talk about variance inflation.

We might do this by simply increasing the observed standard errors of the observational studies, but a more Bayesian way of thinking about it is to add or adjust a prior.

We might add an additional term to the relationship between the unknown efficacy of the intervention (θ) and the observed estimate in the observational studies, which has a normal prior with a certain variance, which is a multiple of the observed study standard error. Because the sum of two random variables has a variance which is the sum of the two individual variances (Equation 1.12), this just acts to inflate the uncertainty.

If an observational study reports $\hat{\theta}_j = 0.6$, $\widehat{SE}(\hat{\theta}_j) = 0.2$, and we want all the observational studies to have their variance boosted by 50%, then we must calculate $\hat{V}(\hat{\theta}_j) = \left(\widehat{SE}(\hat{\theta}_j)\right)^2 = 0.04$ and set the extra term's prior to have a variance of 0.02, therefore a standard deviation of $\sqrt{0.02} = 0.14$.

We should not be surprised to find the extra term to be negatively correlated, perhaps strongly, with θ in the posterior, and as there is an extra term for every observational study, this will place a heavy computational load on software based on the Gibbs sampler or random-walk Metropolis-Hastings; Stan, or other Hamiltonian Monte Carlo implementations, will be preferable.

Another way to do this, without adding new terms, is to have a different heterogeneity standard deviation for the observational studies, and require it to be larger than that of the RCTs. We could multiply τ by some positive unknown, say $\gamma\tau$, and use that for the observational heterogeneity standard deviation. This assumes that the RCTs are not very different to one another in PICO, time scale, and so on, otherwise they might actually be worse than the observational studies!

Such a model aims to honestly reflect the uncertainty around the observational estimates compared to the randomised estimates, albeit in a heuristic way. Their $\hat{\theta}_j$ is able to move a little way further from θ, as long as that difference is counter-balanced by the extra term. This places more importance on matching θ to the estimates from the randomised studies. The prior for this extra term should be subject to sensitivity analysis and thorough justification, even if that is expert opinion.

15.3.4   Bias adjustment

The second potential problem with non-randomised studies is that their estimates may not just be perturbed randomly from the causal unknown, but may be asymmetrically so, because confounders might be suspected of acting mainly in one direction. This is the sort of problem where we add a bias term to θ_j for the observational studies, and use either an elicited expert opinion prior, or an empirical prior from comparable evidence on the effect of confounding [213].

The bias terms are themselves drawn from a heterogeneity distribution with non-zero mean [56, 279]. In Equation 15.4, γ_j is the bias term, which is removed from any studies deemed to be unbiased by multiplication by a study-level bias variable, x_j, which is zero for no bias.

$$\hat{\theta}_j \sim \mathrm{N}(\theta_j + \gamma_j, \mathrm{SE}(\hat{\theta}_j))$$
$$\theta_j \sim \mathrm{N}(\theta, \tau) \tag{15.4}$$
$$\gamma_j \sim \mathrm{N}(\gamma, \tau_\gamma)$$

15.3.5 Risk of bias

Systematic reviews should have a risk of bias (RoB) assessment using a standardised tool. This often leads to categories of low, medium and high bias, and it would be appropriate to set the bias term, for both RCTs and observational studies, to be likewise low, medium and high. We can constrain these to rise in value (or drop) by adding, or subtracting, a positive real number, γ.

Suppose that we send the data to our Bayesian software with an indicator variable for each study, $x_{\mathbf{medhigh}}$, that is 0 for low risk, and 1 for medium or high risk, and another variable, $x_{\mathbf{high}}$, that is 1 for high risk only. We can multiply these by the unknown positive real numbers for the bias:

$$\theta_j \sim \mathrm{N}(\theta, \tau)$$
$$\hat{\theta}_j \sim \mathrm{N}(\theta_j + \gamma_{\mathbf{medhigh}} x_{\mathbf{medhigh}} + \gamma_{\mathbf{high}} x_{\mathbf{high}}, \widehat{SE}(\hat{\theta}_j)) \tag{15.5}$$
$$\gamma_{\mathbf{medhigh}}, \ \gamma_{\mathbf{high}} \in \mathbb{R}^+$$

As above, we should anticipate strong negative correlations among the unknowns, and Stan or brms will outperform BUGS, JAGS, and Stata in this setting. Including multiple heterogeneities on the γs is likely to be asking too much of the data, unless there are plenty of studies in each risk category.

An alternative would be to remove the high risk studies, and this should probably be done to compare with a bias-adjusted analysis as a sensitivity analysis, although the objective of bias-adjustment is not to mimic exclusion of studies. They are two approaches to getting a better estimate, with no guarantee of which, if either, is "correct".

16

Informing Policy and Economic Evaluation

Learning objectives

After reading this chapter, you will:

1. understand the opportunities and challenges of influencing policy through meta-analysis

2. recognise the potential for meta-analysis in evidence-based policy beyond health care

3. know the connections between the meta-analyst's outputs and the required inputs of health economics

4. understand how health economic measures, such as utilities, can be combined in meta-analysis

In this chapter, we want to step back from the calculations and see the bigger picture. As a meta-analyst, you will work within an environment of other people and organisations. Hopefully, that environment will allow evidence-based decision-making to flourish and to lead to demonstrable positive impact in your field. Achieving that will depend on many inter-connecting relationships, and is likely to need constant care and maintenance. It is certainly not guaranteed, and many good meta-analysts and systematic reviewers have seen their hard work go on to gather dust on shelves, while decision-makers follow "gut instinct".

Section 16.1 considers how we can play our part in the care and maintenance of an effective evidence-based policy environment. It also reflects on the application of evidence synthesis, and meta-analysis in particular, to other fields and the potential growth areas in the near future.

Section 16.3 takes a look at what is currently one of the most important information flows from meta-analysts: providing information for economists, whether in health or other subject areas.

16.1 Policy

"Evidence-based policy" is increasingly regarded as a desirable feature of government and NGO decision-making. Public awareness of the role of scientific evidence and its value has been enhanced during the COVID-19 years but also challenged by the proliferation of fake news, political polarisation, and erosion of trust in institutions [10]. To what extent evidence-based policy is feasible will depend in large part on the flow of information, from

DOI: 10.1201/9781003375821-16

good research, through good evidence synthesis, to the decision maker. The meta-analyst has—you have!—an influential role in this process [39, 183].

16.1.1 Work environments to nurture good decision-making

In the UK, the Royal Society and the Academy of Medical Sciences published a report in 2018 into evidence synthesis for policy, which provides a concise overview of the state of the art in evidence-based policy [252]. They point out that "Despite examples of good practice and successful working relationships between evidence synthesis providers, brokers and policymakers, there remain significant challenges with both the supply of, and demand for, evidence synthesis".

The report goes on: "...the means of overcoming [these challenges] generally require collaboration and co-production rather than action solely by synthesis providers or synthesis users".

We agree with this. In our teaching, we emphasise the need for interdisciplinary partnership. The meta-analyst works in the centre of a sandwich of information flows. On one side is the data source, which you must understand to be able to use it while minimising bias. On the other side is the decision-maker, the destination of information. Analysis can only be effective if it is communicated clearly, and if it addresses the decision-maker's needs. Given that the analyst is neither the data collector, nor the decision-maker, this means that communication skills should be front and centre in the CVs of any meta-analyst who wants to get ahead. We heartily recommend taking any opportunity to test those skills in safe, supported ways, and to build a portfolio of effective communication.

To answer the decision-maker's question, the meta-analyst and their team need to be seen as the decision-maker's partners, not a helpdesk. Taking a little time to understand the needs should be presented as the way to provide ultimately better outcomes. We must also recognise that decision-makers will not be well-placed to know what question they need to ask of a statistical team, and we can help them to pin down the needs precisely. Here, Bayesian methods are especially helpful, by allowing probabilistic inferences and clear communication of uncertainty [269]

Some policy interventions are intended to be tweaked as time goes by. Manski describes this as adaptive policy [159], and in this case we should plan for ongoing engagement. Evaluating and communicating the effectiveness of policies that are already implemented has its own challenges [201].

Many interventions that policy considers take place inside complex systems [43]. By *complexity*, we mean that the system has many interacting parts, some of which are intelligent agents that can adapt to circumstance and learn from the past. This means that the whole system changes over time, and even in response to interventions, pilots, or research taking place in it. A consequence of this inter-connectedness is that the relationship between intervention input and effect output can be non-linear: a small input might cause a large output change, or the opposite. The combination of adaptation and non-linearity make the system unpredictable, and what we learn from past studies might tell us very little about future results.

We would characterise health and social care systems as complex, along with economies or markets [98]. At this macro level of intervention research, the meta-analyst should work as part of an interdisciplinary team, looking at the question in a number of ways, including qualitative research. Realist evaluation is a useful framework in this context [190].

Bayesian networks are a method to apply Bayesian probabilities to connected graphs that model options for decision makers and seek to quantify the probabilities of benefits and harms [11]. The meta-analyst can make a valuable contribution to this overarching method for policy evaluation by supplying good estimates of the probabilities at various points in the network, along with probabilty densities representing the uncertainty in them.

16.1.2 Estimands

The quantity that we aim to estimate is called an *estimand*, a term that has become popular in recent years with the rise of interest in causal inference methods. For us, it means what the decision-maker needs. We already mentioned the difficulty that some decision-makers may have in pinning down what they actually need. Another, related problem is that years of working with certain statistical outputs (p-values, for example) may have effectively trained the decision-maker to make do with them and make leaps to their real estimand.

Another problem, less easily addressed, is the frequent situation where there are several different audiences for your work, perhaps doctors, and health system managers, and the public. Although you cannot anticipate what everyone might wish they could learn from your work, you can at least be very clear about what estimands it shows and what it does not, and about how it is intended to be used. This will guard against it being taken out of context (and you being blamed when the future does not turn out as someone hoped).

The most familiar question to most meta-analysts in a biomedical setting will be that of per-protocol or intention to treat analyses in trials. In reality, studies often have to make more decisions about inclusion of exclusion *from the statistical analysis* than the classic question of adherence to recommended treatment. For example, inclusion in the study might be based on preliminary test findings, which are later revised after randomisation and commencement of treatment [257]. Stephen Senn summarises it: "Inevitably some are treated who cannot benefit from the treatment. Should one only consider the effect in those who were infected?" [224].

Some of the literature on estimands is useful background reading for the Bayesian meta-analyst who wishes to communicate effectively, for example in causal inference [110] and econometrics [40]. These fields are quite advanced at defining exactly what is shown, or not, by an analysis.

As an example of estimands and decision-making, consider how a meta-analysis of the prevalence of long COVID symptoms might report a point estimate number per 10,000 population, and confidence or credible interval. Imagine, as a decision maker, a health service manager or politician, deciding on this basis in 2021 whether to invest resources into preparing for more cases. Then, imagine how much more useful it would be to receive output such as the probability of prevalence exceeding a threshold where the current health system resources could absorb it.

16.1.3 Econometric examples

Econometrics and the evaluation of socio-economic interventions is one of the main growth areas for meta-analysis today [40]. Some examples of meta-analytic methods in this field will shed light on opportunities for the meta-analyst to contribute.

The characteristic of econometric work, which make these papers and others look unfamiliar to anyone from a health research background, include the heavy use of linear formulas for multivariate relationships, presentation of results principally (sometimes solely) as coefficients of those formulas and their standard errors, and different conventions in mathematical notation. The difficulty of interpretation is that each coefficient is the impact of one predictor if everything else stays the same*, which is perhaps implausible.

---

*Economists frequently have to make this assumption with limited data, or by habit, and give it the Latin term *ceteris paribus*.

16.1.3.1 Use and abuse of research and development tax policy

Belz and colleagues carried out meta-regressions to help understand how companies use research and development (R&D) expenditure [18]. Many countries and regions try to encourage R&D activities by offering tax breaks and other incentives. However, these can also be abused, for example by spending money buying in R&D or intellectual property from a subsidiary company based in a low-tax country. In this way, multinationals can shift profits to the country with the lowest tax rate on profits, while also claiming tax credits for R&D in the country with the higher tax rate.

To understand this, the authors carried out an impressive and complicated series of connected analyses, including meta-regressions, to unpick the effect of R&D expenditure (which is recorded in tax accounts but was also obtained from studies) on various forms of taxation and on profits. The papers that they synthesize include various definitions of variables, for example the "effective tax rate" paid by firms; including these various definitions in one meta-regression is always challenging because we do not know, and perhaps cannot know, what mathematical formulation will represent the effect of the definitions.

This paper was not Bayesian but we can see ways in which it might have benefitted through more flexible modelling and model comparison, as well as predictive distributions for changes in policy (the "so what?" factor is addressed by offering readers a connection from findings to the next evolution of policy). The question of focusing on the distribution of outcomes is taken up in our next example.

16.1.3.2 Impact of microcredit

Meager assessed the impact of expanding the availability of microcredit[†] in two papers [167, 168]. These are Bayesian hierarchical analyses, which we would call IPD meta-analyses, of data from seven primary studies.

The first paper has some modelling differences to the models we have set out in this book, though we suspect these do not impact much. For example, in their formula 2 [167], the control mean and intervention effect are modelled with a bivariate normal likelihood, including the possibility of correlation (we tend to assume zero correlation). An interesting elaboration is the "LKJ" prior distribution for correlation matrices in their formula 5 [167]; we have not discussed matrix-valued prior distributions in this book; usually the first one that Bayesian analysts encounter is the Wishart distribution for precision matrices. There are also some charts that usefully compare the frequentist analysis with the Bayesian.

The second paper takes a more innovative approach, and is more methodological in its focus [168]. It aims to estimate not just the average treatment effect, as shown in the published paper, but the effect on the shape of the distribution of outcome variables. The way to make this tractable is to deal with a vector of quantiles, which obtain correlated posterior distributions. These are plotted in the pre-print in a way that powerfully makes the case in a way that policy decision-makers can easily grasp and recall. The abstract summarises this:

> "...there is strong evidence that microcredit typically does not lead to worse outcomes at the group level, but no generalizable evidence on whether it improves group outcomes. Households with previous business experience account for the majority of the impact in the tails and see large increases in the upper tail of the consumption distribution in particular". [168]

[†]Microcredit is an intervention where very small loans are made to support entrepreneurship among people in poverty who are unable to access traditional forms of business credit.

This is a more nuanced conclusion than an average treatment effect, and might inform policy for just this reason. How it translates to a decision is then a matter of ethical choice and programme-wide goals. We can imagine some governments deciding to press on with microcredit expansion, as it appears to reward the most capable, while others might view it as a new form of inequality and decide against it, but the value of the analysis is in allowing that level of informed decision-making.

16.1.3.3 "Sugar tax" on sweetened beverages

We can now compare and contrast three published reviews of sugar tax [5, 100, 250]. Evaluations of tax policy changes, or pilots, have been done in various ways, and the meta-analyse draw on different study designs, including pre-post comparisons and natural experiments.

Another vital consideration is how to incorporate different tax levels and different definitions of what products are eligible. Tax levels in percentage terms could be modelled by meta-regression or subgroups, though some policies introduce multiple tax rates for different products or at different times. In a complex system, knowledge of the other tax rates, or future plans and debates, can influence response, but would generally be beyond the scope of a meta-analysis [98]. The shape of the relationship might not be linear, and it would be useful to know more about it, though we are unlikely to obtain enough studies to do this in most cases. This is also the case in the sugar tax literature.

Of particular interest here, the three papers have developed ideas in ways that together give a deep understanding of the current evidence base on this emerging topic. The first to be published, by Teng and colleagues [250], was a classic biomedical meta-analysis of 17 studies, with the familiar format that does not expand much beyond the comparison of control and intervention to consider context and systems.

Building usefully on this, Hagenaars and colleagues published a narrative review that took a more theoretical approach, to consider the content, process and context of the interventions [100]. They use the findings of Teng and colleagues, but go beyond to comment on heterogeneity and implications for future policy, and to draw on a much wider range of research methods. This is a valuable additional layer of insight for the decision maker.

Most recent is a meta-analysis by Andreyeva and colleagues [5], which included 62 studies and more outcome variables. Like Teng and colleagues, the method was not Bayesian, and for this reason, any papers with unreported statistics "and those without statistical testing" were not included in the meta-analysis but described in the systematic review. They adopted a three-level hierarchical model, where studies were nested within jurisdictions. Despite the many facets of this work, the impression is of the paper having been squeezed to fit a word count limit, which is a concern for influencing future policy.

Bayesian methods may have been helpful to allow inclusion of unreported statistics, selection models for publication bias, and correlated outcomes.

16.1.4 Reflections

We have written about doing a meta-analysis, assuming that the evidence base is sufficient. However, meta-analysis is merely the optional culmination of systematic reviews of evidence, and there are many occasions when they reveal that the evidence base does not permit meta-analysis. Knowing this is in some ways as valuable as having the results of the meta-analysis, because it shows the priority areas where work should be done next, to fill the gaps. In Section 3.7.5, we described posterior predictive inference for a putative future trial, which can quantify the potential impact on meta-analysis findings.

The pandemic experience also taught us that there are times when we must make decisions before the evidence is mature. It is important to remember that systematic literature review and meta-analysis is at one end of a spectrum of good practice from "fast and frugal" decision making [92, 159] to a slow, comprehensive, and peer-reviewed project requiring perhaps time to seek funding, recruit staff, and so on. There are times when the case for meta-analysis can be examined quickly by an experienced meta-analyst, and its pros and cons discussed with decision-makers before the choice is made about what point on that spectrum is right for the circumstances.

Your experience will be very useful here. Those who have not done it for themselves may not understand the challenges and time needed, or the potential benefits compared to, for example, a rapid narrative review. At the same time, you can have even greater influence—and enjoyment of your role—if you acquire some knowledge and experience of other research approaches such as qualitative research [48].

The experienced meta-analyst who has also been involved in close scrutiny of the evidence base, to the enhanced level that we describe in this book, will be very well placed to assist in the decision about what methods to use to inform policy, constrained by the *quality* of the evidence available. Your skills and knowledge are likely to be in ever greater demand in the near future.

16.2   Causal Inference

Meta-analyses of randomised controlled trials (RCTs) are considered the highest level of evidence in evidence-based medicine. However, the causal interpretation of the results from such meta-analyses is often overlooked. This section reviews methodologies that implement a causally explicit framework for meta-analysis of RCTs and discusses their scientific relevance and interpretation, mainly related to the seminal paper by Markozannes and colleagues, which reports the findings of a survey of methodologies on causal inference methods in meta-analyses of RCTs [161].

We aim to achieve higher levels of evidence (less bias with respect to the causal truth) when performing a meta-analysis based on multiple RCTs. However, while individual study estimates might have causal interpretations, their aggregation can obscure this because of the variability in study characteristics. The goal is to identify and compute effect estimates that have causally relevant interpretations for the populations sampled by the trials.

Markozannes identified three main methodologies that describe a causal inference framework for the meta-analysis of RCTs. Two of these approaches required individual participant data (IPD) from the RCTs, while the third approach utilised summary data from a network meta-analysis. Each methodology provides a framework for obtaining causally interpretable meta-analytical estimates, although they present conceptual limitations regarding the data-generation process.

The methodologies that used IPD data provided a set of causal assumptions, such as the stable unit treatment value assumption (SUTVA), unconfounded treatment assignment, and equivalence of treatment effects across trials. These assumptions aim to ensure that the meta-analytical estimate has valid causal interpretation. One methodology using summary data from a network meta-analysis adopted an arm-based approach and employed methods such as G-computation, inverse probability of treatment weighting (IPTW), and targeted minimum loss-based estimation (TMLE) to derive causal estimates [40, 110].

Although all three methodologies provide valid causal estimates, there are important limitations in the assumptions regarding the data generation process and sampling of the RCTs to be included in the meta-analysis. Specifically, the assumption that trials are random samples from a well-defined superpopulation may often be unrealistic. The generalisability and scientific relevance of the derived causal effects are challenging, as the structure of the superpopulation defined by the meta-analytical approaches may differ substantially from that of a naturally occurring population.

The causal inference framework is based on the Rubin causal model, which uses potential outcomes to define treatment effects. The methodologies identified include the following:

1. Sobel and colleagues described a framework in which causal estimates can be derived from a meta-analysis of RCTs when individual participant data (IPD) are available [235]. The authors focused on identifying and accounting for possible sources of heterogeneity across trials. They restricted their focus to four possible sources of heterogeneity across trials: response inconsistency, non-equivalent treatments, non-ignorable treatment assignment, and variability in the composition of units in different studies or settings. The identifiability conditions considered in this approach include an extended version of the SUTVA and conditional exchangeability. This framework does not use a complex analytical approach, but is based on the plausibility of the assumptions and a correct model specification using study-level covariates and possibly treatment, study, and covariate interactions.

2. Dahabreh and colleagues proposed a causal inference framework under which meta-analysis estimates are causally interpretable and transportable ATEs to a target population [51]. This approach requires IPD from randomised trials, along with baseline covariate data from a random sample from the target population, to account for differences in distributions. They provided a set of assumptions for identifiability conditions and propose an estimand that takes into account the distributional differences between trials and the target population. This framework assumes that the observed data are obtained by random sampling from an infinite superpopulation of individuals, which is stratified by study. The authors denote this sampling method as "biased" sampling, since the proportion of the sampled population is not expected to be equal to the superpopulation due to convenience sampling in the majority of the RCTs.

3. Schnitzer and colleagues described a framework in which causal estimates can be derived in a network meta-analysis setting using aggregate data from multiple RCTs [221]. This approach focuses on estimating the average treatment effect in the presence of heterogeneity arising from the differences in study-level characteristics. The authors defined a marginal and model-independent causal estimand and outline the key assumptions required for this estimand to be identifiable under measured study-level confounding. An arm-based network meta-analysis approach is adopted, which estimates the arm-specific effects, in contrast to the study-based approach, which estimates study-specific effects. The estimation methods presented and compared in a simulation study include G-computation, IPTW, and TMLE.

The data generation process and sampling assumptions for common, fixed, and random effects are crucial to the methodologies reviewed. Sobel and colleagues did not make explicit remarks on the choice of trials included in their meta-analysis, but considered that each trial sampled from its distinct population, implying that the superpopulation is a mixture of each trial's population. Schnitzer and colleagues explicitly stated that the subjects in each trial were assumed to be random samples of their populations, and defined their superpopulation ("metapopulation") as the union of each trial population.

The external validity of the results, which would provide a pertinent causal interpretation for the superpopulation, is critical. While it is often reasonable to assume that each trial samples randomly from their respective populations, it is implausible that these trials are random samples of a population of trials. Conducting a trial is largely a function of specific motives and aims, and a random sample of trials may not occur naturally. Without considering the potential differences between the structure of the superpopulation and that of a naturally occurring population, the external validity of meta-analytical causal estimates would be hindered. Dahabreh and colleagues' approach partially addresses this issue by focusing on assumptions for trial populations rather than assumptions of trial effects.

In conclusion, while combining causal inference with meta-analysis is promising, further research is needed to develop more robust methods that address the limitations of the assumptions and improve the external validity of the results. Future efforts should focus on refining these methodologies and exploring new approaches to enhance the causal interpretability of the meta-analytical evidence.

16.3   Health Economic Evaluation

Meta-analysis in health economics involves synthesising data from various economic evaluations to derive overall estimates of cost-effectiveness. This process typically involves a systematic review of the health economics literature to identify and review relevant studies that evaluate the economic impact of healthcare interventions. This includes assessing study quality, extracting data on costs and outcomes, and summarising the findings.

However, the pooling of costs is not advocated due to structural variation between systems rather than differences in monetary units and time assessments. The same caution applies to summaries based on cost-effectiveness analyses (CEA), which evaluate the cost and effectiveness of healthcare interventions to determine their value. Outputs from CEA, such as the incremental cost-effectiveness ratio (ICER) or Incremental Net Monetary Benefits (INB), can technically be pooled via meta-analytic methods, but the results could potentially be misleading if taken as fact without careful consideration in context. Instead, it is suggested to visually present individual estimates and facilitate the discussion of findings and interpretation by decision-makers.

16.3.1   Subgroup-specific cost-effectiveness profiling

Subgroup-specific cost-effectiveness profiling enhances decision-making in healthcare by providing more nuanced and patient-specific economic evaluations. This approach acknowledges that patient characteristics, such as age, sex, disease severity, and comorbidities, can significantly influence the cost-effectiveness of treatments. By incorporating subgroup analysis into economic evaluations, researchers can identify variations in treatment effects and cost-effectiveness across different segments of the population. This is particularly important in personalised medicine, where tailored interventions are designed to optimize outcomes for individual patients.

One of the primary methods for conducting subgroup-specific cost-effectiveness analysis is through meta-regression models. Meta-regression models can handle continuous and categorical covariates, allowing for a flexible examination of how various factors influence the cost-effectiveness of interventions. For example, in the context of treating a chronic condition like multiple sclerosis, meta-regression can assess how the cost-effectiveness of disease-modifying therapies varies by baseline disability score, age at diagnosis, or presence of comorbid conditions.

Personalised economic evaluation goes further by tailoring economic analyses to individual patient characteristics, offering a high-resolution perspective on the value of healthcare interventions. This approach leverages advanced modelling techniques to integrate individual patient data (IPD) into cost-effectiveness analyses, providing personalised estimates that can guide clinical decision-making.

Risk stratification involves categorising patients based on their risk profiles using prognostic models, which can then inform the economic evaluation. Predictive modelling develops models that estimate the expected costs and health outcomes for individual patients based on specific characteristics, using techniques such as regression analysis, machine learning, and Bayesian hierarchical models.

An essential aspect of personalised economic evaluation is the use of Bayesian hierarchical models, which allow for the incorporation of prior knowledge and the estimation of treatment effects across different levels of hierarchy, such as individual patients, clinical sites, and populations. These models are particularly useful in health economics, where there is often substantial heterogeneity in patient responses and treatment effects.

Bayesian meta-regression models (see Section 4.7) facilitate the integration of diverse data sources, including clinical trials, observational studies, and real-world evidence, generating robust estimates of treatment effects that account for variability in patient characteristics and clinical settings.

Meta-regression has numerous applications in health economics, such as evaluating the impact of intervention characteristics, exploring population heterogeneity, and assessing study quality and design. By incorporating these elements, meta-regression provides a nuanced understanding of the factors driving variability in economic evaluations, thereby enhancing the precision and relevance of meta-analytic findings in health economics.

16.3.2   Meta-analysis of utilities

Health economic analysis requires not only inputs on effectiveness or efficacy of interventions but also on costs, risks, the value of various health states, and the probability or rate of transitioning from one health state to another. Meta-analysis can therefore play a role in supplying reliable information to all aspects of health economics. However, not all these measures are asymptotically normal, unlike most of our statistics for effectiveness or efficacy.

Bayesian meta-analysis provides a robust framework for synthesising health state utility values, essential components in economic evaluations and health technology assessments (HTA). Health state utility values quantify the quality of life associated with different health states, typically ranging from 0 (death) to 1 (full health). These values are crucial for calculating quality-adjusted life years (QALYs) and assessing the economic value of healthcare interventions. Given the variability and methodological differences across studies, Bayesian meta-analysis leverages prior knowledge and explicitly handles heterogeneity to produce more reliable estimates.

It is possible to carry out utilities meta-analysis using standard Bayesian software tools; a tutorial paper with `brms` is available [218]. One consideration is that the utility is expected to lie in the range $[0, 1]$ and the mode may be at one of the extremes, in which case no transformation will make the shape approximately normal. A beta prior and truncated likelihood may be required.

Another consideration is that some studies may define utilities so as to permit the possibilities of small negative values, which will require different truncation limits for those studies, or a decision by your project team to enforce a common range.

16.3.3 Posterior samples are useful

Many health economic models simulate data from a large number of "patients" with given demographic and clinical characteristics, estimates of intervention effectiveness, risks of adverse events, and probabilities of moving from one health state (characterised by a utility value) to another. The simulations provide a distribution of outcomes in terms of cost-effectiveness, cost-utility, and other metrics.

It is very common for health economists to carry out *probabilistic sensitivity analysis* by running multiple possible vectors ($\boldsymbol{\theta}$) of inputs through such a model. Each $\boldsymbol{\theta}$ might produce thousands of simulated patients so that uncertainty about the inputs *propagates* through the model.

Traditionally, these inputs are drawn from pseudo-random number generators, given the reported univariate (marginal) distributions of the inputs. However, this presents two possible problems: it assumes a distributional form, which may not have been tested, and it ignores any correlations among the inputs.

Posterior samples from Bayesian meta-analysis are a natural source of these vectors of inputs, and will avoid the two problems above. If you supply the health economist with a matrix of the posterior sample, they can select individual draws at random and feed each one into the model as $\boldsymbol{\theta}$. It might not be necessary to use all the posterior draws in order to obtain clarity about the model outputs.

17

Emerging Topics in Bayesian Meta-Analysis

Learning objectives

After reading this chapter, you will:

1. recognise the terminology and concepts around some topics of current active development

2. identify those topics of interest to you, either for methodological work, or to apply in your setting

3. be able to start reading further, and directing your own professional development

The goal of this chapter is simply to list some topics that we think are likely to be impactful on Bayesian meta-analysis in the next ten years after publication. As with most emerging methodological work, publications tend to be heavy on mathematics and sometimes lacking in readily implementable code.

Bearing in mind our intended audience for this book, and that we do not expect you to have a strong mathematical or computational background, we use this chapter simply to identify the topics and familiarise you with the names and what the central concept behind them is.

17.1 Dose-Response

One of the most important insights that we can gain from exploring and explaining heterogeneity is that different intervention effects might be observed for different "doses". When the intervention is a drug, exercise class, or tax rate, this is fairly easy to quantify and use in meta-regression [83]. However, there are other interventions that are not so easily summarised, and many that are multi-faceted, where not all the facets are necessarily increased or decreased in "dose" together.

In an ideal world, our meta-regression would lead to a clear curve, showing the dose associated with the optimal benefit. In reality, this would require a great number of studies, which use a wide range of doses, yet are comparable in all other aspects. Too much uncertainty is likely to persist in the meta-regression for any firm conclusion to be drawn.

Nevertheless, it may be possible to explore the association and generate hypotheses for future primary research. Pitchforth and Mengersen describe just such a Bayesian

DOI: 10.1201/9781003375821-17

meta-analysis [197] of the association in epidemiological studies between red meat consumption and breast cancer incidence.

17.2 Floor and Ceiling Effects

We have seen standardisation of mean differences and means done in different ways in this book. A remaining, and open, question, which arose in Section 15.1, is how best to deal with multiple outcome scales, which may have different levels of sensitivity and may be affected differently by floor and ceiling effects [2, 174].

Non-linear transformations such as the inverse logistic function or the inverse normal cumulative distribution function (often called the *probit*) are one option, although it is hard to justify one over another given the usual lack of information about relative sensitivity in outcome scales.

Another potential approach is to model outcome scales with a floor and a ceiling using the beta distribution, or generalized versions of it. To our knowledge, there has been no work on this in Bayesian meta-analysis.

17.3 Targeting a Specific Population

It can be useful to make predictions for a specific population that lies within the range of the evidence base [3, 195]. The population in this sense will defined by covariates such as age, sex, socio-economic deprivation, work status, and so forth. What would the impact be if this intervention were rolled out in this particular setting? What could we expect to find if we did a new large randomised controlled trial in this particular setting?

The latter question, of predicting trials, falls under the method of posterior predictive distributions (see Section 2.5.4), and is increasingly used in the pharmaceutical and medical devices industries to design future studies for maximum insight.

As with the question of dose-response, this relies on there being sufficient evidence across studies to give us information about not just a curve but a surface, relating all the relevant covariates to the intervention effect, with sufficient certainty.

Not all studies will report all the same covariates, making full Bayesian inference with missing statistics the most feasible way of addressing this problem. However, if individual participant data (IPD) are available, then the prospect becomes much brighter. This is because the covariates vary at the level of the participants, while dose typically varies at the level of the study arm. IPD can therefore give us much finer detail about the location of the surface and its uncertainty.

Methods are not yet well-developed and tested for this targeted analysis in general, particularly without IPD and in heterogeneous evidence bases [73]. In network meta-analysis, some methods have been published [32, 193].

One interesting case study reweights randomised controlled trials of a treatment for schizophrenia, with the aim of matching the population of people with schizophrenia in "usual care settings" in the USA [117]. To define the population, statistics from a large pragmatic clinical trial were used.

17.4   Population-Adjusted Indirect Comparison Methods

Population-adjusted indirect comparison (PAIC) methods, such as matching-adjusted indirect comparison, simulated treatment comparison, multilevel network meta-regression, and augmented inverse probability weighted estimator, are increasingly popular in health technology assessment, particularly when direct head-to-head trials are unavailable.

These methods adjust for imbalances in covariate distributions across studies. Their goal is robust treatment comparisons in scenarios where traditional network meta-analysis is not reliable. This section will provide a conceptual overview with some references for further reading.

17.4.1   Matching-adjusted indirect comparison

Matching-adjusted indirect comparison (MAIC) uses individual participant data from an index trial, which evaluates the new treatment, and aggregate data from the comparator trial. By reweighting the individual participant data to match the baseline characteristics of the comparator trial population, this method addresses the heterogeneity between participant populations and mitigates potential biases [134].

Reweighting gives more or less weight in calculations to different participants in the index trial, and this allows it to apply flexible covariate adjustment, to make populations as comparable as possible. The weighted outcomes from the index trial are then compared with the aggregate outcomes from the comparator trial. Reweighting methods, though common in causal analysis [110], are often not amenable to Bayesian implementations because the weights are derived at an individual participant level and not necessarily from a likelihood-based model.

This approach has several advantages. It provides indirect comparisons when direct trials are not feasible, reduces bias arising from population heterogeneity, and is feasible as long as individual participant data from one trial is available.

However, this method can only adjust for observed baseline characteristics, and cannot account for unmeasured variables (confounders) that may influence the outcomes. The reweighting process can lead to a loss of statistical precision, especially if substantial differences exist between the trial populations. Additionally, it assumes that the relationship between adjusted characteristics and outcomes is consistent across trials, which may not always be true.

Its performance is also sensitive to the selection of baseline characteristics used for matching. Simulation studies have shown that it may be more susceptible to increased bias, compared to other population-adjusted indirect comparison methods, when assumptions are violated [195].

17.4.2   Simulated treatment comparison

Simulated treatment comparison (STC) serves as an alternative approach to indirect treatment comparisons when standard NMA methods are not feasible [198]. It may be useful when:

- individual participant data are available for at least one treatment, and

- trials are comparable in design, but

- they differ in the distributions of measured risk factors.

STC involves modelling the relationship between patient characteristics and outcomes using IPD from one study. The model is then used to simulate outcomes for a population matching the baseline characteristics of the comparator study. Like MAIC, STC aims to reduce the bias resulting from population heterogeneity and enhance the validity of indirect comparisons [123].

The methodology of STC continues to evolve significantly. Zhang and colleagues [287], for example, proposed new simulation methods for improved robustness. STC's application in health technology assessment submissions has also faced criticism. Limitations include the potential for residual confounding due to unmeasured variables, and sensitivity to modelling techniques. Critics have emphasised the importance of careful implementation and transparency in methodological choices during the process [16, 129].

17.4.3 Multilevel network meta-regression

Multilevel network meta-regression includes IPD from one or more studies, and aggregate data from other studies, in one model [194]. This flexibility enables researchers to maximise the use of available data regardless of its format, thereby enhancing the robustness of comparative analyses. Its modelling approach makes it readily adaptable to Bayesian implementation.

Multilevel network meta-regression allows adjustments for effect modifiers [110] and prognostic factors that affect outcomes irrespective of the treatment. This comprehensive adjustment is particularly valuable when standard NMA is not feasible, for example with a very sparse network.

The model can include nonlinear effects and interactions between covariates where the evidence and theory supports it. However, multilevel network meta-regression requires thorough modelling and rigorous assumption checks, as it relies heavily on the correct specification of the relationship between outcomes and covariates, more so than reweighting.

17.4.4 Augmented inverse probability weighting (AIPW)

The Augmented Inverse Probability Weighting (AIPW) paradigm combines weighting and regression to estimate treatment effects, particularly in observational studies [143]. The objective is to adjust for differences in baseline characteristics between treatment groups, while also quantifying the relationship between these characteristics and the outcome of interest.

A notable feature of AIPW is its *double robustness* property, which leads to unbiased estimates if either of two conditions are met:

1. the propensity score model used for weighting is correctly specified

2. the outcome regression model is correctly specified

This reduces the risk of bias, making AIPW more robust than the isolated application of either (re)weighting (for example, in MAIC) or outcome regression alone.

17.4.5 Summary

It is vital to select an appropriate PAIC approach based on context and data availability. MAIC is now widely used in the pharmaceutical industry, especially when only aggregate data are available for the comparator. However, methods such as multilevel network meta-regression, STC, and AIPW may offer more robust alternatives.

The choice should consider factors such as the availability of IPD, the degree of heterogeneity between studies, and the underlying assumptions of each method. Selecting the most suitable method is crucial for ensuring valid and reliable treatment effect estimates, particularly in complex or sparse evidence networks.

Bayesian methods can be useful in conjunction with these methods, because of the flexibility in incorporating prior knowledge, handling complex hierarchical models, and quantifying uncertainty in a probabilistic manner. For instance, in the context of multilevel network meta-regression, Bayesian implementation can enhance model robustness by efficiently managing sparse data without resorting to approximate sampling distributions in the likelihood.

17.5   Model Averaging

Bayesian statistical inference allows us to use all information about the relationship between the unknowns and the knowns in our model. Some writers and teachers describe this as the joint distribution of the data and the parameters. We can extend this concept even further and consider multiple models, giving more weight to those that fit the data more closely. This leads to established methods called stacking and model averaging [12].

In the context of meta-analysis, model averaging has been developed for publication bias in particular [13]. This has been implemented in an R package called RoBMA, which calls JAGS, and can also be used from JASP [19].

The range of models that can be accessed this way are limited to some presets. The broader question of best practice in inference over not just parameter space but model space too, in the context of meta-analysis, when data are likely to be limited and heterogeneous, remains a developing area. There is the potential to explore not just competing plausible models for publication bias but additional "dimensions" of model space for other problems detailed in Part 3 of this book.

17.6   Time-Effects

As we described a curve relating dose to intervention effect, we might also find it helpful to understand the way that the effect changes over time [3]. In some settings, the intervention is a single, short-lived event (a vaccination or training course), and then studies might report multiple time points following the intervention.

This could help to answer questions such as whether it takes time for benefit to build up, and if so how long before it is optimal? On the other hand, the effect might be immediate and then fall away after a while, or a combination of the two. Other interventions might be protracted, and the time points reported by studies might be a combination of interim statistics and post-intervention follow-up. (Earlier in the book, we tended to refer to "end of intervention", hoping to give you some simplicity, though in practice it is not always so clear.)

Larose describes a Bayesian meta-analysis of studies of estrogen use and endometrial cancer incidence [146], using a multivariate normal likelihood over the multiple time points within each study.

A more flexible approach has emerged recently from a programme of methodological work led by Welton, where non-linear functions of time can be compared and the best chosen, within the context of network meta-analysis [191].

17.7 Survival or Time-To-Event Data

The combination of evidence on time-to-event, or survival, data, has in this book been limited to the asymptotic sampling distribution of the log hazard ratio, or IPD meta-analysis. There is no approach at present which would allow combination of study statistics (aggregate data) that are a mixture of hazard ratios, restricted mean survival times, or parametric survival time models. It could be useful to use the Kaplan-Meier curve, which shows "survival" evolving over time, rather than a single statistic. Each study would have its own curves, a non-parametric summary of the survival or censoring times. These are, by definition, arm-based summaries.

To make a Bayesian model for these study-arm curves requires either a parametric or non-parametric representation of them [56]. The parametric approach is taken via common distributions of survival times [186], or more flexible curve-fitting methods such as fractional polynomials [77, 130]. Bayesian non-parametric methods, such as the Dirichlet process, are much harder to learn as they are computationally intensive and quite new, but offer potentially flexible methods for the future.

It might always be possible to reconstruct data from Kaplan-Meier curves and work with that [169]. Such data may not be strictly at IPD level, because there could be more than one participant with coinciding event or censoring times. A number of censorings or events at each time point is indicated by a step in the vertical height of the curve. We discussed the digital or manual extraction of graphical data in Section 5.5.1, and this could be a simpler option than a cutting-edge and bespoke model.

17.8 Gaussian Processes

All the topics mentioned so far have had some element of curve- or surface-fitting. These are regression tasks, but we want them to be flexible. Recently, Bayesian modellers have increasingly worked with Gaussian processes. These are a conceptually distinct way of conceiving of the regression task. They recast multiple time points as generating data from a multivariate normal distribution, where each element, or dimension, of the multivariate distribution relates to one of the time points. The means and covariance matrix of the multivariate distribution will be constrained by some hyper-priors: the smoothness of the curve, for example, or how quickly it returns to the mean from an unusual value.

There are no tutorial papers or books that we know of that introduce Gaussian processes for our audience, but the book by Rasmussen and Williams is regarded as the best introduction for those with a mathematical and machine learning background [200]. We expect that some combination of Gaussian processes and meta-regression will be a helpful addition to the toolbox in the near future.

17.9   Simulation-Based Inference

Simulation-based inference (SBI) is a wide class of methods where pseudo-data are simulated, rather than assessing the likelihood of the real data, usually because it will be easier. Approximate Bayesian Computation (ABC) is an alternative to MCMC methods, and the best known of the SBI methods [160, 232], where a vector of unknowns is proposed, and then pseudo-data are generated using the presumed data generating process (likelihood, in other words). The similarity of the pseudo-data and the real data is quantified, and this is repeated

We feel that ABC is most likely to be used for problems of unreported stats. There are few examples of ABC in practical meta-analysis [144, 243].

More advanced ABC practitioners might seek to infer the unknown statistics and the rest of the meta-analytic model's unknowns at the same time. However, a simpler and more practical starting point for many might be first to carry out a marginal ABC for the unknown stats. For example, if a study provides only quartiles, but we require means and standard deviations, then we can simulate data from an assumed distribution at IPD level (informed, hopefully, by exogenous information from other large studies of the variables).

We might compare the simulated quartiles and the reported ones, and keep the pseudo-datasets that are reasonable matches*, and this will give us a collection of means and standard deviations, one from each pseudo-dataset.

This is then a prior for the missing statistic that we can plug into the rest of our meta-analysis, in various ways as shown in Chapter 11.

17.10   Data Privacy and Meta-Analysis

In recent years, many new approaches have been proposed to preserve individual's privacy when data are published or shared [80], balancing the good of privacy against the good of discovery [17]. Related to this is increasing interest in artificial intelligence ethics and regulation, and the use of the individual's preferences [121].

It is important to recognise that anonymisation of data, the removal of variables that directly identify the individuals, is not actually the measure of whether their privacy and confidentiality has been protected. The word "anonymisation" makes the issue appear binary, but instead, it is the risk of re-identification that matters, considering what other, external information a malicious actor may have. This risk is a spectrum, not binary.

As research institutions adopt various technologies for more active control over data sharing, we expect this to have an effect on IPD meta-analysis. We hope that more data will be available to meta-analysts in the future, but we should also expect it to be altered in some ways to protect privacy. Some of the techniques involve perturbing or coarsening the data so as to balance the competing needs and control the risk of re-identifying an individual.

---

*The devil is in the detail. How, exactly, we propose new vectors of desired statistics, compare vectors of reported and simulated statistics, and what criterion we use to accept or reject, is critical [160, 232], not only for the accuracy of the method, but for it not taking a prohibitively long time.

A particularly promising area of active development by academics, governments, and private enterprise is that of *synthetic data*. In this approach, the joint distribution of all the variables in the IPD are modelled closely, and new pseudo-data are randomly drawn from this joint distribution.

Such modified IPD will possibly require some new models or algorithms, to ensure that posterior distributions remain accurate. Methodological work is ongoing.

Appendix: Software

The table below summarises some features of software that can be used for Bayesian meta-analysis. The list here is not exhaustive and may be updated at the book website.

Software	Language interfaces	GUI	Open source	Algorithm	Variance parameter
BUGS	stand-alone (Windows), R, Python, Stata, Julia	yes (Windows only)	OpenBUGS but not WinBUGS	Gibbs	precision
JAGS	R, Python, Stata, Julia	no	yes	Gibbs	precision
Stan	stand-alone (command line), R, Python, Stata, Julia, etc.	no	yes	Hamiltonian, variational	standard deviation
bayesmeta	R	no	yes	no sampling, analytic distributions	standard deviation
brms	R	no	yes	front end for Stan	standard deviation
Stata	stand-alone, Python	yes	partly	RWMH, Gibbs	variance
JASP	stand-alone	yes	yes	front end for various R packages	standard deviation
MLwiN	stand-alone	yes	no	RWMH, Gibbs	any
SAS	stand-alone	no	no	RWMH	standard deviation
PyMC	Python	no	yes	RMWH, Gibbs, Hamiltonian, variational	standard deviation

Bibliography

[1] A E Ades, D M Caldwell, S Reken, N J Welton, A J Sutton, et al. Evidence synthesis for decision making 7: A reviewer's checklist. *Medical Decision Making*, 33(5):679–691, 2013.

[2] A E Ades, G Lu, S Dias, E Mayo-Wilson, and D Kounali. Simultaneous synthesis of treatment effects and mapping to a common scale: an alternative to standardisation. *Research Synthesis Methods*, 6(1):96–107, 2015.

[3] A E Ades, N J Welton, S Dias, D M Phillippo, and D M Caldwell. Twenty years of network meta-analysis: Continuing controversies and recent developments. *Research Synthesis Methods*, 15(5):702–727, 2024.

[4] D Adigbli, Y Li, N Hammond, R Chatoor, A G Devaux, et al. A patient-level meta-analysis of intensive glucose control in critically ill adults. *NEJM Evidence*, 3(8):EVIDoa2400082, 2024.

[5] T Andreyeva, K Marple, S Marinello, T E Moore, and L M Powell. Outcomes following taxation of sugar-sweetened beverages a systematic review and meta-analysis. *JAMA Network Open*, 5(6):e2215276, 2022.

[6] R R Andridge and R J A Little. A review of hot deck imputation for survey non-response. *International Statistical Review*, 78(1):40–64, 2010.

[7] R Avram, G H Tison, K Aschbacher, P Kuhar, E Vittinghoff, et al. Real-world heart rate norms in the Health eHeart study. *NPJ Digital Medicine*, 2:58, 2019.

[8] C Axfors, A M Schmitt, P Janiaud, J van't Hooft, S Abd-Elsalam, et al. Mortality outcomes with hydroxychloroquine and chloroquine in COVID-19 from an international collaborative meta-analysis of randomized trials. *Nature Communications*, 12:2349, 2021.

[9] P G Bagos and G K Nikolopoulos. Mixed-effects Poisson regression models for meta-analysis of follow-up studies with constant or varying durations. *International Journal of Biostatistics*, 5(1):21, 2009.

[10] P Ball. What the COVID-19 pandemic reveals about science, policy and society. *Interface Focus*, 11:20210022, 2021.

[11] D Barber. *Bayesian Reasoning and Machine Learning*. Cambridge University Press, 2012.

[12] F Bartoš, Q F Gronau, B Timmers, W M Otte, A Ly, et al. Bayesian model-averaged meta-analysis in medicine. *Statistics in Medicine*, 40(30):6743–6761, 2021.

[13] F Bartoš, M Maier, D S Quintana, and E J Wagenmakers. Adjusting for publication bias in JASP and R: Selection models, PET-PEESE, and robust bayesian meta-analysis. *Advances in Methods and Practices in Psychological Science*, 5(3), 2022.

[14] BaSiS Group. BaSiS guidelines for reporting Bayesian analyses, 2001. `http://lib.stat.cmu.edu/bayesworkshop/2001/BaSisGuideline.htm`.

[15] D Bassler, V M Montori, M Briel, P Glasziou, S D Walter, et al. Reflections on meta-analyses involving trials stopped early for benefit: is there a problem and if so, what is it? *Statistical Methods in Medical Research*, 22(2):159–168, 2013.

[16] S Batson, S A Mitchell, and D King. PRM190 — the use and acceptance of novel statistical analyses to support technology submissions to HTA authorities. *Value in Health*, 17(7):A576–A577, 2014.

[17] H Bauchner, M Golub, and P B Fontanarosa. Data sharing: An ethical and scientific imperative. *Journal of the American Medical Association*, 315(12):1238–1240, 2016.

[18] T Belz, D von Hagen, and C Steffens. R&D intensity and the effective tax rate: a meta-regression analysis. *Journal of Economic Surveys*, 31(4):988–1010, 2017.

[19] S W Berkhout, J M Haaf, Q F Gronau, D W Heck, and E J Wagenmakers. A tutorial on Bayesian model-averaged meta-analysis in JASP. *Behavior Research Methods*, 56:1260–1282, 2024.

[20] N Black, M Murphy, D Lamping, M McKee, C Sanderson, J Askham, and T Marteau. Consensus development methods: A review of best practice in creating clinical guidelines. *Journal of Health Services Research and Policy*, 4(4):236–248, 1999.

[21] D Blázquez-Rincón, J Sánchez-Meca, J Botella, and M Suero. Heterogeneity estimation in meta-analysis of standardized mean differences when the distribution of random effects departs from normal: A Monte Carlo simulation study. *BMC Medical Research Methodology*, 23:19, 2023.

[22] L Bojke, M Soares, K Claxton, A Colson, A Fox, et al. Developing a reference protocol for structured expert elicitation in health-care decision-making: a mixed-methods study. *Health Technology Assessment*, 25(37), 2021.

[23] M Borenstein. *Common Mistakes in Meta-Analysis and How To Avoid Them*. Biostat, Inc., 2019.

[24] M Borenstein, L V Hedges, J P T Higgins, and H R Rothstein. *Introduction to Meta-Analysis*. Wiley, 2009.

[25] C Breuer, J J Meerpohl, and W Siemens. From standard systematic reviews to living systematic reviews. *Zeitschrift für Evidenz, Fortbildung und Qualität im Gesundheitswesen*, 176:76–81, 2023.

[26] J Brok, K Thorlund, J Wetterslev, and C Gluud. Apparently conclusive meta-analyses may be inconclusive - trial sequential analysis adjustment of random error risk due to repetitive testing of accumulating data in apparently conclusive neonatal meta-analyses. *International Journal of Epidemiology*, 38(1):287–298, 2008.

[27] S Brooks, A Gelman, G L Jones, and X L Meng. *Handbook of Markov Chain Monte Carlo*. CRC Press, 2011.

[28] C J Bryan, E Tipton, and D S Yeager. Behavioural science is unlikely to change the world without a heterogeneity revolution. *Nature Human Behaviour*, 5:980–989, 2021.

[29] S Bujkiewicz, F Achana, T Papanikos, R D Riley, and K R Abrams. Technical support document 20: Multivariate meta-analysis of summary data for combining treatment effects on correlated outcomes and evaluating surrogate endpoints. Technical report, National Institute for Health and Care Excellence, Decision Support Unit, UK, 2019. `https://www.sheffield.ac.uk/nice-dsu/tsds/multivariate-meta-analysis`.

[30] S Bujkiewicz, J R Thompson, A J Sutton, N J Cooper, M J Harrison, et al. Multivariate meta-analysis of mixed outcomes: a Bayesian approach. *Statistics in Medicine*, 32:3926–3943, 2013.

[31] N Buscemi, L Hartling, B Vandermeer, L Tjosvold, and T P Klassen. Single data extraction generated more errors than double data extraction in systematic reviews. *Journal of Clinical Epidemiology*, 59:697–703, 2006.

[32] E Butterly, L Wei, A I Adler, S A M Almazam, K Alsallumi, et al. Calibrating a network meta-analysis of diabetes trials of sodium glucose cotransporter 2 inhibitors, glucagon-like peptide-1 receptor analogues and dipeptidyl peptidase-4 inhibitors to a representative routine population: a systematic review protocol. *BMJ Open*, 12:e066491, 2022.

[33] P C Bürkner. Brms: An R package for Bayesian multilevel models using Stan. *Journal of Statistical Software*, 80:1–28, 2017.

[34] L Candelise and A Ciccone. Gangliosides for acute ischaemic stroke. *Cochrane Database of Systematic Reviews*, 1:CD000094, 1997.

[35] J R Carpenter, M G Kenward, J W Bartlett, T P Morris, M Quartagno, et al. *Multiple Imputation and its Applications*. Wiley, second edition, 2023.

[36] C Carroll, A Scope, and E Kaltenthaler. A case study of binary outcome data extraction across three systematic reviews of hip arthroplasty: errors and differences of selection. *BMC Research Notes*, 6:539, 2013.

[37] G Casazza, F Casella, and Gruppo di Autoformazione Metodologica (GrAM). Can we trust in trials stopped early for benefit? *Internal and Emergency Medicine*, 7:559–561, 2012.

[38] G Casella and R L Berger. *Statistical Inference*. Duxbury Press, second edition, 2002.

[39] R Caulcutt. How can we help decision-makers? *Significance*, 18(3):34–35, 2021.

[40] G Cerulli. *Econometric Evaluation of Socio-Economic Programs: theory and applications*. Springer, 2015.

[41] D G Chen and K E Peace. *Applied Meta-Analysis with R and Stata*. CRC Press, second edition, 2022.

[42] C Cheurfa, S Tsokani, K M Kontouli, I Boutron, and A Chaimani. Synthesis methods used to combine observational studies and randomised trials in published meta-analyses. *Systematic Reviews*, 13:70, 2024.

[43] P Cilliers. Complexity, deconstruction and relativism. *Theory, Culture & Society*, 22:255–267, 2005.

[44] X Q Cong, Y Li, X Zhao, Y J Dai, and Y Liu. Short-term effect of autologous bone marrow stem cells to treat acute myocardial infarction: A meta-analysis of randomized controlled clinical trials. *Journal of Cardiovascular Translational Research*, 8:221–231, 2015.

[45] P Congdon. *Bayesian Statistical Modelling*. Wiley, second edition, 2006.

[46] H Cooper. *Research Synthesis and Meta-Analysis: A Step-by-Step Approach*. Sage, fifth edition, 2017.

[47] D R Cox and E J Snell. *Analysis of Binary Data*. CRC Press, second edition, 1989.

[48] J W Creswell. *Research Design*. Sage, fourth edition, 2014.

[49] N D Crins, S Ramiro, C Xu, A C Verhoeven, and Y Yazici. Reliability of treatment rankings derived from network meta-analyses: Rank probabilities versus sucra values. *Annals of the Rheumatic Diseases*, 78(8):1136–1139, 2019.

[50] B R da Costa, A W Rutjes, B C Johnston, S Reichenbach, E Nüesch, et al. Methods to convert continuous outcomes into odds ratios of treatment response and numbers needed to treat: meta-epidemiological study. *International Journal of Epidemiology*, 41(5):1445–1459, 2012.

[51] I J Dahabreh, L C Petito, S E Robertson, M A Hernán, and J A Steingrimsson. Toward causally interpretable meta-analysis: transporting inferences from multiple randomized trials to a new target population. *Epidemiology*, 31(3):334–344, 2020.

[52] S Depaoli and R van de Schoot. Improving transparency and replication in Bayesian statistics: The WAMBS-Checklist. *Psychological Methods*, 22(2):240–261, 2017.

[53] R DerSimonian and N Laird. Meta-analysis in clinical trials. *Controlled Clinical Trials*, 7(3):177–188, 1986.

[54] N J DeVito and B Goldacre. Catalogue of bias: publication bias. *BMJ Evidence-Based Medicine*, 24(2):53–54, 2019.

[55] S Dias and A E Ades. Absolute or relative effects? arm-based synthesis of trial data. *Research Synthesis Methods*, 7(1):23–28, 2016.

[56] S Dias, A E Ades, N J Welton, J P Jansen, and A J Sutton. *Network Meta-Analysis for Decision-Making*. Wiley, 2018.

[57] S Dias, N J Welton, A J Sutton, and A E Ades. A generalized linear modelling framework for pairwise and network meta-analysis of randomized controlled trials, updated 2016. Technical report, National Institute for Health and Clinical Excellence, Decision Support Unit, 2016. `https://www.sheffield.ac.uk/nice-dsu/tsds/evidence-synthesis`.

[58] S Dias, N J Welton, A J Sutton, D M Caldwell, G Lu, et al. Evidence synthesis for decision making 4: Inconsistency in networks of evidence based on randomized controlled trials. *Medical Decision Making*, 33(5):641–656, 2013.

[59] F Dominici, G Parmigiani, R L Wolpert, and V Hasselblad. Meta-analysis of migraine headache treatments: combining information from heterogeneous designs. *Journal of the American Statistical Association*, 94(445):16–28, 1999.

[60] S Donegan, P Williamson, C Gamble, and C Tudur-Smith. Indirect comparisons: a review of reporting and methodological quality. *PLOS One*, 5:e11054, 2010.

[61] V A dos Santos Valsecchi, L F Souza Dias, R Riera, and R L Pacheco. Network of uncertainties: Network meta-analyses often does not mention methodological components. *Journal of Evaluation in Clinical Practice*, 2024.

[62] W DuMouchel and S L Normand. Computer modelling and graphical strategies for meta-analysis. In D K Stangl and D A Berry, editors, *Meta-Analysis in Medicine and Health Policy*, chapter 6. CRC Press, 2000.

[63] D M Eddy, V Hasselblad, and R Shachter. *Meta-Analysis by the Confidence Profile Method: The Statistical Synthesis of Evidence*. Academic Press, 1992.

[64] M Egger, G Davey Smith, and D G Altman. *Systematic Reviews in Health Care: Meta-Analysis in Context*. BMJ Books, second edition, 2001.

[65] J H Elliott, A Synnot, T Turner, M Simmonds, E A Akl, et al. Living systematic review: 1. introduction — the why, what, when, and how. *Journal of Clinical Epidemiology*, 91:23–30, 2017.

[66] J H Elliott, T Turner, O Clavisi, J Thomas, J P Higgins, et al. Living systematic reviews: an emerging opportunity to narrow the evidence-practice gap. *PLoS Medicine*, 11:2, 2014.

[67] EQUATOR Network. Preferred reporting items for systematic reviews and meta-analyses (PRISMA), 2020. `https://www.equator-network.org/reporting-guidelines/prisma/`.

[68] EQUATOR Network. Home page, 2024. `https://www.equator-network.org`.

[69] C Esson, L F Skerratt, L Berger, J Malmsten, T Strand, et al. Health and zoonotic infections of snow leopards, *Panthera unica* in the South Gobi desert of Mongolia. *Infection, Ecology and Epidemiology*, 9(1):1604063, 2019.

[70] H J Eysenck. An exercise in mega-silliness. *American Psychologist*, 33(5):517, 1978.

[71] H J Eysenck. Problems with meta-analysis. In I Chalmers and D G Altman, editors, *Systematic Reviews*, chapter 6. BMJ Publications, 1995.

[72] S Finfer, L Billot, P Young, L Navarra, N Hammond, et al. Balanced multielectrolyte solution versus saline in critically ill adults. *New England Journal of Medicine*, 386(9):EVIDoa2100010, 2022.

[73] D J Fisher, J R Carpenter, T P Morris, S C Freeman, and J F Tierney. Meta-analytical methods to identify who benefits most from treatments: daft, deluded or deft approach? *British Medical Journal*, 356:j573, 2017.

[74] C Fonnesbeck. GitHub repository, 2017. `https://github.com/fonnesbeck/uterine_fibroids_MA`.

[75] National Collaborating Centre for Chronic Conditions. Osteoarthritis: national clinical guideline for care and management in adults. Technical report, Royal College of Physicians of London, 2008.

[76] D P Francis, M Mielewczik, D Zargaran, and G D Cole. Autologous bone marrow-derived stem cell therapy in heart disease: Discrepancies and contradictions. *International Journal of Cardiology*, 168:3381–3403, 2013.

[77] S C Freeman, A J Sutton, N J Cooper, A Gasparini, M J Crowther, et al. Bayesian pairwise meta-analysis of time-to-event outcomes in the presence of non-proportional hazards: A simulation study of flexible parametric, piecewise exponential and fractional polynomial models. *Research Synthesis Methods*, 15(5):780–801, 2024.

[78] H P French, T Cusack, A Brennan, A Caffrey, R Conroy, et al. Exercise and manual physiotherapy arthritis research trial (EMPART) for osteoarthritis of the hip: a multicenter randomized controlled trial. *Archives of Physical Medicine and Rehabilitation*, 94:302–314, 2013.

[79] T Friede, C Röver, S Wandel, and B Neuenschwander. Meta-analysis of two studies in the presence of heterogeneity with applications in rare diseases. *Biometrical Journal*, 59(4):658–671, 2017.

[80] B C M Fung, K Wang, A W C Fu, and P S Yu. *Introduction to Privacy-preserving Data Publishing: Concepts and Techniques*. CRC Press, 2011.

[81] T A Furukawa, C Barbui, A Cipriani, P Brambilla, and N Watanabe. Imputing missing standard deviations in meta-analyses can provide accurate results. *Journal of Clinical Epidemiology*, 59:7–10, 2006.

[82] GAISE College Report ASA Revision Committee. Guidelines for assessment and instruction in statistics education (GAISE) college report 2016. Technical report, Americal Statistical Association, 2016. Available from http://www.amstat.org/education/gaise.

[83] D Gallardo-Gómez, J del Pozo-Cruz, H Pedder, R M Alfonso-Rosa, F Álvarez-Barbosa, et al. Optimal dose and type of physical activity to improve functional capacity and minimise adverse events in acutely hospitalised older adults: a systematic review with dose-response network meta-analysis of randomised controlled trials. *British Journal of Sports Medicine*, 57(19):1272–1278, 2023.

[84] M Gechter and R Meager. Combining experimental and observational studies in meta-analysis: A mutual debiasing approach. Technical report, Pennsylvania State University & London School of Economics and Political Science, 2021.

[85] A Gelman. Prior distributions for variance parameters in hierarchical models. *Bayesian Analysis*, 1(3):515–533, 2006.

[86] A Gelman. Bayesian inference completely solves the multiple comparisons problem, 2016.

[87] A Gelman, J B Carlin, H S Stern, D B Dunson, A Vehtari, et al. *Bayesian Data Analysis*. CRC Press, third edition, 2013.

[88] A Gelman, J Hill, and A Vehtari. *Regression and Other Stories*. Cambridge University Press, 2021.

[89] A Gelman and E Loken. The garden of forking paths: Why multiple comparisons can be a problem, even when there is no "fishing expedition" or "p-hacking" and the research hypothesis was posited ahead of time, 2013. http://www.stat.columbia.edu/~gelman/research/unpublished/p_hacking.pdf.

[90] A Gelman and Y L Yao. Holes in Bayesian statistics. *Journal of Physics G: Nuclear and Particle Physics*, 48:014002, 2021.

[91] J E Gentle. *Matrix Algebra: Theory, Computations and Applications in Statistics.* Springer, third edition, 2024.

[92] G Gigerenzer. *Adaptive Thinking: Rationality in the Real World.* Oxford University Press, 2002.

[93] R L Grant. Converting odds ratios to a range of plausible relative risks for better communication of research findings. *British Medical Journal*, 348:f7450, 2014.

[94] R L Grant. The uptake of Bayesian methods in biomedical meta-analyses: a scoping review, 2005-2016. *Journal of Evidence-Based Medicine*, 12(1):69–75, 2019.

[95] R L Grant. A taxonomy of thresholds used to dichotomise outcomes, and their inclusion in bayesian meta-analysis, 2022. `http://www.robertgrantstats.co.uk/papers/Taxonomy-MA-dichotomised-studies.pdf`.

[96] R L Grant. Kudzu density functions and non-parametric Bayesian updating, 2024. `http://www.robertgrantstats.co.uk/kudzu`.

[97] R L Grant, R Carpenter, D C Furr, and A Gelman. Introducing the StataStan interface for fast, complex Bayesian modeling using Stan. *The Stata Journal*, 17(2):330–342, 2017.

[98] R L Grant and R Hood. Complex systems, explanation and policy: implications of the crisis of replication for public health research. *Critical Public Health*, 27(5):525–532, 2017.

[99] P J Green, K Łatuszyński, M Pereyra, and C P Robert. Bayesian computation: a summary of the current state, and samples backwards and forwards. *Statistical Computing*, 25:835–862, 2015.

[100] L L Hagenaars, P P T Jeurissen, N S Klazinga, S Listl, and M Jevdjevic. Effectiveness and policy determinants of sugar-sweetened beverage taxes. *Journal of Dental Research*, 100(13):1444–1451, 2021.

[101] N E Hammond, F R Machado, S Micallef, B Venkatesh, P J Young, et al. Balanced crystalloids versus saline in critically ill adults — a systematic review with meta-analysis. *NEJM Evidence*, 1(2):951–985, 2022.

[102] F Harrell. Statistical thinking: Statistical errors in the medical literature: dichotomania, 2017. `https://www.fharrell.com/post/errmed/#catg`.

[103] K E Hartmann, C Fonnesbeck, T Surawicz, S Krishnaswami, J C Andrews, et al. Management of uterine fibroids. Technical Report 195, Agency for Healthcare Research and Quality, 2017.

[104] J Hartung and G Knapp. On tests of the overall treatment effect in meta-analysis with normally distributed responses. *Statistics in Medicine*, 20(12):1771–1782, 2001.

[105] J Hartung and G Knapp. A refined method for the meta-analysis of controlled clinical trials with binary outcome. *Statistics in Medicine*, 20(24):3875–3889, 2001.

[106] M Hattle, D L Burke, T Trikalinos, C H Schmid, Y Chen, et al. Multivariate meta-analysis of multiple outcomes: characteristics and predictors of borrowing of strength from Cochrane reviews. *Systematic Reviews*, 11:149, 2022.

[107] T Havránek, T D Stanley, H Doucouliagos, P Bom, J Geyer-Klingeberg, et al. Reporting guidelines for meta-analysis in economics. *Journal of Economic Surveys*, 34(3):469–475, 2020.

[108] P Hazell and M Mirzaie. Tricyclic drugs for depression in children and adolescents. *Cochrane Database of Systematic Reviews*, 6:CD002317, 2013.

[109] HEDCO Institute. Four-day school week research database, 2023.

[110] M A Hernan and J M Robins. *Causal Inference: What If?* CRC Press, 2024.

[111] J P T Higgins. Commentary: Heterogeneity in meta-analysis should be expected and appropriately quantified. *International Journal of Epidemiology*, 37:1158–1160, 2008.

[112] J P T Higgins, J Thomas, J Chandler, M Cumpston, T Li, et al. *Cochrane Handbook for Systematic Reviews of Interventions version 6.4 (updated August 2023)*. Cochrane Collaboration, 2023. `https://www.training.cochrane.org/handbook`.

[113] J P T Higgins and A Whitehead. Borrowing strength from external trials in a meta-analysis. *Statistics in Medicine*, 15:2733–2749, 1996.

[114] J P T Higgins, A Whitehead, and M Simmonds. Sequential methods for random-effects meta-analysis. *Statistics in Medicine*, 30(9):903–921, 2011.

[115] H Hong, H Chu, J Zhang, and B P Carlin. A Bayesian missing data framework for generalized multiple outcome mixed treatment comparisons. *Research Synthesis Methods*, 7:6–22, 2016.

[116] H Hong, H Chu, J Zhang, and B P Carlin. Rejoinder to the discussion of "A Bayesian missing data framework for generalized multiple outcome mixed treatment comparisons" by S. Dias and A.E. Ades. *Research Synthesis Methods*, 7:29–33, 2016.

[117] H Hong, L Liu, R Mojtabai, and E A Stuart. Calibrated meta-analysis to estimate the efficacy of mental health treatments in target populations: an application to paliperidone trials for treatment of schizophrenia. *BMC Medical Research Methodology*, 23:150, 2023.

[118] R Horton. From star signs to trial guidelines. *The Lancet*, 355(9209):1033–1034, 2000.

[119] M Hurley, K Dickson, R Hallett, R Grant, H Hauari, et al. Exercise interventions and patient beliefs for people with hip, knee or hip and knee osteoarthritis: a mixed methods review. *Cochrane Database of Systematic Reviews*, 4, 2018.

[120] B Hutton, G Salanti, D M Caldwell, A Chaimani, C H Schmid, et al. PRISMA for Network Meta-Analyses (PRISMA-NMA), 2015. `https://www.prisma-statement.org/nma`.

[121] Ada Lovelace Institute. Rethinking data and rebalancing digital power. Technical report, Ada Lovelace Institute, 2022. `https://www.adalovelaceinstitute.org/report/rethinking-data/`.

[122] P Irwing, T Booth, and D J Hughes. *The Wiley Handbook of Psychometric Testing: A Multidisciplinary Reference on Survey, Scale and Test Development*. Wiley, 2018.

[123] K J Ishak, I Proskorovsky, and A Benedict. Simulation and matching-based approaches for indirect comparison of treatments. *Pharmacoeconomics*, 33(6):537–549, 2015.

[124] E R Ivimey-Cook, D W A Noble, S Nakagawa, M J Lajeunesse, and J L Pick. Advice for improving the reproducibility of data extraction in meta-analysis. *Research Synthesis Methods*, 14(6):911–915, 2023.

[125] D Jackson, M Law, T Stijnen, W Viechtbauer, and I R White. A comparison of seven random-effects models for meta-analyses that estimate the summary odds ratio. *Statistics in Medicine*, 37(7):1059–1085, 2018.

[126] D Jackson, G Rücker, M Law, and G Schwarzer. The Hartung-Knapp modification for random-effects meta-analysis: A useful refinement but are there any residual concerns? *Statistics in Medicine*, 36(25):3923–3934, 2017.

[127] D Jackson and I R White. When should meta-analysis avoid making hidden normality assumptions? *Biometrical Journal*, 60:1040–1058, 2018.

[128] A R Jadad, D J Cook, and G P Browman. A guide to interpreting discordant systematic reviews. *Canadian Medical Association Journal*, 156:1411–1416, 1997.

[129] D James, S Toupin, N Schoenherr, R Wickstead, and D Tyas. PRM252 — simulated treatment comparison: implications and challenges of an alternative approach to estimating the relative efficacy of nivolumab versus relevant comparator chemotherapy treatments for advanced/metastatic urothelial carcinoma in the UK. *Value in Health*, 21:S399, 2018.

[130] J P Jansen. Network meta-analysis of survival data with fractional polynomials. *BMC Medical Research Methodology*, 11:61, 2011.

[131] K Jansen and H Holling. Rare events meta-analysis using the Bayesian beta-binomial model. *Research Synthesis Methods*, 14(6):853–873, 2023.

[132] S Janssens, C Dubois, J Bogaert, K Theunissen, C Deroose, et al. Autologous bone marrow-derived stem-cell transfer in patients with ST-segment elevation myocardial infarction: double-blind, randomised controlled trial. *The Lancet*, 367:113–121, 2006.

[133] JASP Team. JASP (Version 0.18.3). `https://jasp-stats.org/`, 2024.

[134] Z Jiang, Y Chen, J C Cappelleri, N Thomas, M Gamalo, et al. A comprehensive review and Shiny application on the matching-adjusted indirect comparison. *Research Synthesis Methods*, 15(4):671–686, 2024.

[135] Project Jupyter. Home page, 2024. `https://jupyter.org`.

[136] T M Jurgens, A M Whelan, L Killian, S Doucette, S Kirk, et al. Green tea for weight loss and weight maintenance in overweight or obese adults. Technical Report 12, Cochrane Database of Systematic Reviews, 2012.

[137] S Juul, N Nielsen, P Bentzer, A A Veroniki, L Thabane, et al. Interventions for treatment of COVID-19: a protocol for a living systematic review with network meta-analysis including individual patient data (The LIVING Project). *Systematic Reviews*, 9(1):108, 2020.

[138] H A Kahn and C T Sempos. *Statistical Methods in Epidemiology*. Oxford University Press, 1989.

[139] S Kaner. *Facilitator's Guide to Participatory Decision-Making.* Wiley, 2014.

[140] R E Kass and A E Raftery. Bayes factors. *Journal of the American Statistical Association*, 90(430):773–795, 1995.

[141] E Kontopantelis and D Reeves. Performance of statistical methods for meta-analysis when true study effects are non-normally distributed: A simulation study. *Statistical Methods in Medical Research*, 21(4):409–426, 2010.

[142] J K Kruschke. Bayesian analysis reporting guidelines. *Nature Human Behaviour*, 5:1282–1291, 2021.

[143] C F Kurz. Augmented inverse probability weighting and the double robustness property. *Medical Decision Making*, 42(2):156–167, 2021.

[144] D Kwon and I M Reis. Simulation-based estimation of mean and standard deviation for meta-analysis via Approximate Bayesian Computation (ABC). *BMC Medical Research Methodology*, 15:61, 2015.

[145] D Lakens. Calculating and reporting effect sizes to facilitate cumulative science: a practical primer for t-tests and ANOVAs. *Frontiers in Psychology*, 4:863, 2013.

[146] D T Larose. A Bayesian meta-analysis of the relationship between estrogen exposure and occurence of endometrial cancer. In D K Stangl and D A Berry, editors, *Meta-Analysis in Medicine and Health Policy*, chapter 8. CRC Press, 2000.

[147] P M Lee. *Bayesian Statistics: An Introduction.* Hodder Arnold, third edition, 2004.

[148] T C Lee, E G McDonald, G Butler-Laporte, L B Harrison, M P Cheng, et al. Remdesivir and systemic corticosteroids for the treatment of COVID-19: a Bayesian re-analysis. *International Journal of Infectious Diseases*, 104:671–676, 2021.

[149] E C K Li, B S Heran, and J M Wright. Angiotensin converting enzyme (ACE) inhibitors versus angiotensin receptor blockers for primary hypertension. Technical Report 8, Cochrane Database of Systematic Reviews, 2014.

[150] N Li, Y G Lao, and S W Leung. Multilevel models for network meta-analysis. *Proceedings of the 2013 ISI World Statistics Congress, Hong Kong*, 2013.

[151] L Lin and C Xu. Arcsine-based transformations for meta-analysis of proportions: Pros, cons, and alternatives. *Health Science Reports*, 3(3):e178, 2020.

[152] L F Lin and H T Chu. Quantifying publication bias in meta-analysis. *Biometrics*, 74(3):785–794, 2018.

[153] Z Y Liu, F M al Amer, M L Xiao, C Xu, L Furuya-Kanamori, et al. The normality assumption on between-study random effects was questionable in a considerable number of Cochrane meta-analyses. *BMC Medicine*, 21:112, 2023.

[154] S Low-Choy. Priors: slient or active partners of Bayesian inference? In C L Alston, K L Mengersen, and A N Pettitt, editors, *Case studies in Bayesian Statistical Modelling and Analysis*, chapter 3. Wiley, 2013.

[155] G Lu, A E Ades, A J Sutton, N J Cooper, A H Briggs, et al. Meta-analysis of mixed treatment comparisons at multiple follow-up times. *Statistics in Medicine*, 26(20):3681–3699, 2007.

[156] D Lunn, C Jackson, N Best, A Thomas, and D Spiegelhalter. *The BUGS Book: A Practical Introduction to Bayesian Analysis*. CRC Press, 2013.

[157] C Lunny, S S Thirugnanasampanthar, S Kanji, N Ferri, D Pieper, et al. How can clinicians choose between conflicting and discordant systematic reviews? a replication study of the Jadad algorithm. *BMC Medical Research Methodology*, 22:276, 2022.

[158] C Mansilla, Q Wang, T Piggott, P Bragge, K Waddell, et al. A living critical interpretive synthesis to yield a framework on the production and dissemination of living evidence syntheses for decision-making. *Implementation Science*, 19:67, 2024.

[159] C Manski. *Public Policy in an Uncertain World: Analysis and Decisions*. Harvard University Press, 2013.

[160] J M Marin, P Pudlo, C P Robert, and R J Ryder. Approximate Bayesian computational methods. *Statistics and Computing*, 22:1167–1180, 2012.

[161] G Markozannes, G Vourli, and E Ntzani. A survey of methodologies on causal inference methods in meta-analyses of randomized controlled trials. *Systematic Reviews*, 10(1):170, 2021.

[162] D Mavridis and I R White. Dealing with missing outcome data in meta-analysis. *Research Synthesis Methods*, 11:2–13, 2020.

[163] D M Mayo. *Statistical Inference as Severe Testing*. Cambridge University Press, 2018.

[164] C E McCulloch and J M Neuhaus. Misspecifying the shape of a random effects distribution: Why getting it wrong may not matter. *Statistical Science*, 26(3):388–402, 2011.

[165] M S McDonagh, S Iyer, B J Morasco, R Chou, A Y Ahmed, et al. Living systematic reviews: Practical considerations for the agency for healthcare research and quality evidence-based practice center program. Technical report, Agency for Healthcare Research and Quality, 2022.

[166] R McElreath. *Statistical Rethinking*. CRC Press, second edition, 2020.

[167] R Meager. Understanding the average impact of microcredit expansions: A Bayesian hierarchical analysis of seven randomized experiments. *American Economic Journal: Applied Economics*, 11(1):57–91, 2019.

[168] R Meager. Aggregating distributional treatment effects: a Bayesian hierarchical analysis of the microcredit literature. *American Economic Review*, 112(6):1818–1847, 2022.

[169] A Messori. Synthesizing published evidence on survival by reconstruction of patient-level data and generation of a multi-trial Kaplan-Meier curve. *Cureus*, 13(11):e19422, 2021.

[170] A E Mikesky, S A Mazzuca, K D Brandt, S M Perkins, T Damush, et al. Effects of strength training on the incidence and progression of knee osteoarthritis. *Arthritis Care and Research*, 55(5):690–699, 2006.

[171] P P Morgan. The literature jungle. *Canadian Medical Association Journal*, 134:98–99, 1986.

[172] T P Morris, D J Fisher, M G Kenward, and J R Carpenter. Meta-analysis of Gaussian individual patient data: Two-stage or not two-stage? *Statistics in Medicine*, 37(9):1419–1438, 2018.

[173] T P Morris, I R White, and M J Crowther. Using simulation studies to evaluate statistical methods. *Statistics in Medicine*, 38(11):2074–2102, 2019.

[174] M H Murad, Z Wang, H Chu, and L Lin. When continuous outcomes are measured using different scales: guide for meta-analysis and interpretation. *British Medical Journal*, 364:k4817, 2019.

[175] H Naci. Communication of treatment rankings obtained from network meta-analysis using data visualization. *Circulation: Cardiovascular Quality and Outcomes*, 9(5):605–608, 2016.

[176] H Neave. *Elementary Statistics Tables*. Routledge, second edition, 2011.

[177] B Neuenschwander and H Schmidli. Use of historical data. In E Lesaffre, G Baio, and B Boulanger, editors, *Bayesian Methods in Pharmaceutical Research*. CRC Press, 2020.

[178] J Le Noury, J M Nardo, D Healy, J Jureidini, M Raven, et al. Restoring study 329: efficacy and harms of paroxetine and imipramine in treatment of major depression in adolescence. *British Medical Journal*, 351:h4320, 2015.

[179] R Nuzzo. Scientific method: Statistical errors. *Nature*, 506:150–152, 2014.

[180] A O'Hagan, C E Buck, A Daneshkhah, J R Eiser, P H Garthwaite, et al. *Uncertain Judgements: Eliciting Experts' Probabilities*. Wiley, 2006.

[181] A O'Hagan and B Luce. A primer on Bayesian statistics in health economics and outcomes research: Bayesian initiative in health economics and outcomes research. Technical report, Centre for Bayesian Statistics in Health Economics, 2003.

[182] A O'Hagan and J Oakley. SHELF: the Sheffield Elicitation Framework. `https://shelf.sites.sheffield.ac.uk/`, 2022.

[183] K Oliver and P Cairney. The dos and don'ts of influencing policy: a systematic review of advice to academics. *Palgrave Communications*, 5:21, 2019.

[184] K O'Rourke. The combining of information: Investigating and synthesizing what is possibly common in clinical observations or studies via likelihood., 2003. D.Phil. thesis, Department of Statistics, University of Oxford, UK.

[185] S Ostrowski and M Gilbert. Diseases of free-ranging snow leopards and primary prey species. *Snow Leopards*, 15:97–112, 2016.

[186] M J N M Ouwens, Z Philips, and J P Jansen. Network meta-analysis of parametric survival curves. *Research Synthesis Methods*, 1:258–271, 2010.

[187] A B Owen. Refiltering hypothesis tests to control sign error, 2019. `https://arxiv.org/pdf/1610.10028`.

[188] S Pawel, F Aust, L Held, and E J Wagenmakers. Normalized power priors always discount historical data. *Stat*, 12(1):e591, 2023.

[189] Y Pawitan. *In All Likelihood: Statistical Modelling and Inference Using Likelihood.* Oxford University Press, 2001.

[190] R Pawson. *The Science of Evaluation: A Realist Manifesto.* Sage, 2013.

[191] H Pedder, S Dias, M Bennetts, M Boucher, and N Welton. Modelling time-course relationships with multiple treatments: Model-based network meta-analysis for continuous summary outcomes. *Research Synthesis Methods*, 10(2):267–286, 2019.

[192] J Pek and D B Flora. Reporting effect sizes in original psychological research: A discussion and tutorial. *Psychological Methods*, 23(2):208–225, 2018.

[193] D M Phillippo, A E Ades, S Dias, S Palmer, K R Abrams, et al. Methods for population-adjusted indirect comparisons in health technology appraisal. *Medical Decision Making*, 38(2):200–211, 2018.

[194] D M Phillippo, S Dias, A E Ades, M Belger, A Brnabic, et al. Validating the assumptions of population adjustment: Application of multilevel network meta-regression to a network of treatments for plaque psoriasis. *Medical Decision Making*, 43(1):53–67, 2022.

[195] D M Phillippo, S Dias, A E Ades, and N J Welton. Assessing the performance of population adjustment methods for anchored indirect comparisons: A simulation study. *Statistics in Medicine*, 39(30):4885–4911, 2020.

[196] D Piccolo and R Simone. The class of CUB models: statistical foundations, inferential issues and empirical evidence. *Statistical Methods and Applications*, 28:389–435, 2019.

[197] J O Pitchforth and K L Mengersen. Bayesian meta-analysis. In C L Alston, K L Mengersen, and A N Pettitt, editors, *Case Studies in Bayesian Statistical Modelling and Analysis*, chapter 7. Wiley, 2013.

[198] N Pooley, R Payne, C Papageorgakopoulou, and E Adkins. The use of matching adjusted indirect comparison (MAIC) and simulated treatment comparison (STC) in HTA submissions; learnings from recent submissions. *Value in Health*, 20(9):A769–A770, 2017.

[199] PyMC Development Team. PyMC 4.0 release announcement, 2022. `https://www.pymc.io/blog/v4_announcement.html`.

[200] C E Rasmussen and C K I Williams. *Gaussian Processes for Machine Learning.* MIT Press, 2006.

[201] J P Reynolds, K Stautz, M Pilling, S van der Linden, and T M Marteau. Communicating the effectiveness and ineffectiveness of government policies and their impact on public support: a systematic review with meta-analysis. *Royal Society Open Science*, 7:190522, 2020.

[202] R Riley, J Tierney, and L Stewart. *Individual Participant Data Meta-Analysis: A Handbook for Healthcare Research.* Wiley, 2021.

[203] R D Riley, J Ensor, M Hattle, K Papadimitropoulou, and T P Morris. Two-stage or not two-stage? that is the question for IPD meta-analysis projects. *Research Synthesis Methods*, 14(6):903–910, 2023.

[204] HR Rothstein, A Sutton, and M Borenstein. *Publication Bias in Meta-Analysis: Prevention, Assessment and Adjustments.* Wiley, 2005.

[205] C Röver, T Friede, and G Knapp. Hartung-Knapp-Sidik-Jonkman approach and its modification for random-effects meta-analysis with few studies. *BMC Medical Research Methodology*, 15:99, 2015.

[206] C Röver, S Sturtz, J Lilienthal, R Bender, and T Friede. Summarizing empirical information on between-study heterogeneity for Bayesian random-effects meta-analysis. *Statistics in Medicine*, 42:2439–2454, 2023.

[207] P Royston and M K B Parmar. Restricted mean survival time: an alternative to the hazard ratio for the design and analysis of randomized trials with a time-to-event outcome. *BMC Medical Research Methodology*, 13:152, 2013.

[208] D B Rubin and R J A Little. *Statistical Analysis with Missing Data*. Wiley, third edition, 2019.

[209] M Rubio-Aparicio, J A López-López, J Sánchez-Meca, F Marín-Martínez, W Viechtbauer, et al. Estimation of an overall standardized mean difference in random-effects meta-analysis if the distribution of random effects departs from normal. *Research Synthesis Methods*, 9(3):489–503, 2018.

[210] C Röver. Bayesian random-effects meta-analysis using the bayesmeta R package. *Journal of Statistical Software*, 93:1–51, 2020.

[211] C Röver and T Friede. Discrete approximation of a mixture distribution via restricted divergence. *Journal of Computational and Graphical Statistics*, 26(1):217–222, 2017.

[212] C Röver and T Friede. Double arcsine transform not appropriate for meta-analysis. *Research Synthesis Methods*, 13(5):645–648, 2022.

[213] Dias S, A J Sutton, N J Welton, and A E Ades. Evidence synthesis for decision making 3: Heterogeneity—subgroups, meta-regression, bias, and bias-adjustment. *Medical Decision Making*, 33(5):618–640, 2013.

[214] D L Sackett, J J Deeks, and D G Altman. Down with odds ratios! *Evidence-Based Medicine*, 1(6):164–166, 1996.

[215] J A Sacristán, A Aguarón, C Avendaño-Solá, P Garrido, J Carrión, et al. Patient involvement in clinical research: why, when, and how. *Patient Preference and Adherence*, 10:631–640, 2016.

[216] M Salcher-Konrad, M Nguyen, J Savović, J P T Higgins, and H Naci. Treatment effects in randomised and non-randomised studies of pharmacological interventions: a meta-analysis. *JAMA Network Open*, 7(9):e2436230, 2024.

[217] F De Santis. Power priors and their use in clinical trials. *The American Statistician*, 60(2):122–129, 2006.

[218] J A Santos, E Riggi, R Grant, S Ingale, S Bhaumik, et al. Bayesian approach for meta-analyses in biomedical research: a scoping review protocol. *JBI Evidence Synthesis*, 22(3):447–452, 2024.

[219] SAS Institute Inc. Introduction to Bayesian analysis procedures, 2024. `https://support.sas.com/documentation/cdl/en/statug/68162/HTML/default/viewer.htm#statug_introbayes_toc.htm`.

[220] C H Schmid, T T Stijnen, and I R White. *Handbook of Meta-Analysis*. CRC Press, 2021.

[221] M Schnitzer, R Steele, M Bally, and I Shrier. A causal inference approach to network meta-analysis. *Journal of Causal Inference*, 4(2):20160014, 2016.

[222] D W Scott. *Multivariate Density Estimation*. Wiley, second edition, 2015.

[223] A L Seidler, K E Hunter, S Cheyne, D Ghersi, J A Berlin, et al. A guide to prospective meta-analysis. *British Medical Journal*, 367:l5342, 2019.

[224] S Senn. Comment on LinkedIn, 2024.

[225] S Senn. Comment on "Using Randomization Tests to Address Disruptions in Clinical Trials: A Report from the NISS Ingram Olkin Forum Series on Unplanned Clinical Trial Disruptions". *Statistics in Biopharmaceutical Research*, 16(4):414–416, 2024.

[226] A D Sherry, P Msaouel, and E B Ludmir. A meta-epidemiological analysis of post-hoc comparisons and primary endpoint interpretability among randomized noncomparative trials in clinical medicine. *Journal of Clinical Epidemiology*, 175:111540, 2024.

[227] I Shrier, J F Boivin, R J Steele, R W Platt, A Furlan, et al. Should meta-analyses of interventions include observational studies in addition to randomized controlled trials? a critical examination of underlying principles. *American Journal of Epidemiology*, 166:1203–1209, 2007.

[228] K Sidik and J N Jonkman. A simple confidence interval for metaanalysis. *Statistics in Medicine*, 21(21):3153–3159, 2002.

[229] K Sidik and J N Jonkman. Simple heterogeneity variance estimation for meta-analysis. *Journal of the Royal Statistical Society Series C: Applied Statistics*, 54(2):367–384, 2005.

[230] M Simmonds, G Salanti, J McKenzie, and J Elliott. Living systematic reviews. 3. statistical methods for updating meta-analyses. *Journal of Clinical Epidemiology*, 91:38–46, 2017.

[231] J Singh, K R Abrams, and S Bujkiewicz. Incorporating single-arm studies in meta-analysis of randomised controlled trials: a simulation study. *BMC Medical Research Methodology*, 21:114, 2021.

[232] S A Sisson, Y Fan, and M Beaumont. *Handbook of Approximate Bayesian Computation*. CRC Press, 2019.

[233] D D Smith, G H Givens, and R L Tweedie. Adjustment for publication bias and quality bias in Bayesian meta-analysis. In D K Stangl and D A Berry, editors, *Meta-analysis in Medicine and Health Policy*. CRC Press, 2000.

[234] M Soares, A Colson, L Bojke, S Ghabri, O U Garay, et al. Recommendations on the use of structured expert elicitation protocols for healthcare decision making: A good practices report of an ISPOR Task Force. *Value in Health*, 27(11):1469–1478, 2024.

[235] M Sobel, D Madigan, and W Wang. Causal inference for meta-analysis and multilevel data structures, with application to randomized studies of Vioxx. *Psychometrika*, 82(2):459–474, 2017.

[236] X Y Song and S Y Lee. *Basic and Advanced Bayesian Structural Equation Modeling: with Applications in the Medical and Behavioral Sciences*. Wiley, 2012.

[237] M R Spears, N D James, and M R Sydes. "Thursday's child has far to go" — interpreting subgroups and the STAMPEDE trial. *Annals of Oncology*, 28(10):2327–2330, 2017.

[238] D J Spiegelhalter. Incorporating Bayesian ideas into health-care evaluation. *Statistical Science*, 19(1):156–174, 2004.

[239] D J Spiegelhalter, K R Abrams, and J P Myles. *Bayesian Approaches to Clinical Trials and Health-care Evaluation*. Wiley, 2004.

[240] D J Spiegelhalter, J P Myles, D R Jones, and K R Abrams. Bayesian methods in health technology assessment: a review. *Health Technology Assessment*, 4(38), 2000.

[241] M J Spittal, J Pirkis, and L C Gurrin. Meta-analysis of incidence rate data in the presence of zero events. *BMC Medical Research Methodology*, 15:42, 2015.

[242] Stan Development Team. Stan, 2024. `https://mc-stan.org/`.

[243] D K Stangl and D A Berry. *Meta-Analysis in Medicine and Health Policy*. CRC Press, 2000.

[244] J W Stevens. A note on dealing with missing standard errors in meta-analyses of continuous outcome measures in WinBUGS. *Pharmaceutical Statistics*, 10:374–378, 2011.

[245] J Storopoli. Bayesian statistics using Julia and Turing, 2024. `https://storopoli.io/Bayesian-Julia/`.

[246] L Sunga, J Hayden, M L Greenberg, G Koren, B M Feldman, et al. Seven items were identified for inclusion when reporting a Bayesian analysis of a clinical study. *Journal of Clinical Epidemiology*, 58:261–268, 2005.

[247] A J Sutton and K R Abrams. Bayesian methods in meta-analysis and evidence synthesis. *Statistical Methods in Medical Research*, 10:277–303, 2001.

[248] A J Sutton, K R Abrams, D R Jones, T A Sheldon, and F J Song. *Methods for Meta-Analysis in Medical Research*. Wiley, 2000.

[249] J N Tendeiro and H A L Kiers. A review of issues about null hypothesis Bayesian testing. *Psychological Methods*, 24(6):774–795, 2019.

[250] A M Teng, A C Jones, A Mizdrak, L Signal, M Genç, et al. Impact of sugar-sweetened beverage taxes on purchases and dietary intake: Systematic review and meta-analysis. *Obesity Reviews*, 20:1187–1204, 2019.

[251] The Metapsy Collaboration. Meta-analytic database of psychotherapy trials. `https://www.metapsy.org/`.

[252] The Royal Society and the Academy of Medical Sciences. Evidence synthesis for policy. Technical report, The Royal Society and the Academy of Medical Sciences, 2018.

[253] J Thompson. *Bayesian Analysis With Stata*. Stata Press, 2014.

[254] S Thompson, U Ekelund, S Jebb, A K Lindroos, A Mander, et al. A proposed method of bias adjustment for meta-analyses of published observational studies. *International Journal of Epidemiology*, 40(3):765–777, 2011.

[255] S G Thompson and S J Sharp. Explaining heterogeneity in meta-analysis: a comparison of methods. *Statistics in Medicine*, 18:2693–2708, 1999.

[256] Y Thum and S Ahn. Challenges of meta-analysis from the standpoint of latent variable framework. Paper presented at 7th Annual Campbell Collaboration Colloquium, London, UK, 2007.

[257] J F Timsit, E Azoulay, C Schwebel, P E Charles, M Cornet, et al. Empirical micafungin treatment and survival without invasive fungal infection in adults with ICU-acquired sepsis, Candida colonization, and multiple organ failure: The EMPIRICUS randomized clinical trial. *Journal of the American Medical Association*, 316(15):1555–1564, 2016.

[258] A Toloui and M Yousefifard. Observational studies provide insufficient data for a reliable meta-analysis: a call to revise the current guidelines. *Systematic Reviews*, 13:6, 2024.

[259] L Trinquart, G Chatellier, and P Ravaud. Adjustment for reporting bias in network meta-analysis of antidepressant trials. *BMC Medical Research Methodology*, 12:150, 2012.

[260] J Tukey. The future of data analysis. *Annals of Mathematical Statistics*, 33(1):1–67, 1962.

[261] J W Tukey. *Exploratory Data Analysis*, page 10. Addison-Wesley, 1977.

[262] R M Turner, J Davey, M J Clarke, S G Thompson, and J P Higgins. Predicting the extent of heterogeneity in meta-analysis, using empirical data from the Cochrane database of systematic reviews. *International Journal of Epidemiology*, 41(3):818–827, 2012.

[263] R M Turner, C P Domínguez-Islas, D Jackson, K M Rhodes, and I R White. Incorporating external evidence on between-trial heterogeneity in network meta-analysis. *Statistics in Medicine*, 38(8):1321–1335, 2019.

[264] R M Turner, D Jackson, Y H Wei, S G Thompson, and J P T Higgins. Predictive distributions for between-study heterogeneity and simple methods for their application in Bayesian meta-analysis. *Statistics in Medicine*, 34:984–998, 2015.

[265] R M Turner, D J Spiegelhalter, G C S Smith, and S G Thompson. Bias modelling in evidence synthesis. *Journal of the Royal Statistical Society Series A: Statistics in Society*, 172(1):21–47, 2009.

[266] University of Bristol. Centre for multilevel modelling: software, 2024. `https://www.bristol.ac.uk/cmm/software/`.

[267] University of California at Irvine, Machine Learning Repository. Iris dataset. `https://archive.ics.uci.edu/dataset/53/iris`, 1988. Originally published by Anderson (1936). Two known errors in the dataset transcription widely used for teaching both occur in the *Iris setosa* species' data, and so do not affect this book.

[268] R C M van Aert and D Jackson. A new justification of the Hartung-Knapp method for random-effects meta-analysis based on weighted least squares regression. *Research Synthesis Methods*, 10(4):515–527, 2019.

[269] A M van der Bles, S van der Linden, A L J Freeman, J Mitchell, A B Galvao, et al. Communicating uncertainty about facts, numbers and science. *Royal Society Open Science*, 6:181870, 2019.

[270] A A Veroniki, S E Straus, A Fyraridis, and A C Tricco. The rank-heat plot is a novel way to present the results from a network meta-analysis including multiple outcomes. *Journal of Clinical Epidemiology*, 93:84–91, 2018.

[271] E J Wagenmakers. A practical solution to the pervasive problems of p values. *Psychonomic Bulleting and Review*, 14(5):779–804, 2007.

[272] S D Walter, H Han, G H Guyatt, D Bassler, N Bhatnagar, et al. A systematic survey of randomised trials that stopped early for reasons of futility. *BMC Medical Research Methodology*, 20:10, 2020.

[273] C C Wang, C H Schmid, P L Hibberd, R Kalish, R Roubenoff, et al. Tai Chi is effective in treating knee osteoarthritis: A randomized controlled trial. *Arthritis Care & Research*, 61(11):1545–1553, 2009.

[274] D Wang and A Bakhai. *Clinical Trials: A Practical Guide to Design, Analysis and Reporting*. Remedica, 2006.

[275] R L Wasserstein and N A Lazar. The ASA statement on p-values: Context, process, and purpose. *The American Statistician*, 70(2):129–133, 2016.

[276] F Weber, G Kundt, G Knapp, Ä Glass, and K Ickstadt. Interval estimation of the overall treatment effect in random-effects meta-analyses: Recommendations from a simulation study comparing frequentist, Bayesian, and bootstrap methods. *Research Synthesis Methods*, 12(3):291–315, 2020.

[277] Y Wei and J P T Higgins. Estimating within-study covariances in multivariate meta-analysis with multiple outcomes. *Statistics in Medicine*, 32:1191–1205, 2012.

[278] Y Wei, P Royston, J F Tierney, and M K Parmar. Meta-analysis of time-to-event outcomes from randomized trials using restricted mean survival time: application to individual participant data. *Statistics in Medicine*, 34(21):2881–2898, 2015.

[279] N J Welton, A E Ades, J B Carlin, D G Altman, and J A C Sterne. Methods for potentially biased evidence in meta-analysis using empirically based priors. *Journal of the Royal Statistical Society, Series A*, 172:119–136, 2009.

[280] I R White. Network meta-analysis. *Stata Journal*, 15(4):951–985, 2015.

[281] I R White, R M Turner, A Karahalios, and G Salanti. A comparison of arm-based and contrast-based models for network meta-analysis. *Statistics in Medicine*, 38:5197–5213, 2019.

[282] Wikipedia contributors. Probabilistic programming, 2024. `https://en.wikipedia.org/wiki/Probabilistic_programming`.

[283] D Wu, K S Goldfeld, and E Petkova. Developing a Bayesian hierarchical model for a prospective individual patient data meta-analysis with continuous monitoring. *BMC Medical Research Methodology*, 23(1):25, 2023.

[284] J Y Xu, D Liu, Y Zhong, and R C Huang. Effects of timing on intracoronary autologous bone marrow-derived cell transplantation in acute myocardial infarction: a meta-analysis of randomized controlled trials. *Stem Cell Research and Therapy*, 8:231, 2017.

[285] T Yarılgaç. The use of prospective meta-analysis. *Middle Black Sea Journal of Health Science*, 4(3):47–52, 2018.

[286] J Zhang, H Fu, and B P Carlin. Detecting outlying trials in network meta-analysis. *Statistics in Medicine*, 34(19):2695–2707, 2015.

[287] L Zhang, D Jackson, and S Bujkiewicz. Four alternative methodologies for simulated treatment comparison: How could the use of simulation be re-invigorated? *Research Synthesis Methods*, 15(2):227–241, 2023.

[288] P Royston and M K B Parmar. Restricted mean survival time: an alternative to the hazard ratio for the design and analysis of randomized trials with a time-to-event outcome, *BMC Medical Research Methodology*, 13:152, 2013.

Index

For Product Safety Concerns and Information please contact our
EU representative GPSR@taylorandfrancis.com Taylor & Francis
Verlag GmbH, Kaufingerstraße 24, 80331 München, Germany